Lung Liquids

*The Ciba Foundation for the promotion of international cooperation in
medical and chemical research is a scientific and educational charity established by
CIBA Limited – now CIBA-GEIGY Limited – of Basle. The Foundation operates
independently in London under English trust law.*

*Ciba Foundation Symposia are published in collaboration with
Elsevier Scientific Publishing Company, Excerpta Medica,
North-Holland Publishing Company, in Amsterdam.*

Elsevier / Excerpta Medica / North-Holland, P.O. Box 211, Amsterdam

Lung Liquids

Ciba Foundation Symposium 38 (new series)

1976

Elsevier · Excerpta Medica · North-Holland
Amsterdam · Oxford · New York

ISBN Excerpta Medica 90 219 4043 4
ISBN American Elsevier 0-444-15204-0

Published in March 1976 by Elsevier/Excerpta Medica/North-Holland, P.O. Box 211, Amsterdam, and
American Elsevier, 52 Vanderbilt Avenue, New York, N.Y. 10017.

Suggested series entry for library catalogues: Ciba Foundation Symposia
Suggested publisher's entry for library catalogues: Elsevier/Excerpta Medica/North-Holland.

Ciba Foundation Symposium 38 (new series)

Library of Congress Cataloging in Publication Data

Symposium on Lung Liquids, London, 1975.
   Lung liquids.

   (Ciba Foundation symposium ; 38 (new ser.))
   "Held at the Ciba Foundation, London, 22-24
April 1975."
   Bibliography: p.
   Includes indexes.
   1. Lungs--Congresses. 2. Body fluids--Con-
gresses. 3. Biological transport--Congresses.
I. Title. II. Series: Ciba Foundation. Symposium ; new ser., 38. [DNLM: 1. Body fluids--Phys-
iology--Congresses. 2. Lung--Physiology--Con-
gresses. 3. Cell membrane permeability--Congresses.

W3 C161F v. 38 1975 / WF600 S987L 1975]
QP121.S95 1975   612'.2   76-870
ISBN 0-444-15204-0

Printed in The Netherlands by Van Gorcum, Assen

Contents

Participants

Symposium on *Lung Liquids* held at the Ciba Foundation, London
22–24 April 1975

*C. J. DICKINSON (*Chairman*) Medical Unit, University College Hospita-
Medical School, Huntley Street, London WClE 6JJ

T. M. ADAMSON Dept of Paediatrics, Monash University, Queen Victoria
Hospital, Melbourne, Victoria, Australia 3000

E. AGOSTONI Istituto di Fisiologia umana, Università di Milano, Via
Mangiagalli 32, 20133 Milano, Italy

W. A. CROSBIE Chest Unit, Dept of Medicine, King's College Hospital Medical
School, Denmark Hill, London SE5 8RX

P. DEJOURS Laboratoire de Physiologie Respiratoire, Centre National de la
Recherche Scientifique, 23 rue Becquerel, 67087 Strasbourg C, France

K. W. DONALD Dept of Medicine, University of Edinburgh, The Royal
Infirmary, Edinburgh EH3 9YW

R. P. DURBIN Cardiovascular Research Institute, University of California
at San Francisco, San Francisco, California 94143, USA

E. A. EGAN Dept of Pediatrics, Division of Neonatology, College of Medicine,
University of Florida, Gainsville, Florida 32610, USA

L. E. FARHI Dept of Physiology, State University of New York, Buffalo, New
York 14214, USA

A. P. FISHMAN Cardiovascular-Pulmonary Division, Dept of Medicine,
Hospital of the University of Pennsylvania, 3400 Spruce Street, Philadelphia,
Pennsylvania 19104, USA

* *Present address:* Dept of Medicine, St Bartholomew's Hospital Medical College, West
Smithfield, London EClA 7BE

J. T. GATZY   Dept of Pharmacology, The School of Medicine, The University of North Carolina at Chapel Hill, North Carolina 27514, USA

A. C. GUYTON   Dept of Physiology & Biophysics, The University of Mississippi Medical Center, 2500 North State Street, Jackson, Mississippi 39216, USA

J. M. B. HUGHES   Dept of Medicine, The Royal Postgraduate Medical School, Hammersmith Hospital, Du Cane Road, London SE5 8RX

P. HUGH-JONES   Dept of Medicine, Chest Unit, King's College Hospital Medical School, Denmark Hill, London SE5 8RX

R. D. KEYNES   Physiological Laboratory, University of Cambridge, Downing Street, Cambridge CB2 3EG

G. de J. LEE   Cardiac Department, Radcliffe Infirmary, Oxford OX2 6HE

J. MAETZ   Groupe de Biologie Marine, Dept de Biologie, Commissariat à l'Energie Atomique, Station Zoologique, 06230 Villefranche-sur-mer, France

C. C. MICHEL   University Laboratory of Physiology, Parks Road, Oxford OX1 3PT

I. C. S. NORMAND   Dept of Child Health, University of Southampton, East Wing, Room E. 159, Southampton General Hospital, Tremona Road, Southampton SO9 4XY

R. E. OLVER   Dept of Paediatrics, University College Hospital Medical School, Huntley Street, London WC1E 6BH

E. D. ROBIN   Dept of Medicine, Stanford University School of Medicine, Stanford, California 94305, USA

E. SCHNEEBERGER   Dept of Pathology, Harvard Medical School and Children's Hospital Medical Center, 300 Longwood Avenue, Boston, Massachusetts 02119, USA

N. C. STAUB   Cardiovascular Research Institute and Dept of Physiology, University of California School of Medicine, Third & Parnassus Avenues, San Francisco, California 94122, USA

L. B. STRANG   Dept of Paediatrics, University College Hospital Medical School, Huntley Street, London WC1E 6DH

B. A. WAALER Institute of Physiology, University of Oslo, Karl Johans Gate, 47 Oslo 1, Norway

J. G. WIDDICOMBE Dept of Physiology, St. George's Hospital Medical School, Tooting, London SW17 0QT

Editors: Ruth Porter (*Organizer*) and Maeve O'Connor

Introduction: goals of the meeting

C. J. DICKINSON

*Medical Unit, University College Hospital Medical School, London**

Those who organize international symposia usually set out with the idea of reviewing a well-defined and much-studied field—presumably in the hope that a star-studded cast, abundant hospitality and an exotic venue will lead to a synthesis of opposing views and to the advancement of knowledge. I am sure that your experience is the same as mine: the synthesis usually proves elusive. All the participants already know each other and each other's opinions.

This symposium is different. We certainly have a star-studded cast; past experience assures us of the Ciba Foundation's abundant hospitality; and I hope that, at least for those who do not live in a metropolis, Portland Place in London can count as an exotic venue! The difference is in our subject. We have one which is neither well defined nor often discussed, and which may appear abstruse.

The human lungs when aerated in adult life contain only a few hundred millilitres of liquid, and most of this is in blood vessels. But we can identify at least three other actual or potential spaces for liquid: the interstitium, the lining of the alveoli, and the pleural space. We may have to consider separately the perivascular spaces and the liquid lining the larger air passages.

In health each of these compartments is small, but each has a characteristic composition and pressure. This symposium will concern itself especially with the endothelial membrane between blood vessels and interstitial space, and with the epithelial membrane between interstitial space and alveolar fluid. We are going to be looking at the differences between the properties of these two membranes and at the effects of these differences on the composition of different liquids and on the pressures in different spaces.

Although the symposium is concerned mainly with the lung, we have people

---

* *Present address:* Dept of Medicine, St Bartholomew's Hospital Medical College, London.

1

present who have studied the pleural fluid and the pleural space, and I hope we may have some time for discussion of this topic as well.

The choice of a little-discussed subject has given us the opportunity to bring together two main groups of scientists who in the ordinary course of events would seldom meet together. On the one hand we have those who have investigated the physiology of membranes and their permeability characteristics, and on the other we have pulmonary physiologists who are more accustomed to looking at lung function as a whole. I hope that each of us can learn from each other. The idea that a conference bringing together these two groups might be fruitful came first from Professor L. B. Strang, and on behalf of all the participants I would like to thank him and also Professor J. G. Widdicombe and Dr R. Porter of the Ciba Foundation, who helped to plan the meeting.

The theme of the first session is the structure and function, at a molecular level, of the two principal membranes; and we are going to start, very properly, with an account by Dr Schneeberger of the structural basis for alveolar-capillary permeability to molecules of different sizes.

Ultrastructural basis for alveolar-capillary permeability to protein

EVELINE E. SCHNEEBERGER

Department of Pathology, Harvard Medical School and Children's Hospital Medical Center, Boston, Massachusetts

Abstract The intravenous injection into mice of small volumes (less than 0.1 ml) of peroxidatic enzymes of molecular weight of 40 000 daltons or greater results in little if any penetration of these probe molecules into endothelial junctions. The injection of cytochrome *c* (12 000 daltons), on the other hand, results in the localization of this tracer in some but not all endothelial junctions. When horseradish peroxidase (EC 1.11.1.7) is injected in a large volume of saline (0.5 ml), reaction product is present in endothelial junctions and basement membrane, but is prevented from entering the alveolar space by zonulae oc-cludentes between epithelial cells. These experiments indicate that although endothelial junctions, under physiological conditions, are largely impermeable to molecules the size of horseradish peroxidase, and presumably most serum proteins, they are labile and susceptible to stretching if intravascular pressure is increased.

Freeze-fracture studies show that pulmonary capillary endothelial junctions are composed of one or at the most two strands which show areas of discontinuity. Epithelial junctions, by contrast, are composed of a continuous, complex network of anastomosing fibres. These observations confirm physiological experiments which indicate that it is the pulmonary epithelium rather than the endothelium which determines the permeability properties of the alveolar-capillary membrane to lipid-insoluble molecules. Bidirectional pinocytic transport is an additional mechanism whereby lipid-insoluble molecules are transported across both endothelial and epithelial layers. The relative contribution of this transport mechanism to the total amount transported remains to be established.

The alveolar-capillary membrane is uniquely adapted to subserve a number of diverse physiological functions. It not only acts as a membrane across which rapid and efficient exchange of oxygen and carbon dioxide takes place; it also serves as a site for two-way pinocytic transport of macromolecules. Furthermore, it provides an effective barrier against the penetration of harmful airborne particulate material and against the leakage of water and solutes from capillaries into alveolar spaces.

3

To maintain the last-mentioned function, a number of complex structural and functional adaptations exist in the lung which prevent the accumulation of excess fluid and protein in alveolar septa. (1) In contrast to the pressure in the systemic circulation, that of the pulmonary capillary system is between 5 and 15 mmHg (0.66–2 kPa), which is well below the osmotic pressure of plasma proteins. Such conditions favour fluid reabsorption and ensure a minimum entry of interstitial fluid into alveolar walls (Landis & Pappenheimer 1963). (2) Direct measurements indicate that interstitial fluid pressure in the lung may be at subatmospheric levels (Meyer *et al.* 1968; Guyton *et al.* 1971). This negative pressure would tend to draw fluid from both pulmonary capillaries and alveoli. Such interstitial fluid is subsequently drained away by pulmonary lymphatics. (3) As will be discussed, the intrinsic permeability properties of the alveolar-capillary membrane are such that they serve to maintain a barrier at the air–blood interface. (4) Finally, the intra-alveolar surfactant, by reducing surface tension, also counters the transudation of fluid into alveoli (Pattle 1965).

Although the permeability of the alveolar-capillary membrane to water and solutes has been the subject of many physiological studies (Cross *et al.* 1960; Schultz *et al.* 1964; Taylor *et al.* 1965; Chinard *et al.* 1962; Chinard 1966), it has only recently become possible to delineate the ultrastructural basis for the permeability barriers to proteins in the lung (Schneeberger-Keeley & Karnovsky 1968). The dimensions of such barriers have been elucidated by use of a cytochemical technique for the visualization of injected peroxidatic enzymes of different molecular weights (Graham & Karnovsky 1966). By using peroxidatic probe molecules of different sizes, investigators have defined the anatomical basis of a variety of tissue permeability barriers, and have shown that intercellular junctions play an important part in determining the permeability properties of epithelia to lipid-insoluble solutes. More recently, the technique of freeze-fracturing has provided a means of examining the detailed structure of such intercellular junctions (as reviewed by Staehelin 1974), and of correlating this structure with measured transepithelial resistance (Claude & Goodenough 1973). Both macromolecular tracer and freeze-fracture techniques have been applied to the alveolar-capillary membrane and have defined which of the layers in this multilayered structure is the chief anatomical permeability barrier to circulating proteins (Schneeberger-Keeley & Karnovsky 1968; Schneeberger & Karnovsky 1971, and unpublished). It is the purpose of this presentation to review these morphological findings, and to report on some new observations.

ULTRASTRUCTURE OF THE ALVEOLAR-CAPILLARY MEMBRANE

The ultrastructure of the alveolar-capillary membrane was examined in mouse lungs after the intratracheal instillation of formaldehyde–glutaraldehyde fixative (Fig. 1). A continuous non-fenestrated endothelium containing large numbers of pinocytic vesicles surrounds the capillary lumen. Many of these vesicles open on either the luminal or abluminal surface. In contrast to the large arterial vessels of the bronchial and pulmonary circulation (Pietra *et al.* 1971), pulmonary capillary endothelial cells contain few myofibrils (Smith & Ryan 1973), and therefore may be incapable of contracting. Pulmonary endothelial cells are held together by sites of adhesion which alternate with areas in which a gap of about 4 nm separates adjacent endothelial cells (Fig. 2a).

In the thinnest portions of the alveolar-capillary membrane, the alveolar interstitial space contains only the fused endothelial and epithelial basement membranes. These, after heavy metal staining, appear as a uniform dense meshwork of fine filaments which are separated from endothelial and epithelial cells, respectively, by a narrow, more electron-lucent layer.

The alveolar epithelium is heterogeneous in that it is composed of a continuous layer of membranous (type I) pneumocytes interspersed with granular (type II) pneumocytes. The former are flattened cells which cover a large expanse of alveolar surface with a thin smooth layer of cytoplasm. With the exception of relatively numerous pinocytic vesicles, their cellular organelles are inconspicuous. The cuboidal granular pneumocytes, by contrast, contain multivesicular bodies, multilamellar bodies (Sorokin 1966), mitochondria, peroxisomes (Petrik 1971; Schneeberger 1972a,b), rough endoplasmic reticulum and a prominent Golgi apparatus, and they appear to be involved in the synthesis and secretion of surfactant (Askin & Kuhn 1971). Unlike endothelial cell clefts, those between alveolar epithelial cells are obliterated towards the alveolar lumen by fusion of the outer leaflet of the bounding unit membranes (Fig. 2b).

Because it is removed by intracheal infusion of fixative, the extracellular alveolar layer is best seen after intravascular perfusion fixation (Gil 1974), or after freeze-substitution (Kuhn 1972). It is a flocculent or granular material with an electron-dense line about 4 nm thick at its surface.

PERMEABILITY OF THE ALVEOLAR-CAPILLARY MEMBRANE TO CIRCULATING PROTEIN

Extensive physiological studies (Landis & Pappenheimer 1963) have established that non-fenestrated capillary walls function as though they were semipermeable membranes penetrated by water-filled pores through which small,

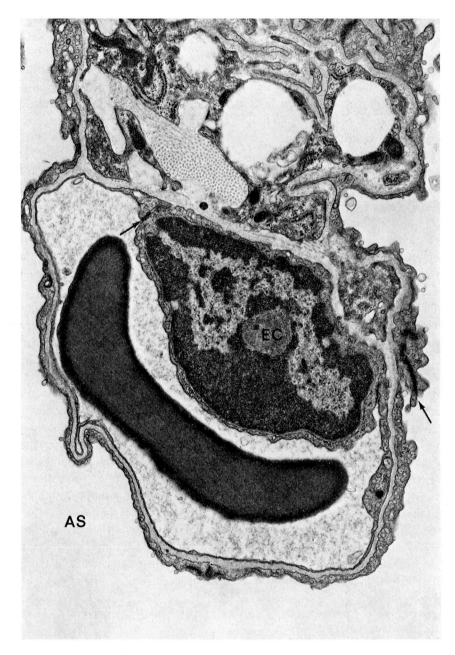

FIG. 1. An alveolar capillary showing the cell body of an endothelial cell (EC). The alveolar space (AS) is lined by type I pneumocytes. Endothelial and epithelial cell junctions are indicated by small arrows. × 17 000.

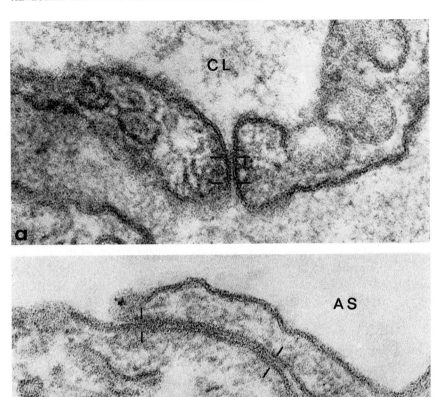

F<small>IG</small>. 2. (*a*) An endothelial cell junction showing a close approximation but no fusion of the bounding unit membranes in the area between the four small black lines. The capillary lumen (CL) is at the top. × 175 000.

(*b*) An epithelial cell junction between two type I pneumocytes. There is an apparent fusion of the bounding unit membranes in the area indicated between the small black lines. The alveolar space (AS) is at the top. × 175 000.

lipid-insoluble molecules exchange by diffusion. When lipid-insoluble molecules were injected into animals the pores resembled cylindrical water-filled channels of 4–4.5 nm radius and occupied not more than 0.1 % of the capillary surface area. There was moderate restriction to diffusion through this 'small pore' system in the molecular weight range of 1–10 000, and progressively greater restriction with increase in molecular weight. Thus molecules larger than

90 000 daltons were completely restricted at normal filtration rates. Further experiments (Grotte 1956; Renkin 1964) indicated that in addition to this 'small pore' system there was a so-called 'large pore' system which accounted for the slow passage of substances of high molecular weight ($> 90 000$ daltons) across the capillary walls. Because there was little restriction to diffusion with the molecular weights used, a vesicular transport system was suggested to be most compatible with the findings. Although this is still controversial (Simionescu *et al.* 1973, 1975), the 'small pore' system in non-fenestrated capillaries has been identified morphologically with intercellular junctions between adjacent endothelial cells (Karnovsky 1967, 1968), and the 'large pore' system with pinocytic vesicles (Bruns & Palade 1968).

In the alveolar-capillary membrane, physiological studies have indicated that it is the alveolar epithelium rather than the endothelium which restricts the passage of water-soluble solutes from the capillary lumen to the alveolar space (Taylor *et al.* 1965). Indeed, from experimentally determined reflection coefficients (Taylor & Gaar 1970), it was calculated that pulmonary endothelial pores have a radius of 4–5.8 nm and pulmonary epithelial pores a radius of 0.6–1 nm.

A clearer understanding of the ultrastructural basis for these results was obtained by using peroxidatic enzymes of different molecular weights as probe molecules. Briefly, the location of the intravenously injected peroxidatic enzyme is demonstrated by incubating aldehyde-fixed tissue with diaminobenzidine (DAB) and hydrogen peroxide. Reduced DAB forms an electron-dense reaction product after it has reacted with osmium tetroxide (Graham & Karnovsky 1966). The peroxidatic probe molecules used to study alveolar–capillary membrane permeability included cytochrome c (12 000 daltons, $a_e = 1.5$ nm) (Karnovsky & Rice 1969), horseradish peroxidase (EC 1.11.1.7) (40 000 daltons, $a_e = 3$ nm) (Graham & Karnovsky 1966), haemoglobin (64 500 daltons, $a_o = 3.5$ nm) (Pietra *et al.* 1969), lactoperoxidase (82 000 daltons, $a_e = 3.6$ nm (Graham & Kellermeyer 1968) and catalase (EC 1.11.1.6) (240 000 daltons, $a_e = 5.2$ nm) (Venkatachalam & Fahimi 1969). The effective hydrodynamic radius (a_e) was calculated using the Stokes–Einstein formula and the published diffusion coefficient for each molecule. The radius of uniform sphere of equal molecular weight (a_o) was calculated according to Renkin & Gilmore (1974).

Within one minute after intravenous injection of cytochrome c (12 000 daltons) into adult mice, the tracer was observed in endothelial junctions and the basement membrane (Fig. 3a). In some endothelial junctions reaction product was not visible in areas where the junctional space was narrowed by the proximity of the bounding unit membranes (Fig. 4a), while in other junctions

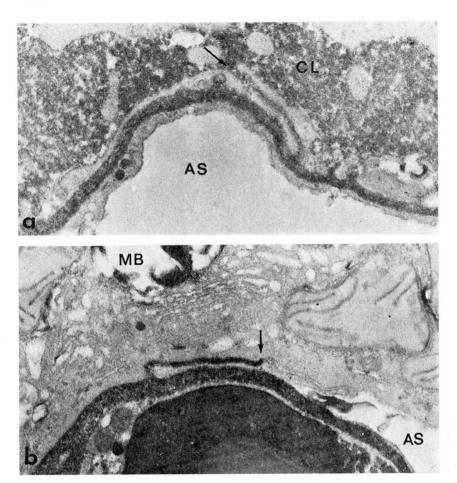

Fig. 3. (a) Lung from a mouse injected with cytochrome c in 0.2 ml saline 90 s before being killed. Reaction product fills the capillary lumen (CL), the endothelial junctions (arrow) and the basement membrane. The alveolar space (AS) is at the bottom. × 50 000.
(b) Lung from the same animal as in (a). Reaction product fills the basement membrane, a portion of the junction between a type I and a type II pneumocyte, but is prevented from diffusing beyond the point indicated by an arrow. A multilamellar body (MB) is indicated. × 50 000.

reaction product was present throughout the entire length of the junction (Fig. 4b). Cytochrome c was prevented from leaking into the alveolar space by tight junctions between both types of alveolar epithelial cells (Fig. 3b).

The intravenous injection of horseradish peroxidase (40 000 daltons) in a large volume of saline (0.5 ml) resulted, within 90 s, in a similar distribution of reaction product as was observed with cytochrome c (Schneeberger-Keeley &

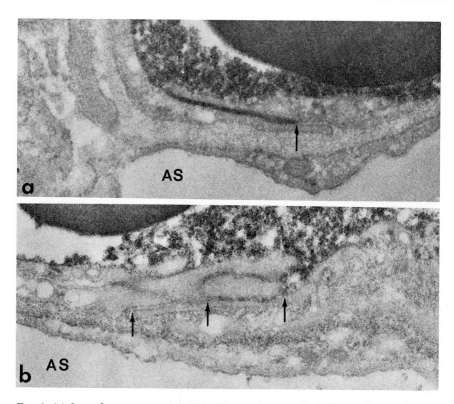

FIG. 4. (a) Lung from a mouse injected with cytochrome c in 0.05 ml saline 1 min before being killed. Reaction product fills the endothelial cleft but is prevented from entering into the basement membrane by a narrowed area within the junction (arrow). × 50 000.
(b) Lung from the same animal as in (a). A small amount of reaction product is visible throughout the length of the endothelial junction (arrows), as well as in the basement membrane. The alveolar space (AS) is at the bottom of both electron micrographs. × 50 000.

Karnovsky 1968). However, when the same dose was administered in the same small volume as was used for the injection of cytochrome c (0.05–0.1 ml), the reaction product remained confined to capillary lumens and pinocytic vesicles up to 6 min after injection, and none could be detected in endothelial junctions (Fig. 5) (Schneeberger & Karnovsky 1971). A similar effect of the injection volume on the distribution of reaction product was observed in the lungs of newborn mice, where the permeability of the alveolar-capillary membrane to peroxidatic tracers resembled that observed in adult mice (Schneeberger & Karnovsky 1971). The observation that horseradish peroxidase leaked through endothelial junctions only when injected in a large volume of saline was interpreted as indicating that a transient increase in intravascular fluid volume

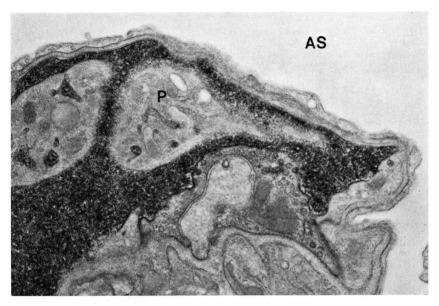

FIG. 5. Lung from a mouse injected with horseradish peroxidase in 0.05 ml saline 6 min before being killed. Note that reaction product is confined to the capillary lumen, vacuoles of platelets (P), and endothelial pinocytic vesicles. None is present in the basement membrane. The alveolar space (AS) is indicated. × 25 000.

widened endothelial junctions and permitted the passage of horseradish peroxidase. However, the extent of junctional widening was limited, since none of the high molecular weight tracers, including lactoperoxidase, catalase and ferritin, diffused through endothelial junctions even when injected in large volumes of saline (Schneeberger & Karnovsky 1971).

These observations are consistent with experiments carried out on isolated perfused dog lungs in which at normal perfusion pressure (15–20 mmHg) (2–2.66 kPa) both horseradish peroxidase and haemoglobin remained confined to the capillary lumen (Pietra et al. 1969). It was only when perfusion pressures were increased to 30 mmHg (4 kPa) for horseradish peroxidase and 50 mmHg (6.65 kPa) for haemoglobin that these two tracers leaked through endothelial junctions. These morphological observations lend support to the concept that endothelial pores may be labile and susceptible to stretching by increased intravascular pressure (Shirley et al. 1957). They also indicate that while endothelial junctions represent the site of diffusion of small water-soluble molecules, at normal capillary pressures, molecules the size of horseradish peroxidase and serum proteins are chiefly transported by pinocytic vesicles.

ROLE OF PINOCYTIC TRANSPORT IN THE ALVEOLAR-CAPILLARY
MEMBRANE

Evidence for the role of pinocytic vesicles in transendothelial transport was
largely obtained from time-sequence studies after the intravenous injection of
particulate electron-opaque tracers such as ferritin (600 000 daltons) (Bruns &
Palade 1968). With the passage of time after administration, endothelial
pinocytic vesicles from the luminal to the abluminal side of the cell gradually
became labelled. Furthermore, vesicular transport did not appear to be
unidirectional since tracer particles could apparently pass from the extracellular
spaces, go through the basement membrane, and then label pinocytic vesicles
(Brandt 1962; Wissig 1964). Although transport of markers from the tissue
towards the capillary lumen has not been directly demonstrated in pulmonary
capillaries, it is likely that pinocytic transport in pulmonary capillary endothelium is bidirectional as it is in other endothelia.

Type II pneumocytes do not participate in vesicular transport but there is
direct evidence for bidirectional pinocytic transport of protein across type I
pneumocytes. When horseradish peroxidase was injected in a large volume of
saline, reaction product was present in large amounts in the basement membrane
and epithelial pinocytic vesicles. Although much of the enzyme released onto
the alveolar surface was washed away by the intratracheal instillation of
fixative, evidence for the release of tracer into the alveolar lumen was provided
when reaction product was found within alveolar macrophages (Fig. 6). As
can be seen, tracer containing pinocytic vesicles at various stages of formation
is present on the surface of the macrophage as well as in the interior of the cell.
That the surface pinocytic vesicles are taking up rather than releasing tracer is
suggested by the fact that the tissue was fixed within two minutes of the enzyme
being injected. Furthermore, the presence of reaction product in the alveolar
macrophage does not represent endogenous peroxidase, since macrophages of
mice do not have any demonstrable endogenous peroxidase activity (Fedorko
& Hirsch 1970).

Epithelial transport appears to be important for delivering small quantities
of serum albumin and immunoglobulins to the alveolar space. Indeed, the
presence of IgG, IgA (Hand et al. 1974) and albumin (Klass 1973; Scarpelli
et al. 1973) has recently been demonstrated in secretions of the lower respiratory
tract. Pinocytic transport may also explain the presence of α_1-antitrypsin
(60 000 daltons) in human alveolar macrophages (Cohen 1973). Admittedly,
the inhibitor may have been taken up by macrophages before their migration
into the alveolar space; however, its presence in normal alveolar secretion has
recently been reported (Tuttle & Westerberg 1974).

Net transport of protein from the alveolar space into capillaries takes place

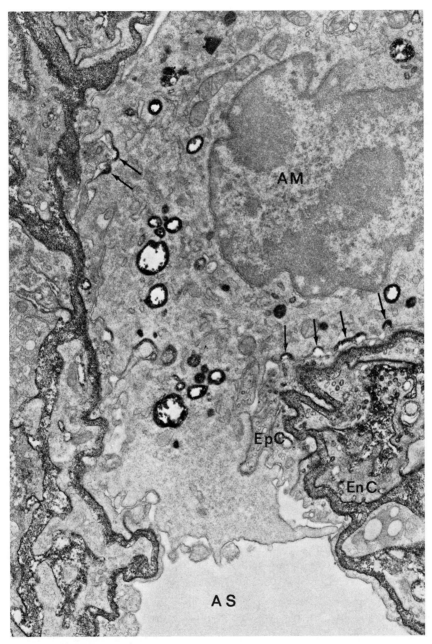

FIG. 6. Lung from a mouse injected with horseradish peroxidase in 0.6 ml saline, 2 min before being killed. Reaction product is present in basement membrane and pinocytic vesicles of endothelial cells (EnC) and epithelial cells (EpC). An alveolar macrophage (AM) is closely apposed to two alveolar surfaces. The small arrows indicate reaction product containing pinocytic vesicles at various stages of formation. Large vacuoles containing reaction product are present in the interior of the alveolar macrophage. × 17 000. Reprinted from Lenfant (1975), with permission.

not only during the resorption of intra-alveolar oedema fluid, but also during removal of lung liquid in the newborn period. That this is by means of pinocytic vesicles was shown after the intranasal administration of small quantities of horseradish peroxidase to adult or newborn mice (Schneeberger & Karnovsky 1971). In these animals, epithelial intercellular junctions remained impermeable to the tracer, and instead small quantities of the enzyme were taken up by vesicles of type I pneumocytes (Fig. 7). The pinocytic transport of protein across epithelium appeared to be relatively slow. Even one hour after administration of the enzyme, easily visualized quantities of tracer remained in the alveolar space. However, it is possible that drying of the tracer deposits at the air–tissue interface precluded a more efficient uptake of protein by epithelial cells. Similar observations have been made in lungs of newborn rabbits (Gonzalez-Crussi & Boston 1972).

FREEZE–FRACTURE STUDIES OF ENDOTHELIAL AND EPITHELIAL JUNCTIONS OF THE ALVEOLAR-CAPILLARY MEMBRANE

The evidence from physiological and morphological studies with tracers suggests that the permeability of the alveolar epithelial junctions differs from that of endothelial junctions. We therefore compared the freeze–fracture images of these two types of junctions. In brief, the technique of freeze–fracture involves the freezing of tissue in liquid nitrogen followed by the cleaving of the frozen specimen with a blade under high vacuum. This fracture surface is then coated with platinum and carbon. Tissue is subsequently removed from the replica with hypochlorite, and the replica is picked up on a copper grid for examination in the electron microscope. By convention the A face of the membrane is on the cytoplasmic side and the B face on the luminal side of the cell.

Endothelial junctions. Preliminary observations show that the A face of pulmonary endothelial junctions is composed of one or at the most two strands, which in some regions have a beaded appearance (Fig. 8*a*). In many areas these strands are continuous and run along a considerable length of the endothelial surface, but there are areas of discontinuity (Fig. 8*b*). Except for the discontinuities, these images are similar to those described in very leaky proximal convoluted tubular junctions of mouse kidney (Claude & Goodenough 1973). In some regions, a small gap junction is associated with the strands of the endothelial junctions. It has been reported that the microvasculature of the rat mesentery and omentum contains gap junctions in the arteriolar and venular portions of this vascular network, but not in the capillaries themselves

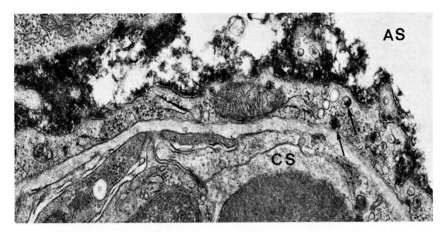

Fig. 7. Lung from a newborn mouse given horseradish peroxidase one hour before being killed. Epithelial pinocytic vesicles (arrows) contain reaction product, but the epithelial junctions (not shown) are free of any detectable reaction product. × 31 300. Reprinted from Lenfant (1975), with permission.

(Simionescu *et al.* 1974). It is possible, therefore, that in the lung those endothelial junctions having an associated gap junction are in fact in either the arteriolar or venular segment of the alveolar vascular bed.

Epithelial junctions. In contrast to the endothelial junctions, those of the epithelium form, on the A fracture face, a complex network of interconnecting junctional strands (Fig. 9). Complementary grooves are present on the B fracture face. These junctions are continuous and form a belt-like region surrounding both type I and type II pneumocytes. Their structure is similar to that described in other 'tight' epithelial junctions (Claude & Goodenough 1973). In the toad urinary bladder and gall bladder it has been shown that the ridges seen in A fracture faces are in fact single fibrils shared by adjacent cells, rather than a double set of fibrils with one set belonging to each cell (Wade & Karnovsky 1974). The single-fibre model provides a more plausible structural explanation than the double-fibre model for the role of these tight junctions in restricting permeability and forming cell-to-cell attachments.

The freeze-fracture observations of the cellular junctions present in the alveolar–capillary membrane lend additional morphological support to reported physiological measurements. They are compatible with the concept that it is the epithelial rather than the endothelial layer which is the chief barrier to diffusion of water-soluble solutes across the alveolar–capillary membrane.

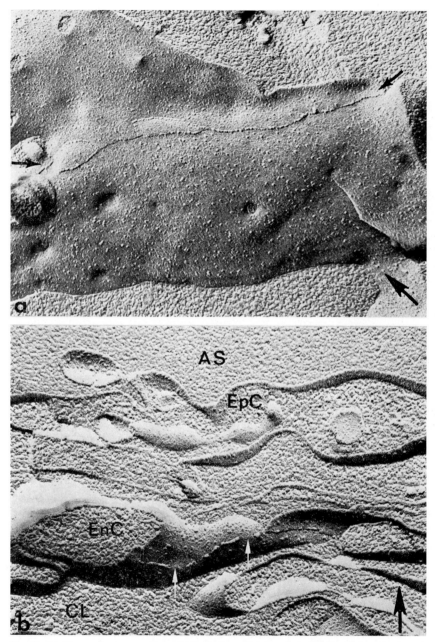

FIG. 8. (a) Freeze-fracture replica of the A face of an endothelial junction. The junction (between the two small arrows) is composed of one or at the most two strands which have a beaded appearance. The large arrow indicates the direction of shadowing. × 69 300.
(b) Freeze-fracture replica of the A face of an endothelial junction showing two areas of discontinuity (white arrows). The alveolar space (AS), epithelial cell (EpC), endothelial cell (EnC) and capillary lumen (CL) are labelled. The large arrow indicates the direction of shadowing. × 82 500.

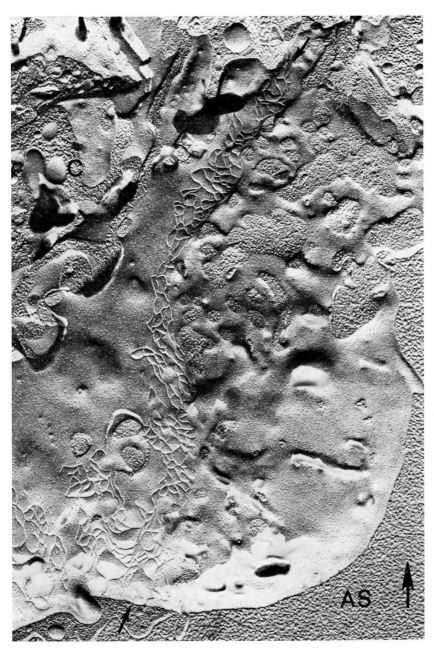

FIG. 9. Freeze-fracture replica of the A face of an epithelial junction (between the two small arrows) which forms a continuous belt-like structure. The junction is composed of an intricate anastomosing network, 3–5 fibres in width. The alveolar space (AS) and a capillary (C) are labelled. The large arrow indicates the direction of shadowing. × 25 000.

DISCUSSION

The ultrastructural and physiological evidence permits a model of the alveolar–capillary membrane to be constructed which reconciles several seemingly contradictory observations. On the one hand the air–blood barrier is relatively impermeable to lipid-insoluble solutes (Chinard 1966), while on the other transport of macromolecules has been shown to occur across this membrane (Klass 1973; Scarpelli *et al.* 1973; Hand *et al.* 1974). This is best explained in the light of both ultrastructural and physiological observations if the intercellular junctions are viewed as the principal barrier to the diffusion of lipid-insoluble molecules. Both tracer and freeze–fracture studies indicate that it is the continuous complex network of fibres of the epithelial junctions which ultimately governs the permeability of the alveolar-capillary membrane. Although the pulmonary endothelial junctions are normally impermeable to proteins the size of horseradish peroxidase, and presumably to most serum proteins, they are susceptible to widening when intravascular pressure is raised (Pietra *et al.* 1969; Schneeberger & Karnovsky 1971), and serum proteins can then diffuse into the underlying basement membrane. This constitutes a possible mechanism for the formation of oedema when hydrostatic pressure is increased.

Recently the role of endothelial junctions as the anatomical equivalent of the 'small pore' system has been questioned, particularly in view of conflicting results obtained with microperoxidase (1900 daltons) in capillaries of mouse diaphragm. While in some studies reaction product was observed to fill the length of endothelial junctions within seconds of injection (Wissig & Williams 1974), in others the tracer was largely confined to pinocytic vesicles and was seen only rarely in endothelial junctions (Simionescu *et al.* 1975). There may be age, species and tissue differences in the permeability of non-fenestrated capillaries which account for these differing observations. In pulmonary capillaries, under physiological conditions, few proteins the size of horseradish peroxidase or larger can be visualized within endothelial junctions, and it is only with increased intravascular pressure that tracer can be demonstrated within the junction. This does not exclude endothelial junctions from being the 'small pore' system in pulmonary capillaries, since the amount of small proteins diffusing through these junctions, under physiological conditions, may be too small to be visualized with the techniques available. Furthermore, the gaps in pulmonary endothelial junctional fibres, as seen by freeze–fracture, suggest that endothelial junctions are not continuous zonulae occludentes, but rather contain sites through which small lipid-insoluble molecules may diffuse.

Both endothelial cells and type I pneumocytes contain pinocytic vesicles which are capable of transporting macromolecules in a bidirectional fashion. That pinocytic vesicles may transport sizeable amounts of protein is suggested by certain theoretical considerations (Shea & Karnovsky 1969). Using data from studies in which ferritin (600 000 daltons) was used as a tracer (Bruns & Palade 1968), Shea & Karnovsky calculated a mean transit time for an endothelial pinocytic vesicle of 1 s, and a traversing flux of nine vesicles/μm^{-2} s^{-1}. Although these calculations were based on cardiac and skeletal muscle capillaries, similar figures may obtain in pulmonary epithelial and endothelial cells. Such pinocytic transport could account for some of the protein present in lung lymph, as well as the presence of albumin, gammaglobulin and α_1-antitrypsin in lung washings (Klass 1973; Scarpelli et al. 1973; Tuttle & Westerberg 1974).

Although recently developed ultrastructural techniques have provided a clearer understanding of the structural basis for the permeability properties of the alveolar-capillary membrane, many questions remain to be answered. For example, what is the magnitude of pinocytic transport across these two cellular layers? Are all endothelial junctions in the pulmonary capillary bed similar or are there some through which diffusion of small macromolecules preferentially takes place? If water and protein leak through endothelial junctions when hydrostatic pressure is increased, by what route do these materials gain access to alveoli during the formation of alveolar oedema fluid? What is the structure and function of the alveolar-capillary membrane during development of the fetal lung? What role does the alveolar-capillary membrane play in the formation of lung liquid? Finally, at birth, what causes the lung to change from a relatively solid, fluid-filled organ to one which is primarily involved in efficient gas exchange? It is evident that much work remains to be done.

ACKNOWLEDGEMENTS

Supported in part by US Public Health Grant No. AM 16392. The excellent technical help of Mrs Monika Leventhal and Miss Joanne Lynch is gratefully acknowledged. Stimulating discussions with Dr Morris J. Karnovsky and the critical review of the manuscript by Dr Robert D. Lynch are greatly appreciated.

References

ASKIN, F. B. & KUHN, C. (1971) The cellular origin of pulmonary surfactant. *Lab. Invest.* 25, 260-268

BRANDT, P. W. (1962) A study of pinocytosis in muscle capillaries. *Anat. Rec. 142*, 219

BRUNS, R. R. & PALADE, G. E. (1968) Studies on blood capillaries. II Transport of ferritin molecules across the wall of muscle capillaries. *J. Cell Biol. 37*, 277-299

CHINARD, F. P. (1966) The permeability characteristics of the pulmonary blood–gas barrier, in *Advances in Respiratory Physiology* (Caro, C. G., ed.), Edward Arnold, London

CHINARD, F. P., ENNS, T. & NOLAN, M. F. (1962) The permeability characteristics of the alveolar capillary barrier. *Trans. Assoc. Am. Physicians Phila.* 75, 253-262

CLAUDE, P. & GOODENOUGH, D. A. (1973) Fracture faces of zonulae occludentes from 'tight' and 'leaky' epithelia. *J. Cell Biol.* 58, 390-400

COHEN, A. B. (1973) Interrelationships between the human alveolar macrophages and alpha-1-antitrypsin. *J. Clin. Invest.* 52, 2793-2799

CROSS, C. E., RIEBEN, P. A. & SALISBURY, P. E. (1960) Urea permeability of alveolar membrane; hemodynamic effects of liquid in the alveolar spaces. *Am. J. Physiol.* 198, 1029-1031

FEDORKO, M. E. & HIRSCH, J. G. (1970) Structure of monocytes and macrophages. *Semin. Hematol.* 7, 109-124

GIL, J. (1974) Ultrastructure of lung fixed under physiologically defined conditions. *Arch. Intern. Med.* 127, 896-902

GONZALEZ-CRUSSI, F. & BOSTON, R. W. (1972) The absorptive function of the neonatal lung. Ultrastructural study of horseradish peroxidase uptake at the onset of ventilation. *Lab. Invest.* 26, 114-121

GRAHAM, R. C. & KARNOVSKY, M. J. (1966) The early stages of absorption of injected horseradish peroxidase in the proximal tubules of mouse kidney. Ultrastructural cytochemistry by a new technique. *J. Histochem. Cytochem.* 14, 291-302

GRAHAM, R. C. & KELLERMEYER, R. W. (1968) Bovine lactoperoxidase as a cytochemical protein tracer for electron microscopy. *J. Histochem. Cytochem.* 16, 275-278

GROTTE, G. (1956) Passage of dextran molecules across the blood-lymph barrier. *Acta Chir. Scand. Suppl.* 211, 5-84

GUYTON, A. C., GRANGER, H. J. & TAYLOR, A. E. (1971) Interstitial fluid pressure. *Physiol. Rev.* 51, 527-563

HAND, W. L., CANTEY, J. R. & HUGHES, C. G. (1974) Antibacterial mechanisms of the lower respiratory tract. *J. Clin. Invest.* 53, 354-362

KARNOVSKY, M. J. (1967) The ultrastructural basis of capillary permeability studied with peroxidase as a tracer. *J. Cell Biol.* 35, 213-236

KARNOVSKY, M. J. (1968) The ultrastructural basis of transcapillary exchange. *J. Gen. Physiol.* 52, 64s-95s

KARNOVSKY, M. J. & RICE, D. F. (1969) Exogenous cytochrome C as an ultrastructural tracer. *J. Histochem. Cytochem.* 17, 751-753

KLASS, D. J. (1973) Immunochemical studies of the protein fraction of pulmonary surface active material. *Am. Rev. Respir. Dis.* 107, 784-789

KUHN, C., III (1972) A comparison of freeze substitution with other methods of preservation of the pulmonary alveolar lining layer. *Am. J. Anat.* 133, 495-508

LANDIS, E. M. & PAPPENHEIMER, J. R. (1963) Exchange of substances through capillary walls, in *Handb. Physiol.* Section 2: *Circulation*, vol. 2 (Hamilton, W. F. & Dow, P., eds.), pp. 961-1034, American Physiological Society, Washington, D.C.

LENFANT, C. (ed.) (1975) *Lung Biology in Health and Disease*, Dekker, New York, in press

MEYER, B. J., MEYER, A. & GUYTON, A. C. (1968) Interstitial fluid pressure. V. Negative pressure in the lungs. *Circ. Res.* 22, 263-271

PATTLE, R. E. (1965) Surface lining of lung alveoli. *Physiol. Rev.* 45, 48-79

PETRIK, P. (1971) Fine structural identification of peroxisomes in mouse and rat bronchiolar and alveolar epithelium. *J. Histochem. Cytochem.* 19, 339-348

PIETRA, G. G., SZIDON, J. P., LEVENTHAL, M. M. & FISHMAN, A. P. (1969) Hemoglobin as a tracer in hemodynamic pulmonary edema. *Science (Wash. D.C.)* 166, 1643-1646

PIETRA, G. G., SZIDON, J. P., LEVENTHAL, M. M. & FISHMAN, A. P. (1971) Histamine and interstitial pulmonary edema in the dog. *Circ. Res.* 29, 323-337

RENKIN, E. M. (1964) Transport of large molecules across capillary walls. *Physiologist 7*, 13-28

RENKIN, E. M. & GILMORE, J. P. (1974) Glomerular filtration, in *Handb. Physiol.* Section 8: *Renal Physiology* (Orloff, J. & Berliner, R. W., eds.), pp. 185-248, American Physiological Society, Washington, D.C.

SCARPELLI, E. M., WOLFSON, D. R. & COLACICCO, G. (1973) Protein and lipid-protein fractions of lung washings: Immunological characterization. *J. Appl. Physiol. 34*, 750-753

SCHNEEBERGER, E. E. (1972a) A comparative cytochemical study of microbodies (peroxisomes) in great alveolar cells of rodents, rabbit and monkey. *J. Histochem. Cytochem. 20*, 180-191

SCHNEEBERGER, E. E. (1972b) Development of peroxisomes in granular pneumocytes during pre- and postnatal growth. *Lab. Invest. 27*, 581-589

SCHNEEBERGER, E. E. & KARNOVSKY, M. J. (1971) The influence of intravascular fluid volume on the permeability of newborn and adult mouse lungs to ultrastructural protein tracers. *J. Cell Biol. 49*, 319-334

SCHNEEBERGER-KEELEY, E. E. & KARNOVSKY, M. J. (1968) The ultrastructural basis of alveolar-capillary membrane permeability to peroxidase used as a tracer. *J. Cell Biol. 37*, 781-793

SCHULTZ, A. L., GRISNER, J. T., WADA, S. & GRANDE, F. (1964) Absorption of albumin from alveoli of perfused dog lungs. *Am. J. Physiol. 207*, 1300-1304

SHEA, S. M. & KARNOVSKY, M. J. (1969). Vesicular transport across endothelium: Simulation of a diffusion model. *J. Theor. Biol. 24*, 30-42

SHIRLEY, H. H., JR, WOLFRAM, C. G., WASSERMAN, K. & MAYERSON, H. S. (1957) Capillary permeability to macro-molecules: Stretched pore phenomenon. *Am. J. Physiol. 190*, 189-193

SIMIONESCU, N., SIMIONESCU, M. & PALADE, G. E. (1973) Permeability of muscle capillaries to exogenous myoglobin. *J. Cell Biol. 57*, 424-452

SIMIONESCU, M., SIMIONESCU, N. & PALADE, G. E. (1974) Characteristic endothelial junctions in sequential segments of the microvasculature. *J. Cell Biol. 63*, 316a

SIMIONESCU, N., SIMIONESCU, M. & PALADE, G. E. (1975) Permeability of muscle capillaries to small heme-peptides. Evidence for the existence of patent transendothelial channels. *J. Cell Biol. 64*, 586-607

SMITH, U. & RYAN, J. W. (1973) Electron microscopy of endothelial and epithelial components of the lung: Correlations of structure and function. *Fed. Proc. 32*, 1957-1966

SOROKIN, S. P. (1966) A morphological and cytochemical study on the great alveolar cell. *J. Histochem. Cytochem. 14*, 884-897

STAEHELIN, L. A. (1974) Structure and function of intercellular junctions. *Int. Rev. Cytol. 39*, 191-283

TAYLOR, A. E. & GAAR, K. A. (1970) Estimation of equivalent pore radii of pulmonary capillary and alveolar membranes. *Am. J. Physiol. 218*, 1133-1140

TAYLOR, C. E., GUYTON, A. C. & BISHOP, V. S. (1965) Permeability of the alveolar membrane to solutes. *Circ. Res. 16*, 353-362

TUTTLE, W. C. & WESTERBERG, S. C. (1974) Alpha-1 globulin trypsin inhibitor in canine surfactant protein. *Proc. Soc. Exp. Biol. Med. 146*, 232-235

VENKATACHALAM, M. A. & FAHIMI, H. D. (1969) The use of beef liver catalase as a protein tracer for electron microscopy. *J. Cell Biol. 42*, 480-489

WADE, J. A. & KARNOVSKY, M. J. (1974) The structure of the zonula occludens. *J. Cell Biol. 60*, 168-180

WISSIG, S. L. (1964) The transport by vesicles of proteins across the endothelium of muscle capillaries. *Anat. Rec. 148*, 411

WISSIG, S. L. & WILLIAMS, M. C. (1974) Passage of microperoxidase across the endothelium of capillaries of the diaphragm. *J. Cell Biol. 63*, 375a

Discussion

Farhi: What is the pattern of charge distribution in ferritin, Dr Schneeberger?

Schneeberger: Native ferritin has a negative charge. We have not used cationic ferritin in the lung and I don't know whether it would produce a difference in the pattern of pinocytic labelling. Positively and negatively charged ferritin molecules are being used to study the permeability of the glomerular capillary membrane (M. A. Venkatachalam and R. S. Cotran, personal communication). In the glomerular capillary wall there appears to be a distinct difference in the distribution of positively as compared to negatively charged ferritin.

Farhi: In general, with negatively charged ferritin, do you see a distribution of charges along either the endothelial or epithelial membrane, such as Skutelsky & Danon (1970) saw with red cell membrane?

Schneeberger: We have not looked at it with that in mind.

Strang: The selective permeation of different electrolytes across fetal pulmonary epithelium indicates that it carries fixed negative charges (Olver & Strang 1974).

Staub: Would the horseradish peroxidase method detect one molecule? Can you give me a published reference to the sensitivity of the method and its limits of detection?

Schneeberger: I don't know how many molecules are required. It is said that enzymic tracers have the advantage over particulate tracers of having an amplifying effect, that is one molecule of enzyme can give rise to many molecules of reaction product. However, the detection of small quantities of reaction product is limited by our ability to discriminate between small variations in electron density on electron micrographs. Peroxidase tracers vary in their sensitivity. Microperoxidase, for example, is considerably more sensitive than horseradish peroxidase.

Fishman: G. G. Pietra and J. Aronson (unpublished observations) have found that the concentration of horseradish peroxidase that can be detected is of the order of 0.05%. Horseradish peroxidase has a greater amplifying effect than myoglobin and haemoglobin, which have to be present in concentrations of 1.0 to 0.5% before they can be detected. Myeloperoxidase has a greater amplifying effect than any of the others.

Dickinson: When you see a slot of 4 nm diameter between two apposed cells in the endothelium presumably what you are seeing is one hole or discontinuity in the single line which shows in the freeze–fracture surface. Since the discontinuities seem to be rather infrequent, are the junctions where you can see a passage right through equally infrequent?

Schneeberger: Yes, they are rather infrequent but I can't yet give you exact figures. However, freeze–fracture studies of diaphragmatic capillaries and muscle capillaries in G. E. Palade's laboratory (Simionescu *et al.* 1974) have shown that the number of strands seen in freeze-fracture images is greater than the number of sites of apposition that can be detected by transmission electron microscopy. At present, therefore, there is no good correlation between the images seen by freeze–fracture and those observed by transmission electron microscopy.

Dickinson: Have you done any comparable morphological investigations on the lung in pulmonary oedema, or are the freezing problems insuperable?

Schneeberger: I have not done that, but we would of course like to study the freeze–fracture image of lungs fixed under increased intravascular pressure. In lungs perfused with EDTA or under increased pressure (Hovig *et al.* 1971) no widening of endothelial junctions was detected. Whether there is widening of the discontinuities in the strands seen by freeze–fracture has yet to be determined.

Maetz: Pinocytic phenomena also occur in the 'chloride cells' of fish gills. Have you ever seen any microfilamentous or microtubular structures associated with the pinocytic vesicles, Dr Schneeberger? In sea water fish, substances such as colchicine block salt secretion within four hours and the microtubules associated with pinocytic vesicles are destroyed. Something similar in your animals might help to answer some of the quantitative questions.

Schneeberger: Are the pinocytic vesicles reduced in number in those conditions?

Maetz: I don't know yet.

Schneeberger: I have not looked at microfilaments carefully myself but Smith & Ryan (1973) reported that, in the lung, microfilaments are more numerous in arteriolar endothelial cells than in capillary endothelial cells.

Durbin: Are you suggesting that these vesicles do not move by Brownian motion but by some other mechanism, Dr Maetz?

Maetz: Calcium as well as ATP is essential for the active movements which produce salt secretion in the gills of the mullet. Without calcium, salt secretion stops. Calcium is also essential in neurosecretion, for example, and exocytosis of the pinocytic vesicles can be blocked with colchicine. The problem is that colchicine may have numerous other effects (see Douglas 1974).

Fishman: The pictures that have been shown suggest that alveolar junctions have little potential for stretching. Indeed, they seem more apt to tear than to enlarge. If this is so, why is alveolar oedema reversible?

Schneeberger: We have yet to find the answer to that question. I am not aware of any systematic studies in which the effect of increased intraluminal pressure on tight intercellular junctions has been studied.

Olver: This has been studied in the frog cornea (Zadunaisky 1971). Hydrostatic pressure expands intercellular junctions, leading to a marked increase in fluid permeability and ionic conductance. After as little as two minutes both ultrastructural and functional changes are back to normal.

Schneeberger: Are those gaps large enough to allow the escape of protein?

Olver: Zadunaisky produced gaps in the intercellular junctions which appeared large enough to allow the passage of proteins. Although these changes were reversible, a stage may be reached at which the epithelium is completely disrupted and has to be repaired before function is restored.

Fishman: I remain puzzled about the implications of your pictures for the mechanisms by which interstitial fluid enters the alveoli, Dr Schneeberger. In our laboratory, the macromolecular tracers seemed to have more difficulty in reaching alveolar spaces from the interstitium than in passing from the capillary lumens into the interstitium. We concluded that alveolar junctions are tighter than endothelial junctions—but not immutable. Your pictures suggest irreversibility even though clinical experience suggests that alveolar oedema is remarkably reversible. How can we reconcile the ultrastructural and clinical observations? The fact that alveolar junctions are tighter than endothelial junctions is entirely consistent with clinical experience. But the suggestion that alveolar junctions must be disrupted in order to open is puzzling.

Schneeberger: Yes, we don't know what factors cause these junctions to come apart, if they come apart at all.

Olver: In the lamb fetus the epithelial junctions may open up as lung liquid is absorbed, but Dr Egan will tell us about that later (this volume, pp. 101–110).

How complex are the tight junctions in the alveolar epithelium in relation to those in other epithelia? Is the correlation between complexity and electrical resistance good enough for us to be able to predict what the electrical resistance of the alveolar epithelium might be?

Schneeberger: Claude & Goodenough (1973) have correlated the number of strands with the transepithelial resistance of epithelia. I think it remains to be established whether this is a really good correlation. As I mentioned, at least in the endothelium we don't find a good correlation between the number of strands and the patency of the junction. Pulmonary epithelium has rather complex tight junctions, although not as complex as those in toad bladder. Gut epithelium has tight junctions similar in appearance to those we have observed in the alveolar epithelium.

Olver: Which part of the gut are you referring to? The small intestine is quite leaky.

Schneeberger: The jejunum (Claude & Goodenough 1973).

Strang: Labelled albumin injected intravenously is detectable about two minutes later in lung lymph.

Robin: Wright & Pietras (1975) have done a lovely series of studies on the ability of large polar solutes, such as sucrose and inulin, to penetrate various epithelial surfaces—rabbit gall bladder, frog choroid plexus and toad urinary bladder. The permeability coefficients (10^{-7}cm/s)were:

	Rabbit gall bladder	*Frog choroid plexus*	*Toad urinary bladder*
Urea	890	120	14
Sucrose	40	16	1.4

We did (similar) experiments in saline-filled dog lungs (Theodore *et al.* 1975) and the permeability coefficients (10^{-7}cm/s) of inulin and dextran, urea and sucrose were:

	Alveolar epithelium
Urea	27
Sucrose	7
Inulin	1
Dextran (mol.wt. 60 000—90 000)	0.8

Macromolecules do get through saline-filled alveolar epithelium. Inulin and relatively large dextran molecules also get through with measurable and reproducible permeability coefficients. The other point is that alveolar epithelium, if a number of assumptions are granted, fits midway between the 'tightest' epithelium, toad urinary bladder, and the 'loosest' epithelium, rabbit gall bladder. We interpreted these findings as suggesting that alveolar epithelium has a system of channels with a small number of wide pores ($>$ 8 nm), permitting permeation of large polar solutes. One can also see, and this is true for inulin as well, that the various epithelial surfaces appear to be either consistently tight or consistently loose. That is to say that the order for urea, sucrose and inulin is the same, with an epithelial surface which is tight for one molecule being consistently tight for other molecules as well.

Dickinson: How big are urea and sucrose molecules?

Olver: The urea molecule is 0.22 nm in radius and sucrose is 0.51 nm. The alveolar epithelium of the saline-filled dog lung is clearly different from fetal alveolar epithelium, which is completely impermeable to inulin and to albumin. The ratio of urea to sucrose permeability is much higher in the fetal lung, at least 100-fold, indicating that the fetal lung epithelium is much tighter than epithelium in this saline-filled dog lung.

Robin: It is interesting that the permeability coefficients for sucrose, inulin and dextran bear the same ratios to each other as the free diffusion coefficients in water. This would suggest that not only is diffusion taking place, but it is taking place through aqueous-filled pores.

Olver: But through large pores. The fact that the ratios of the permeability coefficients are roughly equal to those of the free diffusion coefficients implies that the epithelium may have been damaged in this type of experiment.

Robin: That is possible. Smulders & Wright (1971) obtained evidence that permeation of polar solutes could not be accounted for by edge damage and they went to great lengths to establish this. Such evidence, or such assurance, is much more difficult to get for the lung. The fact that one gets regular reproducibility would suggest either that one is indeed dealing with an intrinsic property of the alveolar epithelium, or that one is producing exactly the same amount of damage each time. The latter is unlikely.

Staub: In the rabbit, EDTA produces a profound pulmonary oedema but there is no evidence, by transmission electron microscopy, of changes in the intercellular junctions (Hovig *et al.* 1971). In the pancreas EDTA appears to break down tight junctions although it has no effect on gap junctions (Amsterdam & Jamieson 1974). It might be profitable to study freeze-fractured material to see whether EDTA alters the number of junctional strands, and to relate that to whether the endothelium is becoming more leaky.

Dejours: The thickness of alveolar capillary walls varies in different mammals, and possibly the structure of pulmonary cells varies too. Does the permeability of the alveolar wall vary with size in mammals? What kind of mice did you study, Dr Schneeberger?

Schneeberger: The Swiss albino mouse.

Dickinson: Can anyone tell us about the ultrastructural appearance of lungs of other species?

Dejours: Weibel (1973) studied mammals ranging in size from the shrew to the dog.

Staub: Those animals all had about the same barrier thickness.

Dejours: They were not identical.

Staub: The differences are trivial. The thickest alveolar membrane that I know of is in the kangaroo rat, because of its thick alveolar epithelium.

Hugh-Jones: Your permeability coefficients were presumably obtained with isotonic saline, Professor Robin. What happens if the osmotic pressure is slightly altered? There must be a critical relationship, with molecules passing or not passing through the epithelium according to whether it is slightly stretched.

Robin: That is true. Lungs filled with isotonic saline have minor ultrastructural abnormalities. On the other hand, they provide reproducible data, and the lung filled with isotonic saline is much more like the lung in pulmonary oedema than an air-filled lung. This suggests that relationships like this indeed provide a valid picture of how alveolar-pulmonary capillary junctions function in pulmonary oedema.

Hugh-Jones: But it is also important in relation to other species. There must be very slight changes in amphibians and in fish in those conditions.

Robin: Yes, that is true, and Dr Maetz has evidence about this. Elasmobranchs with a tonicity of about 1 osmol presumably have cell membranes and sub-cell membranes with relative impermeability to urea. How they function under various osmotic circumstances is, of course, complex.

Hugh-Jones: But is it actually the epithelial holes which alter with osmotic pressure?

Robin: Probably both epithelium and endothelium are affected.

Agostoni: Is there any evidence of pores between the mesothelial cells of the visceral pleura?

Schneeberger: I am not aware of any tracer studies of the visceral pleura. According to Cotran & Karnovsky (1968), the junctions between mesothelial cells of the abdominal cavity are very permeable to horseradish peroxidase.

Staub: Scanning electron microscopy of the parietal pleura shows quite large gaps (Wang 1975).

References

AMSTERDAM, A. & JAMIESON, J. D. (1974) Studies on dispersed pancreatic exocrine cells. I. Dissociation technique and morphologic characteristics of separated cells. *J. Cell Biol. 63*, 1037-1056

CLAUDE, P. & GOODENOUGH, D. A. (1973) Fracture faces of zonulae occludentes from 'tight' and 'leaky' epithelium. *J. Cell Biol. 58*, 390

COTRAN, R. S. & KARNOVSKY, M. J. (1968) Ultrastructural studies on the permeability of the mesothelium to horseradish peroxidase. *J. Cell Biol. 37*, 123

DOUGLAS, W. W. (1974) Exocytosis and the exocytosis-vesiculation sequence with special reference to neurohypophysis, chromaffin and mast cells, calcium and calcium ionophores, in *Secretory Mechanisms of Exocrine Glands* (Thorn, N. A. & Peterson, O. H., eds.), *(Alfred Benzon Symp. 7)*, 116-129, Munksgaard, Copenhagen

HOVIG, T., NICOLAYSEN, A. & NICOLAYSEN, G. (1971) Ultrastructural studies of the alveolar-capillary barrier in isolated plasma-perfused rabbit lungs. Effects of EDTA and of increased capillary pressure. *Acta Physiol. Scand. 82*, 417-431

OLVER, R. E. & STRANG, L. B. (1974) Ion fluxes across the pulmonary epithelium and the secretion of lung liquid in the foetal lamb. *J. Physiol. (Lond.) 241*, 327-357

SIMIONESCU, M., SIMIONESCU, N. & PALADE, G. E. (1974) Characteristic endothelial junctions in sequential segments of the microvasculature. *J. Cell Biol. 63*, 316a

SKUTELSKY, E. & DANON, D. (1970) Electron microscopical analysis of surface charge labelling density at various stages of the erythroid line. *J. Membr. Biol. 2*, 1973

SMITH, U. & RYAN, J. W. (1973) Electron microscopy of endothelial and epithelial components of the lung: correlation of structure and function. *Fed. Proc. 32*, 1957

SMULDERS, A. P. & WRIGHT, E. M. (1971) The magnitude of nonelectrolyte selectivity in the gallbladder epithelium. *J. Membr. Biol. 5*, 297-318

THEODORE, J., ROBIN, E. D., GAUDIO, R. & ACEVEDO, J. (1975) Transalveolar transport of large polar solutes (sucrose, inulin, dextran). *Am. J. Physiol. 229*, 989-996

WANG, N-S. (1975) The preformed stromas connecting the pleural cavity and the lymphatics in the parietal pleura. *Am. Rev. Respir. Dis. 111*, 12-20

WEIBEL, E. R. (1973) Morphological basis of alveolar-capillary gas exchange. *Physiol. Rev. 53*, 419-495

WRIGHT, E. M. & PIETRAS, R. J. (1975) Routes of nonelectrolyte permeation across epithelial membranes. *J. Membr. Biol. 17*, 293-312

ZADUNAISKY, J. A. (1971) Electrophysiology and transparency of the cornea, in *Electrophysiology of Epithelial Cells* (Giebisch, G., ed.) pp. 225-255, Schattayer, Stuttgart

Permeability of pulmonary vascular endothelium

A. P. FISHMAN and G. G. PIETRA

Cardiovascular-Pulmonary Division of the Department of Medicine, and the Department of Pathology, University of Pennsylvania School of Medicine, Philadelphia, Pennsylvania

Abstract   Three aspects of transendothelial exchange in the lungs are considered: stretching of interendothelial junctions of pulmonary microvessels by increase in pulmonary capillary pressures; selective stretching of interendothelial junctions of bronchial venules in response to histamine, bradykinin and endotoxin; active transport of peptides across the body of the endothelial cell after enzymic action at or near the luminal surface of the endothelial cell. Stretching of interendothelial junctions between the cells lining the pulmonary capillaries was demonstrated using a variety of macromolecular tracers under controlled haemodynamic conditions. Selective leakage of bronchial venules, the *systemic* venules of the lungs, was shown using colloidal carbon as a tracer. Transendothelial transport of peptides across the pulmonary capillary lining involved the use of electron microscopic autoradiography after intravenous administration of radioactively-labelled lipoproteins. Different mechanisms appear to provide routes of entry into the perivascular interstitial spaces of the lungs.

More than a decade ago, our laboratory initiated a systematic exploration of the mechanisms by which excess water and proteins accumulate in the lungs (Fishman 1972). A natural point of departure for these studies seemed to be Starling's law of transcapillary exchange: on the one hand, a great deal of information had accumulated by then to show that the 'law' applied to the systemic circulation (Landis & Pappenheimer 1963); on the other hand, initial attempts to see how the law fared in the lungs had suggested the unsettling conclusion that interstitial pressures could be discounted in any explanation of haemodynamic pulmonary oedema (Guyton & Lindsey 1959). We were aware of the formidable problems that would face attempts to measure interstitial fluid and oncotic pressures directly. Consequently, we tried to circumvent this apparently insuperable problem for the lungs by resorting to experimental conditions under which the concentration of interstitial proteins in the lungs could reasonably be assumed to be negligible albeit not directly measurable

(Levine *et al.* 1967). Under experimental conditions involving extreme haemo-
dilution and increments in pulmonary capillary pressures, we found that the
forces identified by Starling's law did indeed apply to water exchange in the
lungs, that interstitial forces did not appear to be negligible, and that the
interstitial fluid pressures in the vicinity of the pulmonary capillaries had to be
subatmospheric if our experimental observations were to be explained (Mellins
et al. 1969).

Then, as now, the concentration of albumin in the interstitial space was a
haunting enigma. Moreover, there was no clear idea of the route by which
albumin managed to reach the interstitial spaces of the lungs. Therefore, when
stroma-free haemoglobin, which was being developed for its possibilities as a
plasma substitute, became available to us, we seized the opportunity to use it
as a macromolecular tracer for ultrastructural studies under controlled haemodynamic conditions, since it was about the same molecular weight as albumin
and its molecular configuration was well understood. In our studies, tracer
quantities of haemoglobin were localized by Karnovsky's technique for the
electron microscopic demonstration of peroxidatic activity (Graham &
Karnovsky 1966). Our results showed that the level of pulmonary capillary
pressure was a major determinant of pulmonary capillary permeability: at
normal pressures, the injected haemoglobin appeared to be confined to the
vascular spaces of the lungs; when pulmonary capillary pressures were greatly
increased—of the order of three times normal—the tracer was readily seen
between the interendothelial clefts, forming an uninterrupted stream between
the vascular lumen and the pericapillary interstitial space (Pietra *et al.* 1969).
Pinocytosis appeared to be playing only a subsidiary role, if any, in this enhanced
passage of the tracer. From these experiments, the conclusion seemed inescapable that the enhanced passage of the tracer was due to the 'stretching' of
interendothelial junctions ('pores') that are closed at ordinary pulmonary
capillary pressures. A similar explanation had been offered previously for
systemic and lung capillaries, to account for otherwise inexplicable transcapillary passage of macromolecules (Shirley *et al.* 1957). This conclusion also
served to reconcile our observations with earlier experiences of others using
horseradish peroxidase (EC 1.11.1.7) in the mouse (Schneeberger & Karnovsky
1968). That more than molecular weight was involved was demonstrated by
using different tracers and finding disparities in the level of pulmonary capillary
pressure that caused leakage. For example, myoglobin (molecular weight,
17 000) failed to escape into the pericapillary interstitial space at levels of
pressure which promoted the ready passage of horseradish peroxidase (molecular
weight, 40 000) across pulmonary capillary walls into the interstitial space
(Pietra *et al.* 1972).

Quite surprising was the lack of effect on pulmonary capillaries of pharmacological agents, such as histamine and bradykinin, which enjoy an apparently well-earned reputation for enhancing permeability of systemic capillaries. Indeed, in the lungs, as in muscles and abdominal viscera, these agents seem to enhance permeability by affecting systemic, rather than pulmonary, blood vessels.

Against this background, the present report will summarize some recent observations on the permeability of the minute pulmonary blood vessels and the passage of tracers across their walls.

STRETCHED PORES

We have reported previously that myoglobin, a smaller molecule than horseradish peroxidase, did not leak at a level of pressure that caused horseradish peroxidase to leak (Pietra *et al.* 1972). We have since continued to explore the behaviour of myoglobin as an ultrastructural tracer. Fig. 1 shows

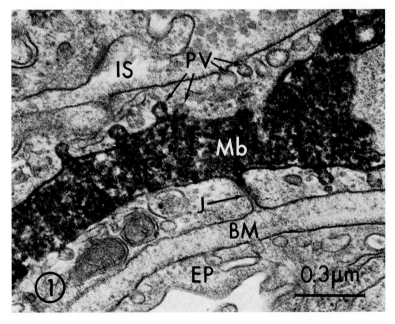

FIG. 1. A pulmonary capillary after injection of a solution of myoglobin (Mb). Pulmonary capillary pressure was normal. The tracer is confined to the capillary lumen and to the plasmalemmal vesicles (PV) that open to the lumen. It extends to the junctional region (J) of the interendothelial cleft, leaving unstained the basement membrane (BM), the interstitial space (IS), the alveolar epithelial cells (EP), and the abluminal plasmalemmal vesicles (PV).

an electron micrograph from a lobe of a dog lung that was perfused with a 3 % myoglobin solution before the lobar vein was tied and the pulmonary artery pressure maintained at 10 mmHg (1.33 kPa) for 5 min. Osmiophilic reaction product (Mb) fills the capillary lumen, the vesicles (PV) that open on to the lumen, and the segment of the interendothelial cleft on the luminal side up to the point of arrest in the region of the junction (J). The pericapillary interstitial space is devoid of reaction product. The apparent limitation of the tracer to the lumen of the capillary and to its direct continuities implies that if any tracer has traversed the capillary wall, it has done so at concentrations that are not detectable by this technique.

In contrast, Fig. 2 illustrates the results obtained when the pulmonary arterial pressure in the lung lobe is maintained at 30 mmHg (4 kPa) for 5 min. This lower magnification shows that the reaction product is no longer confined to the capillary lumen. Instead, it stains the basement membrane and the ground substance of the interstitial space. Two interendothelial clefts (arrows) are filled with reaction product. Some vesicles that are apparently free in the endothelial cytoplasm and others that open on the basement membrane are also filled with reaction product. Close scrutiny of many similar sections reveals that the concentration of tracer in the pericapillary interstitial space is less than in the lumen, indicating restriction to the transcapillary movement of myoglobin. One conclusion seems unavoidable: the movement of myoglobin across the capillary wall was enhanced by the higher pulmonary arterial pressure. However, the route taken by myoglobin in crossing the capillary wall is debatable: it may have passed through the interendothelial junctions, filling the abluminal vesicles by retrograde filling from the interstitial space (Karnovsky 1967); an alternative is accelerated transendothelial movement of vesicles or formation of transendothelial channels by fusion of chains of vesicles, followed by retrograde filling of the interendothelial junctions (Simionescu et al. 1973, 1975). Of the two, our evidence favours passage via stretched interendothelial junctions. In many instances we found interendothelial clefts completely filled with tracers while vesicles free in the endothelial cytoplasm appeared empty; only in one instance did we find a chain of vesicles connecting the lumen with the pericapillary space, suggesting that fusion of vesicles for transport of macromolecular tracers is an infrequent occurrence in pulmonary capillaries.

LEAKY BRONCHIAL VENULES

Histamine, bradykinin and endotoxin (Pietra et al. 1971; Pietra et al. 1974), administered intravenously, caused bronchial venules to become highly

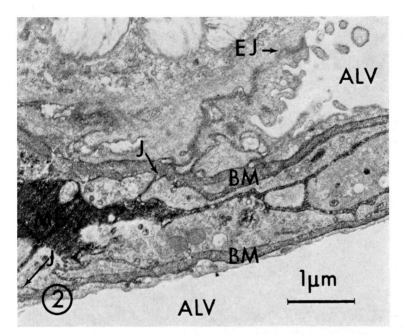

FIG. 2. A pulmonary capillary after injection of a solution of myoglobin at increased pulmonary capillary pressure. The tracer fills two interendothelial clefts (J), stains the basement membrane (BM) and has spread widely throughout the interstitial space. It does not penetrate the epithelial junction (EJ) and does not enter the alveoli (ALV).

permeable to large tracers without apparent effect on pulmonary capillary permeability. Administration of histamine by routes other than intravenously achieved the same effect (Pietra *et al.* 1971). The effect of subpleural injection of 0.1 mg of histamine base on the dog lung is shown in Fig. 3. Colloidal carbon was injected intravenously, 0.5 ml/kg body weight, immediately before the subpleural injection. The lung was fixed one hour later. Carbon deposits are shown between the endothelium and the pericytes of a peribronchial venule. Similar results were obtained by liberation of endogenous histamine by compound 48/80 administered subpleurally (Pietra *et al.* 1971).

The mechanism by which carbon escapes is illustrated in Fig. 4. Carbon is shown in a widened interendothelial junction of a bronchial venule 3 min after subpleural histamine administration. The ground substance in the perivenular space appears unusually electron-lucent, suggesting that excess water has accumulated in the vicinity of the bronchial venule. Not shown are the pulmonary capillaries which retained carbon within their lumens. Consequently, these chemical mediators of permeability caused peribronchial interstitial oedema without affecting the pulmonary circulation. It should be

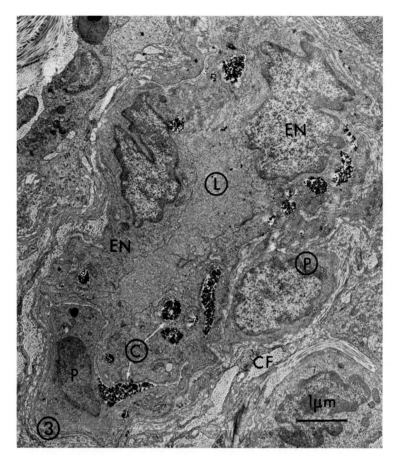

Fig. 3. A bronchial venule about one hour after subpleural injection of histamine base and colloidal carbon. Carbon deposits are found outside the lumen (L), between the endothelium (EN) and pericytes (P). There is no oedema at this time.

noted that the period of increased bronchial venular permeability is transient: leakage consistently stopped within 10 min after histamine or bradykinin administration, leaving trapped tracer (colloidal carbon) in the adventitia of the bronchial venules. Gradually, as in Fig. 3, the oedema fluid is removed and the carbon is left as evidence that leakage had occurred.

The mechanism by which histamine, bradykinin and endotoxin exert this selective effect on the endothelium of the bronchial venules is speculative. Most attractive is the idea of opening of interendothelial junctions by contraction of the endothelial fibrils with which bronchial venular endothelium is richly endowed. In this respect, the systemic venules of the lungs

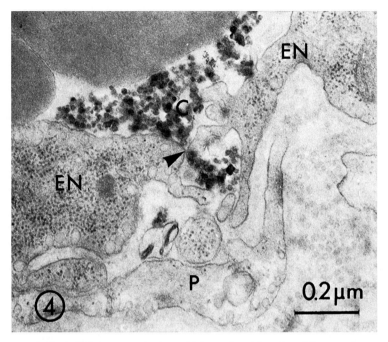

FIG. 4. Endothelial aspect of a bronchial venule, with carbon (C) traversing a widened inter-endothelial junction (arrowhead).

appear to resemble the systemic venules of the cremaster muscle of the rat which also leak selectively in response to histamine (Majno *et al.* 1969). In contrast to the rich concentration of fibrils in bronchial venular endothelium is their sparsity in the endothelium of alveolar capillaries and pulmonary veins. The selective response of the bronchial venules to a wide assortment of biologically active substances, as well as the extraordinary extent and ramifications of the bronchial venular plexus, raises intriguing questions about the possible pathogenic role of this vascular bed in impairing water drainage from the lungs.

TRANSENDOTHELIAL TRANSPORT

The lungs provide the first capillary bed that is encountered by chylomicrons and lipoproteins as they leave the intestine and liver. Chylomicrons and very low density (VLD) lipoproteins constitute a readily available circulating source of energy and may provide substrate for the synthesis of the phospholipid and protein components of the surfactant material (Felts 1964; Hamosh & Hamosh 1975; King 1974). In order to explore how these substances are handled by

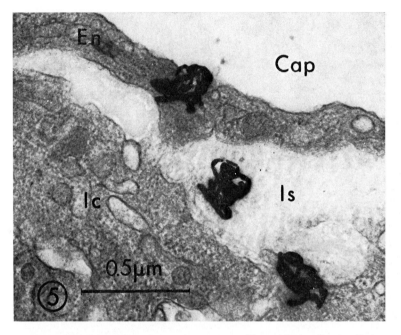

FIG. 5. Endothelial aspect of a pulmonary capillary (Cap) after perfusion with ^{125}I-labelled peptide (VLD lipoprotein) for 60 min. Radioactivity is localized to three areas: endothelial cell (En), interstitial space (Is) and interstitial cell (Ic).

the lung capillaries, in our laboratory Pietra *et al.* (1975) have applied a combination of biochemical ultrastructural and physiological strategies to this problem. Of particular interest to the present report are some results obtained by perfusing isolated rat lungs with radioactively labelled low density (LD) and VLD lipoproteins. Fig. 5 is an electron microscopic autoradiograph from a rat lung that was perfused *in vitro* with ^{125}I-labelled peptide (VLD lipoprotein) for 60 min. Since it was shown separately that 5–30% of the radioactive label disappeared from the perfusate during the 60 min of perfusion and that a lipoprotein lipase (triacylglycerol lipase, EC 3.1.1.3) is located in or near the endothelium, the autoradiograph helps to localize the site of transport of the labelled peptides. Three silver grains are seen: one over the cytoplasm of an endothelial cell, another in the interstitial space, and the third over an interstitial cell. None were found over intercellular junctions. Since the peptides are lipid-insoluble, some active mechanism for their transendothelial transport seems most likely. Whether pinocytosis involving plasmalemmal vesicles or another carrier mechanism is involved is unsettled (Zilversmit 1973).

These observations illustrate the complexity of the transport processes that are responsible for moving constituents of blood across the endothelium into the interstitial space of the lungs. It seems clear that even within the lungs, the endothelium is uniform neither in ultrastructure nor in function and the trans-endothelial transport mechanisms may vary accordingly. Certainly the minute vessels of the lungs that arise from the systemic circulation differ in responses from those of the pulmonary circulation. It would take us far afield at this juncture to attempt to uncover the reasons why histamine and bradykinin appear to be without effect on pulmonary capillary permeability while they are exerting dramatic ultrastructural effects on the permeability of bronchial venules. But it does seem reasonable to wonder whether the lack of effect is related to the rapid inactivation of these (and other) biologically active substances at the endothelial surfaces of the pulmonary capillaries (Fishman & Pietra 1974). As a corollary, does the bronchial venular endothelium lack this ability? Moreover, no matter what the reason for this discrepancy, physiological and pathophysiological implications of the selective responses of the endothelial cells that we have reported above remain to be elucidated.

ACKNOWLEDGEMENTS

The personal research referred to was generously supported by grants from the National Heart and Lung Institute. We are grateful to our associates, Drs L. G. Spagnoli, D. M. Capuzzi and J. B. Marsh, for permission to reproduce Fig. 5.

References

FELTS, J. M. (1964) Biochemistry of the lung. *Health Phys. 10*, 973-979

FISHMAN, A. P. (1972) Pulmonary edema. The water exchanging function of the lung. *Circulation 46*, 390-408

FISHMAN, A. P. & PIETRA, G. G. (1974) The handling of bioactive substances by the lung. *N. Engl. J. Med. 291*, 884-890, 953-959

GRAHAM, R. C. & KARNOVSKY, M. J. (1966) The early stage of absorption of injected horse-radish peroxidase in the proximal tubule of the mouse kidney. Ultrastructural cyto-chemistry by a new technique. *J. Histochem. Cytochem. 14*, 291-302

GUYTON, A. C. & LINDSEY, A. W. (1959) Effect of elevated left atrial pressure and decreased plasma protein concentration on the development of pulmonary edema. *Circ. Res. 7*, 649-657

HAMOSH, M. & HAMOSH, P. (1975) Lipoprotein lipase in rat lung. The effect of fasting. *Biochim. Biophys. Acta 380*, 132-140

KARNOVSKY, M. J. (1967) The ultrastructural basis of capillary permeability studied with peroxidase as a tracer. *J. Cell Biol. 35*, 213-236

KING, R. J. (1974) The surfactant system of the lung. *Fed. Proc. 33*, 2238-2247

LANDIS, E. M. & PAPPENHEIMER, J. R. (1963) Exchange of substances through the capillary wall, in *Handb. Physiol.* Section 2 (Hamilton, W. F. & Dow, P., eds.), pp. 961-1034, American Physiological Society, Washington, D.C.

LEVINE, O. R., MELLINS, R. B., SENIOR, R. M. & FISHMAN, A. P. (1967) The application of Starling's law of capillary exchange to the lungs. *J. Clin. Invest.* 46, 934-944

MAJNO, G., SHEA, S. M. & LEVENTHAL, M. M. (1969) Endothelial contraction induced by histamine-type mediators: an electron microscopy study. *J. Cell Biol.* 42, 647-672

MELLINS, R. B., LEVINE, O. R., SKALAK, R. & FISHMAN, A. P. (1969) Interstitial pressure of the lung. *Circ. Res.* 24, 197-212

PIETRA, G. G., SZIDON, J. P., LEVENTHAL, M. M. & FISHMAN, A. P. (1969) Hemoglobin as a tracer in hemodynamic pulmonary edema. *Science (Wash. D.C.)* 166, 1643-1646

PIETRA, G. G., SZIDON, J. P., LEVENTHAL, M. M. & FISHMAN, A. P. (1971) Histamine and interstitial pulmonary edema in the dog. *Circ. Res.* 29, 323-337

PIETRA, G. G., SZIDON, J. P., & FISHMAN, A. P. (1972) Leaky pulmonary vessels. *Trans. Assoc. Am. Physicians Phila.* 85, 369-376

PIETRA, G. G., SZIDON, J. P., CARPENTER, H. A. & FISHMAN, A. P. (1974) Bronchial venular leakage during endotoxin shock. *Am. J. Pathol.* 77, 387-402

PIETRA, G. G., SPAGNOLI, L. G., CAPUZZI, D. M., MARSH, J. B. & FISHMAN, A. P. (1975) Lipoprotein uptake by the lung. *Am. J. Pathol.* 78, 10a

SCHNEEBERGER, E. E. & KARNOVSKY, M. J. (1968) The ultrastructural basis of alveolar-capillary membrane permeability to peroxidase used as a tracer. *J. Cell Biol.* 37, 781-793

SHIRLEY, H. H. JR., WOLFRAM, C. G., WASSERMAN, K. & MAYERSON, H. S. (1957) Capillary permeability to macromolecules. Stretched pore phenomenon. *Am. J. Physiol.* 190, 189-193

SIMIONESCU, N., SIMIONESCU, M. & PALADE, G. E. (1973) Permeability of muscle capillaries to exogenous myoglobin. *J. Cell Biol.* 57, 424-452

SIMIONESCU, N., SIMIONESCU, M. & PALADE, G. E. (1975) Permeability of muscle capillaries to small heme-peptides. Evidence for the existence of patent transendothelial channels. *J. Cell Biol.* 64, 586-607

ZILVERSMIT, D. B. (1973) A proposal linking atherogenesis to the interaction of endothelial lipoprotein lipase with triglyceride-rich lipoproteins. *Circ. Res.* 33, 633-638

Discussion

Waaler: Are the vascular pressures you referred to in the work on stretched pores, left atrial pressures or calculated capillary pressures?

Fishman: The experimental design was such that capillary pressures could be determined directly from the height of the perfusing column.

Dickinson: Since the circulation is arrested for 10 min when you clamp the pulmonary veins, would any components of the apparent change in pore size be due to shortage of nutrients? Presumably the lung was still ventilated, so that it was oxygenated and carbon dioxide was being removed.

Fishman: The same phenomenon can be observed under more natural conditions while the circulation is intact. The use of a static column in one lobe of the lung allows precise control of capillary pressure and conserves tracer substances. The same picture of stretched pores occurs after much briefer periods of arrest, e.g. 1 min.

Dejours: Were you speaking of steady hydrostatic pressure or of pulsatile pressure in the lung, Dr Fishman?

Fishman: In the experiments that I showed a static column was used and the pressures were mean pressures. However, the same phenomenon occurs during pulsatile flow. Indeed, it seems to us that pulsatile capillary pressures in the pulmonary circulation favour the formation of interstitial fluid. Thus, during strenuous exercise, excess water may enter the interstitial space with each systolic beat as pulmonary capillary systolic pressures reach levels high enough to stretch endothelial pores.

Waaler: Is this a continuous and gradual effect, with signs of the pores being stretched as soon as pressure is raised above the normal level, or does nothing happen until a certain pressure threshold is reached? When we measured hydraulic conductivity in isolated perfused lungs (P. K. Lunde & B. A. Waaler, unpublished work) we got the impression that the extent of capillary filtration was proportional to the increase in capillary pressure, at least up to the level of 30 mmHg (4 kPa).

Fishman: Until pulmonary capillary pressures exceeded levels of about twice normal, the stretched pore phenomenon was not observed. Thereafter, it occurred regularly. Not all pores were stretched at a given pressure level. But, as pressures increased, more and more of the pores appeared to be involved. Since pressures vary in the capillaries from the top to the bottom of the lungs, it seems reasonable to expect that the dependent capillaries would have the higher pressures and be more apt to show the stretched pore phenomenon. But this is still speculative since we have not had the opportunity to do a systematic study of this problem.

Waaler: So there are pressure thresholds for this mechanism?

Fishman: Our experiments suggest that there are thresholds.

Michel: Fluid filtration is a much more sensitive index of pore stretching than permeability. If pores expand continuously as pressure is raised, the rate of filtration increases as a power function of capillary pressure. At first glance, the reported findings suggest that this may happen. Dr Guyton (Guyton & Lindsey 1959; Gaar *et al.* 1967) and Dr Waaler (Lunde & Waaler 1969) believe their findings suggest that filtration increases with left atrial pressure only after left atrial pressure has reached a certain level. I think that your earlier findings (Levine *et al.* 1967) were similar, Dr Fishman, but you drew a curve through them and this curve was of the shape predicted for pore stretching.

I believe that these findings can be used to examine the stretched pore hypothesis more closely (see Fig. 1). Dr Guyton's group lowered the protein concentration of the plasma perfusing the lungs and found that high rates of filtration were then seen at much lower pressure than when the protein was normal; the dependence of fluid accumulation in the lung on left atrial pressure was similar to that seen when plasma protein concentration was normal but

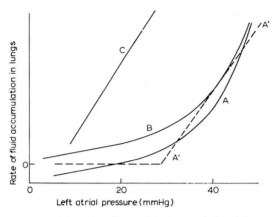

Fɪɢ. 1. (Michel) The effects of changes in left atrial pressure upon fluid accumulation in the lung. Curve A represents the relationship which would be anticipated if fluid moved out of pulmonary capillaries through pores which were stretched as intravascular pressure increased. Curve A is consistent with the reported data though Guyton & Lindsey (1959) and Gaar *et al.* (1967) represented the relationship as a linear one with a threshold (dashed curve A′). Curve B is the relationship which would be anticipated for such a capillary bed when the plasma protein concentration of the perfusate is reduced; the slope of B varies with pressure in the same way as the slope of A. Curve C represents the data of Gaar *et al.* (1967) for lungs perfused with plasma having a lowered protein concentration. These data appear to be inconsistent with the hypothesis that stretched pores are responsible for the increasing rate of fluid accumulation at raised left atrial pressures.

with the relationship displaced in a parallel fashion to a region of low pressure. It is difficult to interpret these findings in terms of the stretched pore hypothesis, for why should the stretching of pores be dependent on protein concentration?

Guyton: You are absolutely correct that, theoretically, when the curve shifts to the left the slope should decrease if the stretched pore phenomenon is operating. If it is not operating, shifting to the left would not affect the slope. Unfortunately, in our studies, when the curve shifted to the left because of decreased colloid osmotic pressure, we also had a much greater scatter of points than with normal colloid osmotic pressure. Therefore, I would not be able to say for certain from those findings whether there was a change in slope or not.

Michel: If haemoglobin cannot get out of pulmonary capillaries at low pressures, but can leak out through stretched pores at high pressures, there must be a significant difference between the filtration coefficient at low pressure and at high pressure.

Fishman: But the all-or-none model that you are describing is hardly realistic. Clearly some of the exchange appears to occur by way of stretched pores. Whether other mechanisms are also operative is unsettled. Among these potential mechanisms are pinocytosis and transendothelial transport via 'large pores'.

Michel: If a few large pores are opened up they will tend to dominate what happens to fluid flow if all the fluid flows through a pore system.

Fishman: Yes, unless they are emptying into circumscribed interstitial pockets that communicate sluggishly with the rest of the interstitial space. A good deal depends on the model that one has in mind.

Robin: Dr Guyton was measuring changes in lung water or, more specifically, in lung weight; and since there is a disposal pathway which is probably not constant, namely the lymphatics, then as filtration increases, the rate at which water is taken out by the lymphatics may well increase too. You are only dealing with net transport, Dr Michel, whereas Dr Fishman—although his results are qualitative—is dealing with gross transport.

Strang: It is one thing to propose various mechanisms for the transport of proteins or molecules across epithelia, but are there any viable proposals for the volume flow of water or filtration occurring by any pathway other than the pore system?

Fishman: Most investigators accept that the bulk of the water flow occurs directly across the endothelial cell. At least that is the impression I gathered from the proceedings of the Benzon conference on capillary permeability (Crone & Lassen 1970).

Michel: I slightly disagree with that. Yudilevich & Alvarez (1967) showed that 50% of the water exchanging in their indicator dilution experiments might be diffusing across the cell, that is by a pathway not available to small hydrophilic solutes. A lot of argument at the Benzon symposium was about whether 50% of the water is or is not going across the cell membrane when there is net fluid flow across the capillary wall. If as much as 50% of the water does pass the capillary wall via the cell membrane under these conditions, then it means that the original analysis of Pappenheimer *et al.* (1951), which neglected the osmotic reflection coefficient, was numerically correct. That is, there was no need for Pappenheimer *et al.* to account for the reflection coefficient because the capillary wall behaved almost as if it were a semi-permeable membrane.

Fishman: Do you think that most of the water flow is through pores or through the body of the cell?

Michel: It is quite possible that a fair fraction of water goes through a pathway—I won't say it is the cell—which is not available to the low molecular weight hydrophilic solutes.

Staub: The net effect can't be significant. We find that the total electrolyte concentration of lung lymph is nearly identical to that of plasma. If any free water filters through the endothelial cells, this changes the plasma concentration of electrolytes so that they diffuse rapidly through the intercellular junctions. For practical purposes, it is as if the water and electrolytes flowed freely through the junctions.

Michel: As Pappenheimer (1953) said many years ago, the rates of diffusion of small molecules are so rapid that one just cannot expect to set up a significant concentration difference during ultrafiltration.

Staub: What is the lowest pressure at which you find any evidence of pore stretching, Dr Fishman? Our studies on steady state, unanaesthetized sheep do not support the view that pores are stretched at left atrial pressures of up to at least 40 cmH$_2$O (3.92 kPa) (Staub 1974). At higher pressures, there may well be pore stretching.

Fishman: Fig. 2 (p. 33) shows what happened when myoglobin was the tracer substance and capillary pressure was maintained at 30 mmHg (4 kPa) for 5 min. It illustrates that a pulmonary capillary pressure of 30 mmHg produced stretched pores.

Michel: In systemic capillaries there is a lot of evidence against pore stretching occurring in the sort of range, i.e. up to 50 mmHg (6.65 kPa), that you are dealing with, Dr Fishman. The capillary wall in many tissues is reasonably well supported and this may prevent the stretching of pores. In the lungs, capillaries may be supported less well and the pores may get stretched.

Staub: Our evidence against pore stretching was based on the lymph/plasma ratios of albumin and gammaglobulin under steady state conditions at various levels of pulmonary microvascular hydrostatic pressure.

Fishman: How would you recognize it by that technique?

Staub: Our conclusion is based on the protein flow, rather than the fluid flow. Every increase in left atrial pressure in our sheep caused an increase in steady state lymph flow, but the protein flow (lymph concentration × lymph flow) did not increase as much. The simplest model that fitted these observations, both for albumin and gammaglobulin over a wide range of capillary hydrostatic pressures in four different sheep, consisted of three equivalent pore populations (Erdmann *et al.* 1975; Blake & Staub 1972).

In sheep given intravenous infusions of *Pseudomonas* bacteria, however, there was a large increase in protein flow as well as fluid flow, indicating a significant increase in the microvascular permeability to proteins (Brigham *et al.* 1974). When we modelled the equivalent pore structure for the microvascular membrane under these conditions, we found that the fluid and protein flow could be accounted for by modest increases in the number and dimensions of the small and intermediate pores. These changes are probably too small to be detected by electron microscopy.

Dickinson: That may be useful in reconciling these two types of experiments.

Fishman: I'm afraid that I remain unreconciled on several accounts. For example, I cannot relate Dr Staub's physiological interpretations to the anatomical changes that Dr Schneeberger and I have shown. Particularly unsettling are the comments about endotoxin. In our laboratory, Pietra and co-workers have shown that histamine and endotoxin cause pulmonary arterioles and venules—not capillaries—to leak. Therefore, it would seem reasonable to wonder whether it is really the pulmonary capillaries that are leaking in Dr Staub's endotoxin experiments.

Finally, I have serious misgivings about modelling on the basis of three pore sizes: given three pore sizes and a good computer, there is not much about pulmonary vascular permeability that cannot be explained. But the biological validity of the explanation could depend heavily on the anatomical assumptions about the size, nature and distribution of the pores.

Waaler: What you said about the permeability of pulmonary vessels not being influenced by histamine and bradykinin agrees completely with what we found several years ago, Dr Fishman. The filtration coefficient didn't change at all when we infused large doses of histamine or bradykinin into the pulmonary circulation of isolated lungs (Hauge *et al.* 1966).

Widdicombe: Have you eliminated effects due to the contraction of bronchiolar smooth muscle which histamine will cause, Dr Fishman? And does histamine act on the pulmonary or bronchial venular muscle? I have the impression that you were interpreting your results entirely as an action on the intracellular matrix and not on the smooth muscle.

Fishman: It is difficult to be sure, especially in the experiments involving intravenous injection of histamine, since they showed considerable changes in pulmonary mechanics. The situation seemed more straightforward when subpleural injections of minute quantities of histamine were used. Histologically, the adjacent bronchioles were unaffected after subpleural injection. But we are less confident about the mechanism that causes the gaps in pulmonary venular endothelium than about the consistent formation of gaps after injection of histamine, bradykinin and endotoxin.

Widdicombe: Did you measure airways resistance to see whether perivascular oedema appeared at the same time as an increase in resistance?

Fishman: We did measure airways resistance and pulmonary compliance after intravenous administration but did not attempt to define the temporal relationship between peribronchial oedema and the change in lung mechanics. Instead we resorted to the subpleural injections, using minute doses of the agent in the attempt to avoid appreciable changes in bronchial calibres.

Staub: Dr K. L. Brigham has perfused the pulmonary artery of unanaesthetized steady-state sheep with histamine for periods of four hours. He found that lung lymph flow increased moderately and that the protein concentration in the lymph did not change. Thus, protein flow increased at the same rate as lymph flow, indicating an increase in vascular permeability. He also perfused histamine at the same rate into the left atrium so that it would enter the bronchial circulation in higher concentration. He found that histamine had much less effect by that route than through the pulmonary circulation. He concluded that the major effect of histamine in low doses was in the pulmonary circulation rather than in the bronchial circulation (Brigham 1975).

Fishman: Wasn't the dose that Dr Brigham used a large one?

Staub: It was about 120 μg kg^{-1} min^{-1} in a 30 kg sheep.

Fishman: The subpleural injections in our experiments were much smaller, e.g. 0.1 μg of histamine.

Durbin: Do you interpret this to mean that the capillary pressure has been raised by histamine?

Staub: No, it is not a pressure effect. Since protein flow increased at the same rate as lymph flow, Dr Brigham concluded that there was a true change in the pulmonary vascular permeability to protein.

Dickinson: Is there any evidence of species differences in the response to histamine?

Michel: I think there is: for example, there is no effect of histamine or bradykinin on permeability of frog capillaries (Renkin *et al.* 1974*a*). There is evidence from other vascular beds that histamine might change permeability in different ways. There is electron microscope evidence that wide gaps are being opened up between the endothelial cells, but there is physiological evidence that this can't be happening in some vascular beds. For example Renkin *et al.* (1974*b*) have looked at the effects of histamine infusion on the capillaries of the dog paw. They have shown, just as Dr Staub did, that as the histamine goes in so lymph flow goes up and protein concentration goes up. But if the venous pressure is then increased, which really is the test of a large pore system opening up, lymph flow goes up and protein concentration comes down. This finding suggests that either there is significant molecular sieving of macromolecules, which is inconsistent with the large leaks seen by the electron microscopists, or there are separate pathways for water and protein across the capillary wall.

Lee: To the uninitiated those electron microscopic studies are not very clear. For instance, I could not see where the lymphatics were in your figures, Dr Fishman. I know, from measuring lung lymph flow, that at very high rates of flow it is quite common to find blood in the lymph. Thus, in your studies, if lymph flow went up for any particular reason, entry points for the lymphatic system could appear from the systemic venous system and there could be back movement of red cells into lymph. So it would look as if your electron-dense marker was coming from the veins when in fact it was mixing backwards into a system which was draining normally into those veins.

Fishman: The observation I referred to was made by Majno *et al.* (1969). They made local applications of histamine to the surface of the cremaster muscle of the rat, using colloidal carbon as tracer. They found that leakage of the carbon was confined to the venular system via gaps such as those in Fig. 4 (p. 35). Thus, in the lungs, the systemic venules (bronchial venules) appear to behave like the cremasteric venules.

Robin: I wonder about two things, one on each side of what is apparently a controversy! One problem is the use of carbon particles as evidence of increased permeability. If permeability is increased substantially, carbon particles would indeed get through, but carbon particles are gigantic in comparison with molecules such as albumin and so on. That part of the titration curve makes one a little uneasy about the possibility of picking up moderate increases in permeability.

The other problem is, can one equate lung lymph flow in a precise way with what is taking place in the interstitial space? There are a large number of lymph nodes interposed between the interstitial space and the pulmonary lymph ducts. Lymph nodes may well be involved in modifying the composition and volume of lymph fluid. There may be important delays in time. Looking at lung lymph and saying that what is taking place there is what takes place in the interstitial space is about equivalent to assessing the state of the British economy by looking at the number of diners at the Mirabelle restaurant. There must be a certain amount of disparity between the precise timing of events in the interstitial space and how closely these events are reflected in lymphatic flow rates and the composition of lymph fluid.

Staub: We use only steady-state experiments so there isn't any time problem.

Widdicombe: Paintal (1974) has postulated that contractions of bronchiolar smooth muscle which can be caused by histamine can adjust the amount of interstitial fluid at the alveolar/bronchiolar level. The evidence is perhaps not yet very convincing but if he is right it will be very important in terms of peribronchial oedema.

Staub: In your experiments on transendothelial transport do you think the iodine is still attached to the protein?

Fishman: The experiments involving lipoprotein handling are at an early stage. To date, albumin and low density lipoproteins have been shown to be handled differently from very low density lipoproteins (D. Capuzzi, G. G. Pietra, L. Spagnoli & A. P. Fishman, unpublished observations, 1975).

Optimism is high that the material in the cell is a peptide derived from very low density lipoprotein and labelled with iodine. But it will have to be tested.

Staub: Does lipoprotein lipase remove the tracer iodine at the same time as it removes the peptide?

Strang: In using iodide-labelled proteins one has to be careful that the label doesn't come loose. We usually confirm the attachment by gel filtration.

Maetz: We used iodide-labelled albumin to study the pathway of blood in the fish gills and we learned that it is essential to perfuse with cold albumin in addition to the label. If we don't use it we get an enormous absorption on the endothelial surface. Therefore the substance may disappear in the perfusing fluid, and it looks as if it is crossing to the other side, whereas it is just clinging to the surface.

Fishman: I do not know how to relate observations on the gill to those on the lung. The gill capillaries, *per se*, appear to be highly permeable to albumin so that it is the tight surface junctions that keep the albumin from running into the sea (Fishman & Pietra 1973). Whether gill and pulmonary capillaries differ in other respects is not clear to me.

Egan: The constant concentration of the labelled proteins in your perfusate is a nice way to perfuse the lung. The assumption is that the albumin normally present in the interstitium and lymphatics of the lung originates from the blood. If labelled proteins are injected *in vivo* a regular decrease in blood concentration is observed which is due to diffusion into interstitial fluids and catabolism. In the isolated perfused lung you have a constant level of labelled protein in the perfusate, and I wonder whether the isolated perfused preparation in itself is somehow changing the normal dynamics?

Fishman: We were concerned about the prospects of pulmonary oedema in the isolated lung. However, we found that after up to two hours of perfusion, the wet weight/dry weight ratio remained unchanged. Therefore, to be sure of avoiding oedema, perfusion was not continued beyond one hour. Another check was the repeated determination of airway pressures. As the lungs start to accumulate excess water, airway pressures go up. This phenomenon was also avoided by one hour of perfusion.

Egan: Yet it seems that one should observe a decrease in the concentration of labelled protein in the perfusate, due to equilibration with the interstitium.

Fishman: If it is carried on long enough there might be a drop, I agree.

Crosbie: Two of your findings correlate fairly well with what we call the shock lung or acute respiratory distress syndrome. Firstly, in stages 2 and 3 which Moore *et al.* (1969) described so well, there is a high cardiac output going through the lungs—sometimes as much as 12–14 l/min. Where the pulmonary artery pressure has also been measured it is normal or only moderately increased. It seems that the whole lung is well perfused. This syndrome is seen in a particularly vicious form where there is also pancreatic damage, possibly because enzymes are being released from that organ which then damage the lung capillaries and pulmonary oedema is produced. Have you seen examples of this?

Fishman: I know of three instances of acute respiratory insufficiency after acute pancreatitis. My impression is that this form of 'shock lung' is generally calamitous. Perhaps its refractoriness to therapy stems from the entry of lytic enzymes into the circulation. Whether these substances increase capillary permeability and compound the haemodynamic contribution to the clinical picture is an important topic for investigation.

References

BLAKE, L. H. & STAUB, N. C. (1972) *Physiologist 5*, 88

BRIGHAM, K. L. (1975) *Chest Suppl. 67*, 50S-52S

BRIGHAM, K. L., WOOLVERTON, W. C., BLAKE, L. H. & STAUB, N. C. (1974) *J. Clin. Invest. 54*, 792-804

CRONE, C. & LASSEN, N. A. (eds.) (1970) *Capillary Permeability (Alfred Benzon Symp. 2)*, Academic Press, New York

ERDMANN, A. J., III, VAUGHAN, T. R. JR, BRIGHAM, K. L., WOOLVERTON, W. C. & STAUB, N. C. (1975) *Circ. Res. 37*, 271-285

FISHMAN, J. A. & PIETRA, G. G. (1973) *Bull. Mt. Desert Isl. Biol. Lab. 13*, 36-38

GAAR, K. A., TAYLOR, A. E., OWENS, L. J. & GUYTON, A. C. (1967) Effect of capillary pressure and plasma protein on development of pulmonary edema. *Am. J. Physiol. 213*, 79-82

GUYTON, A. C. & LINDSEY, A. W. (1959) Effect of elevated left atrial pressure and decreased plasma protein concentration on the development of pulmonary edema. *Circ. Res. 7*, 649-657

HAUGE, A., LUNDE, P. K. M. & WAALER, B. A. (1966) Bradykinin and pulmonary vascular permeability in isolated blood-perfused rabbit lungs, in *Hypotensive Peptides* (Erdös, E. G., Bach, N. & Wilde, A. F., eds.) pp. 385-395, Springer, New York

LEVINE, O. R., MELLINS, R. B., SENIOR, R. M. & FISHMAN, A. P. (1967) The application of Starling's law of capillary exchange to the lungs. *J. Clin. Invest. 46*, 934-944

LUNDE, P. K. M. & WAALER, B. A. (1969) Transvascular fluid balance in the lungs. *J. Physiol. (Lond.) 205*, 1-18

MAJNO, G., SHEA, S. M. & LEVENTHAL, M. M. (1969) Endothelial contraction induced by histamine-type mediators: an electron microscopy study. *J. Cell Biol. 42*, 647-672

MOORE, F. D., LYONS, J. H. & PIERCE, E. C. J. (1969) *Post-Traumatic Insufficiency*, Saunders, Philadelphia

PAINTAL, A. S. (1974) Fluid pump of type J receptors of the cat. *J. Physiol. (Lond.) 238*, 53-54P

PAPPENHEIMER, J. R. (1953) Passage of molecules through capillary walls. *Physiol. Rev. 33*, 387-423

PAPPENHEIMER, J. R., RENKIN, E. M. & BORRERO, L. M. (1951) Filtration, diffusion and molecular sieving through peripheral capillary membranes. *Am. J. Physiol. 167*, 13-46

RENKIN, E. M., CURRY, F. E. & MICHEL, C. C. (1974a) Failure of histamine, 5-hydroxytryptamine, or bradykinin to increase capillary permeability to plasma proteins in frogs: action of compound 48/80. *Microvasc. Res. 8*, 213-217

RENKIN, E. M., CARTER, R. D. & JOYNER, W. L. (1974b) Mechanism of the sustained action of histamine and bradykinin on transport of large molecules across capillary walls in the dog paw. *Microvasc. Res.* *7*, 49-60

STAUB, N. C. (1974) Pulmonary edema. *Physiol. Rev.* *54*, 678-811

YUDILEVICH, D. L. & ALVAREZ, O. A. (1967) Water, sodium and thiourea transcapillary diffusion in the dog heart. *Am. J. Physiol.* *213*, 308-314

The permeability of lung capillary and alveolar walls as determinants of liquid movements in the lung

L. B. STRANG

Department of Paediatrics, University College Hospital Medical School, London

Abstract The lungs of the exteriorized fetal lamb offer an unusually good opportunity for measuring the permeability of lung capillary and alveolar walls, because access to plasma, interstitial fluid and alveolar liquid can be obtained without seriously disturbing their physiological relationships. Although there are probably some differences in permeability between fetal and air-breathing lungs, the underlying pattern appears to be similar. Large water-soluble molecules, including proteins, can penetrate capillary but not alveolar walls. The latter appear to be impermeable to molecules with diffusion radii greater than 0.5–0.6 nm. Pore theory can be used to characterize these permeabilities and to obtain estimates of osmotic reflection coefficients for various water-soluble substances. From them, predictions can be made of the bulk movements of liquid to be expected in a variety of circumstances, including the adaptation of the lungs at birth, lung oedema and drowning in sea water or fresh water.

A complete epithelium covering the fine air spaces of the lung was first demonstrated by Low & Daniels (1952). Blood is separated from air by two cellular barriers—endothelium and epithelium. Both must be very permeable to respiratory gases, yet prevent the net accumulation of solutes and liquid in the air spaces. There is a conflicting need: certain water-soluble substances such as glucose, amino acids and even immunoglobulins must have access to the epithelium from the pulmonary circulation. These requirements are met by differing permeability characteristics of vascular endothelium and alveolar epithelium.

When it comes to examining the permeabilities of these structures in detail, the lungs of the fetal lamb offer substantial advantages. They can be used in the intact animal without interfering with gas exchange (the placenta looks after that) and they are already filled with liquid, which avoids the probably

49

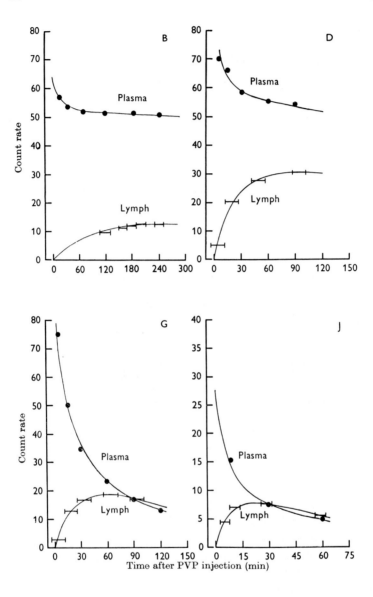

Fig. 1. Counts in plasma and lung lymph of 4 out of 11 gel filtration fractions of ^{125}I-labelled PVP after intravenous injection at zero time. Mean molecular radius of fractions ($\pm$ 0.5 nm): B = 8.9 nm, D = 5.8 nm, G = 3.4 nm, J = 2.1 nm. Rate constants ($K_c$min^{-1}) and steady state lymph/plasma ratios obtained by compartmental analysis. Clearance constant $K = K_c V_i$ where V_i is interstitial volume. Reproduced from Boyd *et al.* (1969), by permission of *J. Physiol. (Lond.)*.

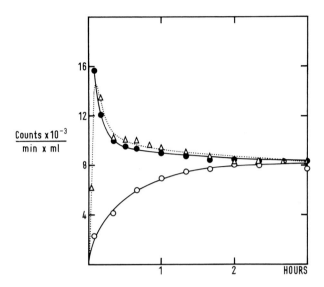

FIG. 2. Counts of [²⁴Na]Cl in plasma (●), lymph (△), and lung liquid (○) after injection of tracer into plasma at zero time. Reproduced from Olver & Strang (1974), by permission of *J. Physiol. (Lond.)*.

important artifacts caused by adding liquid to air-breathing lungs. Samples of fetal lung liquid from the potential air spaces can be obtained simultaneously with plasma and lung lymph. Tracer substances can be injected into plasma and followed in lymph and lung liquid; or they can be mixed into lung liquid through the trachea and then followed in lymph and in plasma. By these means the permeabilities of both the membranes can be measured in the intact animal without the lungs being disturbed or handled. Fig. 1 illustrates an experiment from Boyd *et al.* (1969) in which the polymer ¹²⁵I-labelled PVP (polyvinylpyrrolidone) was injected intravenously and followed in lymph and plasma. We followed 11 fractions of ¹²⁵I-labelled PVP obtained by gel filtration on Sephadex G200. Four of them, with mean values for diffusion radius of 8.9, 5.8, 3.4 and 2.1 nm, are shown in Fig. 1. From such curves of concentration we can calculate, for each molecular size, a rate constant for transcapillary transit and a steady-state lymph/plasma (L/P) concentration ratio (see Boyd *et al.* 1969, for details of calculation).

None of these large molecules crossed the second barrier from interstitial fluid to lung liquid, but smaller, inert, molecular probes and labelled ions did so. Fig. 2 shows an example from Olver & Strang (1974) in which labelled Na⁺ ion was injected intravenously and followed in plasma, lymph and lung liquid. In this case, rate constants for capillary and for alveolar wall transfer

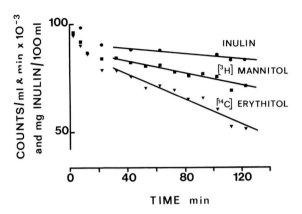

FIG. 3. Unlabelled inulin, [³H]mannitol and [¹⁴C]erythritol added to and mixed with lung liquid at zero time. Since inulin does not penetrate lung epithelium, it can be used to estimate volume and secretion rate of lung liquid. Differences between its slope and those for [³H]mannitol and [¹⁴C]erythritol represent permeation of epithelium by these tracers. Reproduced from Normand *et al.* (1971), by permission of *J. Physiol. (Lond.)*.

can both be obtained from the curves. For ions and small molecules, the rate constant for capillaries is probably suspect because there may be some equilibration with blood plasma in the circulation of lymph vessels and lymph nodes (see Staub 1974); but that criticism does not apply to the results for macromolecules shown in Fig. 1, nor does it apply to transfer across alveolar walls, for which a rate constant can be calculated from the concentration curves of the type shown in Fig. 2.

The other type of experiment we can do is illustrated in Fig. 3. In this case we withdrew, through the trachea, 59 ml of lung liquid (about half the volume actually present), then added a number of substances and returned it to the lung. After a period for mixing, the concentrations of the test substances declined at rates determined by the sum of dilution by newly formed liquid and transfer out of the lung across alveolar walls. An impermeant tracer (inulin in this case) enables us to measure lung liquid volume and secretion rate (Normand *et al.* [1971] showed that inulin and labelled albumin do not cross alveolar walls). From the differences between the slope for the impermeant substance and those for permeant tracers, we can obtain rate constants for transalveolar transfer (see Normand *et al.* [1971] for details of calculation). We were able to eliminate slow diffusion in the lung liquid compartment as a cause of the decline in concentration with time by showing that two impermeant tracers (¹²⁵I-labelled albumin and inulin) with diffusion coefficients that differ by a factor of 2.5 have, nonetheless, closely similar slopes. The values obtained in

LUNG CAPILLARIES

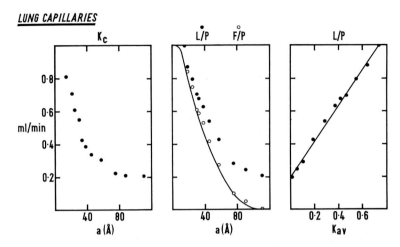

FIG. 4. Permeability of lung capillaries to macromolecules—[125]I-labelled PVP fractions. _Left:_ values of capillary clearance constant K(ml/min) for 11 Sephadex G200 gel filtrations fractions on molecular radius, _a_ (Å). _Centre:_ for the same ^{125}I-labelled PVP fractions, lymph/plasma (L/P, ●) and filtrate/plasma ratios (F/P, ○; F/P values calculated assuming whole of largest fraction reaches lymph through leaks) on molecular radius. The line fitted to the F/P values shows predictions of pore theory for pore radius of 150Å (15 nm). _Right:_ L/P ratios on K_{av} (fraction volume of Sephadex G200 gel occupied by PVP fraction). Data for mature fetal lambs from Boyd _et al._ (1969).

this way for a series of small non-electrolyte and electrolyte tracers agreed very well with the values obtained when the tracer was put into blood.

Results from these two types of experiment have enabled us to relate the rate of permeation of both capillary and alveolar walls to molecular size. For capillary walls, relying only on the results for macromolecules, we find that the clearance constants and the calculated steady-state lymph/plasma ratios (L/P) both decrease with increasing molecular size in the range between 11.0 and 1.7 nm (Fig. 4). One of the most striking features of these findings is the linear relationship that was found between the L/P values and the Sephadex elution volume, K_{av}. The L/P values express fractional capillary wall penetration, and K_{av} values the fractional volumes of Sephadex G200 penetrated. Capillary walls and Sephadex G200 seem to impose a similar degree of restriction on molecular movement. Both function as molecular sieves but for neither is it possible, at present, to establish a definite structure. One of Ackers' (1967) models for Sephadex gel treats it as containing spaces or pores with a random distribution of sizes; and capillary walls could, similarly, contain a range of pore sizes as was suggested long ago by Rous _et al._ (1930). Another view might be that the complex of capillaries and interstitial space could form a gel-like structure which imposes molecular sieving, as does Sephadex G200 gel. If, alternatively, we attempt to analyse the L/P values by applying Pappenheimer's pore theory (Pappenheimer 1953), according to which the restriction to transfer is imposed by uniform pores in capillary walls, we find that the unmodified results do not fit that theory: the L/P ratios of the largest molecules are greater than predicted. Boyd *et al.* (1969), following Grötte's (1956) example, assumed that the largest of these fractions crossed capillary walls, unrestricted, through large leaks more than 100 nm in radius; and when the ratios were adjusted to allow for the leaks, there was rather a good fit for the Pappenheimer theory (see open symbols in centre panel of Fig. 4). Boyd *et al.* (1969) obtained, in mature fetal lambs, the value of 15 nm for pore radius, and for newborn lambs a somewhat smaller value of 9 nm. Since the mean pulmonary artery pressure of the fetal lamb is usually between 50 and 60 mmHg (6.65–8 kPa) and that of the newborn between 20 and 35 mmHg (2.66–4.65 kPa), the higher pore radius in the fetus may be due to pore stretching. With different assumptions the findings could be made to fit models for various combinations of two or more pore sizes, and indeed Staub (1974) has applied a model of two pore sizes and large leaks to similar results with macromolecules. From a functional point of view, however, there is no doubt that, irrespective of the theory by which the findings are interpreted, the passive permeability of capillary walls is such that some substantial transfer, even of large plasma proteins, takes place across them.

With alveolar walls we find that the results for small molecules fit very well with the proposition that transfer takes place only by restricted diffusion through uniform water-filled pores. Fig. 5 shows that there is a large increase in permeability for small reductions in molecular radius, and that the barrier is quite permeable to water itself. By using a statistical procedure for fitting the equation for restricted diffusion to the results (see left-hand panel of Fig. 5), we obtain an estimated value for pore radius of 0.61 nm, only a little different from our previously published value of 0.55 nm (Normand *et al.* 1971). I have included in the diagram values for the rate constants of Na^+ and Ca^{2+} and their hydrated ionic radii. We have reason to believe (Olver & Strang 1974) that these ions move passively across the alveolar epithelium. Cl^-, on the other hand, which is actively transported, has a rate constant about a quarter that for Na^+, despite a smaller hydrated radius. In fitting the curve for restricted diffusion in Fig. 5, we obtain a value of 107 cm^{-2} for the term, pore area per unit path-length and lung liquid volume $((A_p/\Delta_x)/V_L)$. From it and a body weight of 3.5 kg we can calculate $A_p/\Delta_x = 11\,235$ cm ($V_L \approx 30$ ml/kg). Assuming that Δ_x is the length of the tight junction between epithelial cells shown by Weibel (1969, Fig. 5), $\Delta_x = 3.0 \times 10^{-5}$ cm, and $A_p = 0.34$ cm^2. For

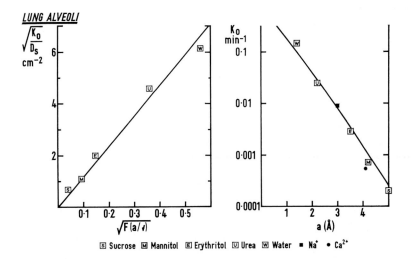

FIG. 5. *Left:* method for computing pore radius. Since according to the theory of restricted diffusion, $K_o = [(A_p/\Delta_x)/V_L]F(\frac{a}{r})D_s$, best fit values of $(A_p/\Delta_x)/V_L$ and $F(\frac{a}{r})$ were found by finding minimum variance for $(K_o/D_s)/(Fa/r)$ of the test substances. $K_o =$ experimentally determined rate constant for transepithelial flux; $D_s =$ free diffusion coefficient; $A_p =$ pore area; $\Delta_x =$ path-length; $V_L =$ lung liquid volume; $F(a/r) =$ Faxen-Ferry function of molecular radius (a) and pore radius (r); see equation 5 in Normand *et al.* (1971). The square root scales are used only as a convenience for the illustration. *Right:* values of K_o (min^{-1}) as a function of estimated molecular radius of non-electrolytes and of hydrated radius for two passively transferred ions, Na$^+$ and Ca^{2+}. Line shows predictions for restricted diffusion through uniform cylindrical pores 6.1 Å (0.61 nm) in radius.

a body weight of 3.5 kg, assuming proportionality to body surface, we can calculate from data in Thurlbeck & Wang (1974) a value for total alveolar area, A, of 1.01×10^5 cm. Hence $A_p/A = 3.3 \times 10^{-6}$.

From these two sets of permeability data, we can see how the lung is set up for solute permeability. The air-breathing lung, no doubt, differs in detail, but the basic pattern is probably similar. There is good access even for large proteins from the blood to the interstitial space and to one surface of the epithelium. Nutritionally speaking, the epithelium is like a man before a fire on a cold night. He is warmed from one side only, but effectively warmed. There is, however, severely restricted access for solutes to the air spaces; and in the absence of net solute movement, the net leakage of water through the epithelium is prevented. In lung oedema, or in hyaline membrane disease, when water and proteins enter the air spaces, some kind of breakdown in the epithelium must take place.

From estimates of pore radius, total membrane area, hydraulic conductivity and permeability, it is possible to calculate, for the two membranes, approximate values for the osmotic reflexion coefficient (σ_s) of various solutes.* Dainty & Ginzburg (1963) derived the expression

$$\sigma_s = 1 - \frac{\omega_s \overline{V}}{L_p} - \frac{A_{sf}}{A_{wf}} \qquad (1)$$

(where ω_s is solute mobility coefficient, $\overline{V}_s$ partial molar volume of solute, L_p hydraulic conductivity, and A_{sf}/A_{wf} the ratio of apparent pore area for solute to that for water in the presence of hydrodynamic flow:

$$\frac{A_{sf}}{A_{wf}} = \frac{[2(1-a_s/r)^2 - (1-a_s/r)^4]\,[1-2.104(a_s/r) +2.09(a_s/r)^3 - 0.95(a_s/r)^5]}{[2(1-a_w/r)^2(1-a-_w/r)^4][1-2.104(a_w/r)+2.09(a_w/r)^3 - 0.95(a_w/r)^5]}$$

a_s and a_w are respectively radii of solute and water molecules; r = pore radius).

For capillary walls, the permeability to small solutes is so high that only albumin is relevant. With a value of 3.4 nm for its diffusion radius, the permeability to ^{125}I-labelled albumin given by Adamson et al. (1970) and the range of capillary hydraulic conductivities for sheep quoted by Staub (1974), the value of σ_{alb} comes out between 0.74 and 0.65 for a pore radius of 10.0 nm and between 0.53 and 0.43 for a pore radius of 15.0 nm. The estimate is, of course, critically dependent on the model used to estimate pore radius. Using a model with two pore sizes of 2.0 and 12.5 nm and large leaks, Staub (1974) has obtained $\sigma_{alb} = 0.8$.

The alveolar wall is impermeable to albumin and the σ_{alb} value for that structure must be 1.0. For alveolar walls it is also relevant to calculate σ_{Na}, since Na is the most abundant plasma solute and one to which alveolar walls have only a low permeability. In obtaining an estimate for σ_{Na} we can use our value for pore radius (0.6 nm), the hydrated radius of a Na^+ ion (say 0.3 nm) and measurements of Na^+ permeability (Olver & Strang 1974); but we lack a value for L_p. We can estimate it approximately from experiments in which the volume flow rate of fetal lung liquid was augmented osmotically by adding measured amounts of sucrose to lung liquid. The result for σ_{Na} turned out to be not very sensitive to the actual value of hydraulic conductivity used within the range suggested by these experiments, because the first term on the right-hand side of the Dainty & Ginzburg (1963) equation is in any case very small. The value of σ_{Na} we obtained was 0.87.

The σ_{alb} value for capillary walls predicts that while osmotic pressure differences will be generated across capillaries depending on the concentrations of

*For a detailed description of σ see House (1974).

albumin in plasma and interstitial fluid, they are likely to be smaller than has often been assumed. From the concentrations of protein in lymph and plasma given by Humphreys *et al.* (1967), the calculated osmotic pressure for absorption into the blood comes out between 3.5 and 5.7 mmHg (0.46–0.76 kPa). The high σ_{Na} value for alveolar walls predicts that large osmotic pressures could be generated by relatively small differences in the concentration of small molecules. The inhalation of fresh water or sea water provides extreme examples. Both are known to cause very large osmotic flows of water. In fresh-water inhalation, absorption will be determined by the NaCl concentration in plasma and not, as often claimed (see Comroe 1974), by its relatively trivial molar concentration of albumin. The σ_{Na} of 0.87 means that the force for absorption should be about 6.6 atmospheres (about 670 kPa). In sea-water inhalation the force extracting liquid from the circulation should be about 21 atmospheres (2130 kPa). These calculations go some way towards explaining the effects of different types of drowning. They also serve as an illustration of the consequences for water movements of the low permeability of the alveolar wall to solutes. For respiratory gases and other lipid-soluble substances such as acetone, alcohol and paraldehyde, the permeability of the lung alveoli is, of course, much greater (see Normand *et al.* [1971] for relationship of alveolar wall permeability to lipid solubility). Indeed, we might well consider that it is in combining a high permeability to non-polar substances and to water with a low permeability to polar solutes that the lung achieves its primary function.

References

ACKERS, G. K. (1967) A new calibration procedure for gel filtration columns. *J. Biol. Chem.* *242*, 3237

ADAMSON, T. M., BOYD, R. D. H., HILL, J. R., NORMAND, I. C. S., REYNOLDS, E. O. R. & STRANG, L. B. (1970) Effect of asphyxia due to umbilical cord occlusion in the foetal lamb on leakage of liquid from the circulation and on permeability of lung capillaries to albumin. *J. Physiol. (Lond.)* *207*, 493-505

BOYD, R. D. H., HILL, J. R., HUMPHREYS, R. W., NORMAND, I. C. S., REYNOLDS, E. O. R. & STRANG, L. B. (1969) Permeability of lung capillary to macromolecules in foetal and newborn lambs and sheep. *J. Physiol. (Lond.)* *201*, 567-588

COMROE, J. H. JNR., (1974) *Physiology of Respiration*, 2nd edn., p. 287, Year Book Medical Publishers, Chicago

DAINTY, J. & GINZBURG, B. Z. (1963) Irreversible thermodynamics and frictional models of membrane processes with particular reference to the cell membrane. *J. Theoret. Biol.* *5*, 256

GRÖTTE, G. (1956) Passage of dextran molecules across the blood-lymph barrier. *Acta Chir. Scand. Suppl.* *211*, 1-84

HOUSE, C. R. (1974) *Water Transport in Cells and Tissues*, ch. 3, Arnold, London

HUMPHREYS, P. W., NORMAND, I. C. S., REYNOLDS, E. O. R. & STRANG, L. B. (1967) Pulmonary lymph flow and the uptake of liquid from the lungs of the lamb at the start of breathing. *J. Physiol. (Lond.)* *193*, 7

Low, F. N. & Daniels, C. W. (1952) Electron microscopy of the rat lung. *Anat. Rec. 113*, 437

Normand, I. C. S., Olver, R. E., Reynolds, E. O. R., Strang, L. B. & Welch, K. (1971) Permeability of lung capillaries and alveoli to non-electrolytes in the foetal lamb. *J. Physiol. (Lond.) 219*, 303-330

Olver, R. E. & Strang, L. B. (1974) Ion fluxes across the pulmonary epithelium and the secretion of lung liquid in the foetal lamb. *J. Physiol. (Lond.) 241*, 327-357

Pappenheimer, J. R. (1953) Passage of molecules through capillary walls. *Physiol. Rev. 33*, 387-423

Rous, P., Gilding, H. P. & Smith, F. (1930) The gradient of vascular permeability. *J. Exp. Med. 51*, 807-830

Staub, N. C. (1974) Pulmonary edema. *Physiol. Rev. 54*, 678-811

Thurlbeck, W. M. & Wang, N. S. (1974) Lung structure, in *MTP International Review of Science, Respiratory Physiology* (Guyton, A. C. & Widdicombe, J. G., eds.), Butterworths, London

Weibel, E. R. (1969) The ultrastructure of the alveolar-capillary membrane or barrier, in *The Pulmonary Circulation and Interstitial Space* (Fishman, A. P. & Hecht, H. H., eds.), University of Chicago Press, Chicago

Discussion

Robin: I am a little worried about electrolytes being handled in the same way as uncharged particles; for example, your plot of how molecular diameters correlate with the ability to get across alveolar epithelium would either suggest that there was no transmembrane potential on the inner surface of the alveolar epithelium which was capable of accelerating or decelerating sodium and calcium movement, or it would suggest that the fit might be coincidental. I think I would be a little worried about calculating a permeability coefficient for a charged particle without knowing the electrical gradient as well as the chemical gradient. Do you have direct information on the transmembrane potential?

Strang: Richard Olver will be discussing permeation of electrolytes through the epithelium later. The evidence that sodium and calcium move from lung liquid to plasma by passive diffusion is excellent and takes full account of all the electrochemical forces acting on the ions. As Dr Olver will show, other ions, notably the halides and K^+, are actively transported.

Olver: You said that in the lamb fetus the pulmonary artery pressure is 50 mmHg (6.6 kPa) but we don't really know what the capillary pressure is. Left atrial pressure is the same in the fetus as in the newborn, isn't it?

Strang: It is slightly higher in the newborn. It is less than 5 mmHg (0.66 kPa) in both. Pulmonary capillary pressure is somewhere between that value and pulmonary artery pressure, which has a mean value in the fetus of about 50 mmHg. In some circumstances a high pulmonary artery pressure seems to be linked to a high rate of filtration from the pulmonary circulation. In altitude oedema, pulmonary artery pressure is high, left atrial pressure is low, and there is a high rate of filtration from the capillary bed. The same is true in the fetus (Humphreys *et al.* 1967).

Durbin: Do you envisage the small pores through the alveolar epithelium as being between cells or through cells?

Strang: I envisage them being between the cells. They are capable of enlargement, according to measurements that Dr Egan is going to present, and also of returning to their original size.

Dickinson: You found zero permeability to albumin?

Strang: Yes, and to inulin; and the permeability to sucrose (molecule radius, 0.51 nm) is very low, about 4.1×10^{-9} cm/s (Normand *et al.* 1971).

Normand: On the other hand these measurements are consistent with the size of pore reported in studies of transfers across red cell membranes (Goldstein & Solomon 1960).

Dickinson: In that case the non-electrolytes might be getting through the membranes themselves rather than through tight junctions.

Strang: Yes, it is perfectly possible that they could be going entirely through the membranes if it weren't for the change which takes place when the fetal lungs are first ventilated. At that time the water-filled pathways apparently expand by a factor of 5–10, which is much too large for the transcellular route (Egan *et al.* 1975). The simplest explanation is that the pathways are paracellular and capable of expansion.

Olver: There can be quite large pores in cell membranes. The oocyte of the frog has pores of 3 nm radius (Dick 1971).

Egan: We have calculated that the total area of all the pores in the fetal lung surface is a very small fraction, about 1×10^{-6}, of the total area for gas diffusion. I think that would support the idea that the pores are between cells but it is not conclusive.

Guyton: You assumed that all the decay in albumin and inulin concentrations was caused by secretion. Did you have any reason for excluding the idea that there are some large pores through which both could diffuse equally well?

Strang: In early experiments we placed labelled inulin in the lung liquid but we were unable to detect any in the lung lymph afterwards. We also infused labelled PVP into the blood and failed to detect it by very sensitive methods in the lung liquid during periods of observation of up to six hours. In neither of those situations is the volume of distribution so large as to prevent one from picking up a little tracer if it is there.

Guyton: Did you ever try measuring the actual volume of secretion?

Strang: Dr Adamson has measured the volume and rate of secretion independently.

Adamson: We studied the fetal lamb *in utero* and measured the effluent from the fetal trachea, for 20 days or more (Adamson *et al.* 1975). Flow rates of around 9 ml/h were obtained, which is close to the rate of secretion obtained in your experiments, Dr Strang.

Strang: The results using the direct collection method and tracer dilution agree well. We were more concerned with the extent to which the slopes of concentration might represent slow mixing within the lung liquid compartment. We were reassured on that by finding that the slopes were similar for two impermeant tracers (albumin and inulin) that differed in their free diffusion coefficients by a factor of 2.5 (Olver & Strang 1974).

Robin: Did you give the inulin by a single bolus or by constant infusion?

Strang: Most of our experiments were done with a single bolus.

Robin: If you had a low rate constant for inulin transport and a high rate constant for the rate of formation of water, then could you not be diluting the appearance of the inulin, so that operationally you could not measure any permeation, whereas if you had maintained a steady-state high concentration of plasma inulin you might have been able to find some?

Strang: We did do infusion experiments but it doesn't make a lot of difference in practice. The levels of inulin or albumin that can be obtained in the interstitial fluid are in any case high in relation to the rate of permeation. The only difference it makes is in the calculation of the rate constants, which is more of a headache if there is a change in plasma concentration, but it can be done (Normand *et al.* 1971).

Staub: Are pleural pressure and alveolar presure in the fetal lung identical, in the intact chest, if the lung is not being expanded?

Strang: They are almost equal. There is a pressure drop of about 1 cmH$_2$O (0.1 kPa) across the lung.

Staub: So there is no significant hydrostatic pressure gradient between fetal alveolar liquid and interstitial fluid?

Strang: I don't know what the hydrostatic pressure of interstitial fluid is.

Dickinson: At present it seems that we have to guess at the interstitial fluid pressure. It might be greater or it might even be less than intra-amniotic pressure, for all we know.

Strang: Lymph from the lungs of the mature fetus which is making no respiratory movements flows freely and steadily at about twice the rate of that in the air-breathing newborn lung more than six hours old (Humphreys *et al.* 1967).

Maetz: Does the permeability of alveolar walls to water differ in the fetus and the adult? Fluid secretion ought to be greater in the fetal lung than in the adult.

Strang: When a bronchus is occluded in the adult lung and air is absorbed from that part of the lung, it doesn't then begin to fill up with liquid, whereas in the fetal lungs of animals weighing about 4 kg the rate of formation is about 10 ml/h. So I am sure you are right that there is a difference, even though one might say that occluding the airway is somewhat pathological.

It was Jost who first showed that the fetal lung actually secretes liquid (Jost & Policard 1948). He showed that when the trachea was occluded the lungs began to swell up. But, to deal with the specific question of water permeability, I don't know of measurements in the adult lung. We find them difficult to make in the fetal lung. The value we obtained was 3.3×10^{-6} cm/s (Normand et al. 1971).

Maetz: I am interested in that because of the comparison with fish. Fish which live in fresh water all the time resist the osmotic invasion of water because branchial water permeability is very low (see Maetz, this volume). So it appears that the one major difference between fetal and adult lungs is in the osmotic permeability of the epithelial surfaces. I would very much like to know the size of the surface available for the diffusion of water, or for the osmotic permeability of water, so that we could get absolute values for permeability in those membranes and see what difference there is. Fish membranes are obviously among the least permeable of any species.

Hugh-Jones: Is anything known about the hydrostatic effect in fetal lungs as opposed to adult lungs? In the air-filled lung, with large alveoli at the top and smaller ones at the bottom, the different stretching from top to bottom should affect the permeability. Have any measurements been made of permeability?

Agostoni: The adult lung has a vertical gradient for transpulmonary pressure. In the fetus it may depend on whether the fetus is kept under liquid, because the compliance of the chest wall in the fetus is high. In the adult dog, if air is replaced with liquid the vertical pleural pressure gradient is -1 cmH$_2$O/cm (-0.1 kPa/cm). This means that all the hydrostatic effect of the liquid in the lung is taken up by the chest wall, which behaves as a rigid but mobile container. If the animal is supine the ribs are rigid relative to the gravitational field, and the diaphragm then faces an equal hydrostatic gradient on both sides. In these conditions the transpulmonary pressure is the same at the top and at the bottom, and the vertical gradient of transpulmonary pressure is not different from zero. Indeed, under these conditions the effect of the abdomen on the vertical gradient of transpulmonary pressure (Agostoni et al. 1970; Agostoni 1972) must disappear.

We have relevant results from five adult dogs in the supine posture (D'Angelo & Agostoni 1975). The relationship between lung height and pleural surface pressure is shown in Fig. 1. With air in the lung, at the resting volume of the respiratory system, the pressure is about -4 cmH$_2$O (-0.4 kPa) at the top

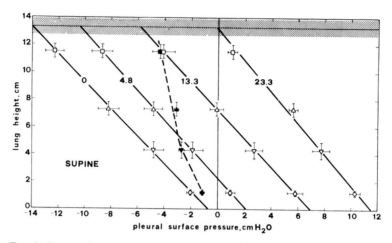

Fig. 1. (Agostoni) Pleural surface pressure plotted against lung height in supine dogs with lungs filled with saline. The numbers on the lines indicate the height (cm) of the level of saline in the filling system relative to the bottom of the lung. The broken line indicates the relationship with air-filled lungs at functional residual capacity. Each point is the average of results from 5 dogs. The horizontal and vertical bars indicate the standard error. The top of the lung is indicated by the horizontal line, the dashed area indicating its s. e. Reproduced from D'Angelo & Agostoni 1975, with permission.

and nearly zero at the bottom (broken line). With saline in the lung the values of pleural surface pressure depend on the level of the liquid in the filling system. The numbers on the lines indicate the height of the level of saline in the filling system relative to the bottom of the lung. The corresponding lung volumes were about 25, 50, 80 and 100% of the total lung capacity. In all cases the vertical gradient of pleural surface pressure was -1 cmH$_2$O/cm. The relationship between lung height and transpulmonary pressure is shown in Fig. 2. With saline in the lung the vertical gradient of transpulmonary pressure is not significantly different from zero. When the animal is in the head-up posture the lower part of the chest wall is more compliant than the upper part and the vertical gradient of pleural surface pressure differs significantly from -1 cmH$_2$O/cm, varying from -0.8 at small lung volume to -0.5 cmH$_2$O/cm at large lung volume. This means that not all the hydrostatic effect of the liquid in the lung is taken up by the chest wall, because the chest wall is now compliant in the direction of gravity. In the adult lung filled with liquid part of this hydrostatic effect is taken up by the lung itself and the vertical gradient of transpulmonary pressure is reversed. That is, the lower part of the lung is more expanded than the upper part. In the fetus, even in the supine position, the rib cage may not be so rigid and the lower part may be more expanded than the upper part.

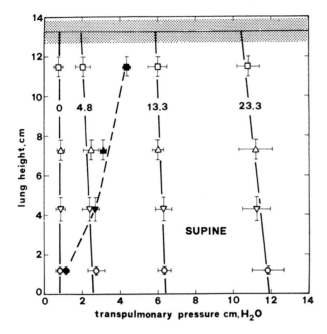

FIG. 2. (Agostoni) Transpulmonary pressure plotted against lung height in supine dogs with the lungs filled with saline. For further explanation see legend to Fig. 1. Reproduced from D'Angelo & Agostoni 1975, with permission.

Adamson: We have been looking at the effect on fetal lung growth of tying the trachea (D. Alcorn *et al.*, unpublished work, 1975). After occlusion the lung gets to five times the normal size, and the liquid pressure is still only about 1 or 2 mmHg (0.13–0.27 kPa) above atrial pressure. I therefore think that the fetal lung is highly compliant.

Michel: The calculation of reflection coefficients on the pore theory has been advanced considerably in the last year, notably by Curry (1974) and also by Anderson & Malone (1974). This would not affect the substance of Dr Strang's argument, although I think that the reflection coefficients would be slightly lower than he gave.

Staub: We have looked at the new calculations according to the Anderson theory in terms of our three equivalent-pore model. The correction did not seem to have much effect on the calculated pore sizes.

Michel: As the ratio of molecular radius to pore radius becomes greater there is a big deviation between the Durbin (1960) theory and the more recent formulations. Such a deviation between the theories was calculated by both Curry (1974) and Anderson & Malone (1974).

Durbin: In testing such a theory, one should use data from well-defined membranes, like the mica membranes introduced by Beck & Schultz (1970).

Michel: Beck & Schultz (1970) didn't report measurements of reflection coefficients on their membranes. But I entirely agree that to test the theories it would be best to work on artificial membranes penetrated by cylindrical pores of accurately known dimensions.

References

ADAMSON, T. M., BRODECKY, V., LAMBERT, T. F., MALONEY, J. E., RITCHIE, B. C. & WALKER, A. M. (1975) Lung liquid production and composition in the 'in utero' foetal lambs. *Aust. J. Exp. Biol. Med. Sci. 53*, 65-75

AGOSTONI, E. (1972) Mechanics of the pleural space. *Physiol. Rev. 52*, 57-128

AGOSTONI, E., D'ANGELO, E. & BONANNI, M. V. (1970) The effect of the abdomen on the vertical gradient of pleural surface pressure. *Respir. Physiol. 8*, 332-346

ANDERSON, J. L. & MALONE, D. M. (1974) Mechanism of osmotic flow in porous membranes. *Biophys. J. 14*, 957-982

BECK, R. E. & SCHULTZ, J. S. (1970) Hindered diffusion in microporous membranes with known pore geometry. *Science (Wash. D.C.) 170*, 1302-1305

CURRY, F. E. (1974) A hydrodynamic description of the osmotic reflection coefficient with application to the pore theory of transcapillary exchange. *Microvasc. Res. 8*, 236-252

D'ANGELO, E. & AGOSTONI, E. (1970) Vertical gradients of pleural and transpulmonary pressure with liquid-filled lungs. *Respir. Physiol. 23*, 159-173

DICK, D. A. T. (1971) Water movements in cells, in *Membranes and Ion Transport* (Bittar, E. E., ed.), pp. 211-250, Wiley, New York

DURBIN, R. P. (1960) Osmotic flow of water across cellulose membranes. *J. Gen. Physiol. 44*, 315-346

EGAN, E. A., OLVER, R. E. & STRANG, L. B. (1975) Changes in non-electrolyte permeability of alveoli and the absorption of lung liquid at the start of breathing in the lamb. *J. Physiol. (Lond.) 244*, 161-179

GOLDSTEIN, D. A. & SOLOMON, A. K. (1960) Determination of equivalent pore radius for human red cells by osmotic pressure measurement. *J. Gen. Physiol. 44*, 1

HUMPHREYS, P. W., NORMAND, I. C. S., REYNOLDS, E. O. R. & STRANG, L. B. (1967) Pulmonary lymph flow and the uptake of liquid from the lungs of the lamb at the start of breathing. *J. Physiol. (Lond.) 193*, 1-29

JOST, A. & POLICARD, A. (1948) Contribution expérimentale à l'étude du développement prénatal du poumon chez le lapin. *Arch. Anat. Microsc. 37*, 323-332

NORMAND, I. C. S., OLVER, R. E., REYNOLDS, E. O. R. & STRANG, L. B. (1971) Permeability of lung capillaries and alveoli to non-electrolytes in the foetal lamb. *J. Physiol. (Lond.) 219*, 303-330

OLVER, R. E. & STRANG, L. B. (1974) Ion fluxes across the pulmonary epithelium and the secretion of lung liquid in the fetal lamb. *J. Physiol. (Lond.) 241*, 327-357

Interstitial fluid and transcapillary fluid balance in the lung

BJARNE A. WAALER and PETTER AARSETH

Institute of Physiology, University of Oslo

Abstract Alterations in extravascular lung water content when capillary pressure or plasma colloid osmotic pressure is increased have been evaluated in isolated, continuously weighed, plasma-perfused pairs of rabbit lungs. After modest increases in left atrial pressure, most preparations rapidly reached a new stable weight, and thus a new transcapillary fluid balance, but no significant increase in extravascular lung water content could be detected. In preparations where there was still a steady, slow gain in weight and thus still some transvascular filtration of fluid 15 min after the increase in pressure, a moderate but significant increase in extravascular water could be detected. It is concluded that only very small transvascular shifts of fluid occur in the lungs when capillary pressure changes, as long as this change is kept below the level that causes oedema. This limitation of pressure-induced transvascular shifts of fluid in the lung could be explained by the existence, close to the capillaries, of a small interstitial space containing fluid with a high protein concentration. Alterations in the colloid osmotic pressure exerted by this fluid would then contribute markedly towards continuous readjustment of the transcapillary fluid balance in the lung.

Experiments by other workers indicate that alveolar pressure can markedly affect the transcapillary fluid balance of the isolated perfused lung.

Physiologists have eagerly studied the pressure-induced transcapillary flux of liquid in several vascular beds. As far as we know, the extent and direction of such fluid shifts are governed by the actual transvascular hydrostatic and colloid osmotic pressures, as outlined by Starling (1896) nearly 80 years ago. The great importance, in this connection, of the interstitial space adjacent to the capillaries has been pointed out more recently. Both the size and structure of this space, as well as the hydrostatic pressure and fluid composition prevailing within it, are of great interest.

Our group in Oslo has attempted to study the transcapillary movements of liquid in the lungs, and in this connection we have also been interested in the size and characteristics of the 'capillary-near' interstitial space in this organ.

How much liquid will be shifted across the walls of the pulmonary exchange vessels as a result of alterations in capillary hydrostatic pressure—and how large are the changes in interstitial volume then involved? On the one hand the huge capillary surface area in the lungs might allow extensive fluid filtration or reabsorption when capillary pressure changes. On the other hand, microstructural studies reveal only minute interstitial spaces adjacent to most capillaries, and it is difficult to envisage that large volumes of fluid could be accommodated here under normal circumstances.

From several series of experiments on isolated lungs we know that during prolonged periods with markedly increased capillary pressure large amounts of liquid will be filtered out of the microvessels and will accumulate somewhere in the tissue (Bø et al. 1975). Eventually such outward filtration leads to definite and visible oedema. We have, however, been equally interested in the pulmonary events occurring when the increase in capillary pressure is less marked, so that oedema development is not seen. How much liquid is then filtered out of the exchange vessels? How much is reabsorbed when capillary pressure goes down? In other words: how much liquid is shifted across the walls of the exchange vessels in the lung by alterations in capillary pressure that are within the 'normal range' for the organ? And consequently, what is the normal range for expansion and reduction of the extravascular space close to the capillaries, with which the capillary blood is in a transcapillary fluid balance?

In this paper we will refer to experimental results achieved by several workers from our group at the Institute of Physiology in Oslo. Some initial studies on lung extravascular water content were carried out by G. Bø, A. Hauge and P. Aarseth (unpublished work) in anaesthetized cats with the chest opened. Here ^{125}I-labelled albumin and ^{51}Cr-labelled erythrocytes were used as blood tracers. The two relatively small upper lung lobes were then removed under different conditions: one lobe of each pair was removed at normal vascular pressures, and the other after left atrial pressure had been raised for 20 min (by 5, 10, 20 or 30 mmHg [0.665, 1.33, 2.66 or 4 kPa]). Extravascular water content was evaluated in the same way as described below for lobes removed from isolated perfused lungs. After these 20-min periods of increased left atrial pressure extravascular lung water increased very little or not at all. At most, extravascular fluid went up some 3% for every 10 mmHg increment in left atrial pressure. In the intact lung, accumulation of tissue fluid is thus very efficiently limited, and probably the outward transcapillary filtration of fluid is similarly limited during such a period with high capillary pressure. Increased lymph drainage, as well as changes in the interstitial space adjacent to the capillaries, may contribute to this limitation to the accumulation of extravascular fluid.

Stimulated by these and similar findings, we studied further the transvascular flux of liquid in isolated perfused lungs, where various important parameters can be controlled. Isolated pairs of rabbit lungs were perfused with homologous plasma. The perfusate, maintained at 37 °C, was pumped into a cannula placed in the pulmonary artery and drained back to a reservoir through a left atrial cannula. A ladder arrangement on the outflow side allowed left atrial pressure to be set at any desired level. Sudden changes in capillary pressure could thereby be induced. The bottom part of the preparation was positioned some 7 cm below the left atrial outflow cannula.

The whole preparation was suspended underneath a force transducer, so allowing preparation weight to be followed continuously, with an accuracy of at least ± 0.05 g. The preparation weighs some 18–20 g. As for lymph drainage from these isolated lungs, the central lymphatic vessels were cut during removal of the lungs from the animal. One would therefore expect all lymph originating from the perfused lungs to drip down (or to evaporate) from the cut lymphatics of the preparation. However, we usually observed no—or only a very sparse— dripping of fluid from such perfused lungs and we concluded from this that only minute amounts of lymph were produced during the experiments. The preparation and the perfusion technique have been further described elsewhere (Lunde & Waaler 1969; Nicolaysen 1971).

When capillary pressure is suddenly raised in such a preparation, there is always an immediate and marked increase in preparation weight. The extent of this sudden increase depends on how much the vascular hydrostatic pressure has been increased. From various types of experiments we know that this early rise in weight is due to vascular distension, with an increase in the blood volume of the lung. This vascular distension appears to take place mainly during the first 30 s and to be completed within 2 min of the increase in pressure. Thereafter one of two trends in weight development might be seen (Lunde & Waaler 1969). If the increase in pressure has been modest (5–10 mmHg), the preparation will soon reach a new stable weight. After such a development the preparation must possess a new transvascular fluid balance. The other trend is that of a continuous but relatively slow gain in weight, usually along a fairly straight slope. This weight gain, which is more marked the greater the increase in left atrial pressure, will eventually lead to a stage where oedema is visible—initially in the lower parts of the lungs.

We were particularly interested in the first type of development—the achievement of a new stable weight for the preparation. How much transvascular filtration of fluid is necessary for this new stable level to be reached? What sort of changes occur in the relevant interstitial space as a result of this filtration?

We consequently attempted to evaluate the extent of the increase in extravascular water when capillary hydrostatic pressure in isolated lungs is changed suddenly. In two experiments we also evaluated the effect on extravascular water content of a sudden change in plasma colloid osmotic pressure. Vascular volume was estimated by the use of ^{125}I-labelled albumin, which was thoroughly mixed with the perfusate. The two small upper lobes of the lungs were then quickly tied off, one after the other, and removed for analyses of intravascular volume and extravascular tissue water. The lobes were rapidly frozen in liquid nitrogen, cut in suitable pieces and weighed; ^{125}I activity was then measured. From the isotope content in each lobe and in a plasma sample, the lobar vascular volume was calculated. The wet weight of the lobar tissue was arrived at by subtracting plasma weight from total lobar wet weight. The lobes as well as the plasma samples were dried at 70 °C and weighed. From the dry weights obtained, net tissue dry weight was calculated. As an expression of tissue water content we then used the ratio, tissue wet weight/tissue dry weight.

In 18 such upper lobes removed under normal low capillary pressures, the tissue wet weight/tissue dry weight ratio was about 5.5 (range 4.4–6.0). This ratio was certainly increased in oedematous lobes. In two lobes with definite oedema when they were removed, the tissue wet weight/tissue dry weight ratio was 14.0 and 16.6, respectively. The ratio also increased in atelectatic lobes. In one lobe with atelectasis in about 60 % of the lobar tissue, the ratio was thus 8.4 (as opposed to 4.4 in the non-atelectatic contralateral lobe in the same preparation).

With these results as background we proceeded to examine the increase in extravascular tissue water when left atrial pressure (and thereby also capillary hydrostatic pressure) was suddenly increased. In each of a series of experiments we compared the conditions in the removed lobe No. 2 with those in a previously removed lobe No. 1. The tissue wet weight/tissue dry weight ratio in each lobe No. 2 was expressed as a percentage of the same ratio in the corresponding lobe No. 1. Table 1 gives the main results. In three control experiments (group 1) No. 1 lobes and No. 2 lobes were removed at 15-min intervals and without any changes in capillary pressure or in perfusate composition. The tissue wet weight/tissue dry weight ratios for these No. 2 lobes were 101, 97 and 94 % of the ratios found for the corresponding No. 1 lobes.

In the next two groups of six and five experiments, lobe No. 1 was removed 5 min before an increase in left atrial pressure, whereas lobe No. 2 was removed 10 min after this increase. Left atrial pressure was raised from an initial value of about 1–2 mmHg and by 5, 10 or 15 mmHg. In six preparations which had completely or very nearly reached a stable weight when lobe No. 2 was removed, the ratios for the No. 2 lobes were 102, 109, 109, 94, 97 and 97 % of those in the corresponding No. 1 lobes. In five preparations which still gained

TABLE 1

Extravascular tissue water in isolated plasma-perfused pairs of rabbit lungs

Group of experiments	Ratio, No. 2 lobe, as % of ratio, No. 1 lobe	Median value in group (%)[a]
1 No pressure increase between removal of lobe No. 1 and lobe No. 2	101, 97, 94	97
2 Left atrial pressure increase after removal of lobe No. 1. New stable, or near-stable, weight at removal of lobe No. 2	102, 109, 109, 94, 97, 97	99.5
3 Left atrial pressure increase after removal of lobe No. 1. Preparation weight increasing at a rate of 0.2–0.25 g/min or more at time of removal of lobe No. 2	134, 113, 118, 100, 117	117
4 Perfusate protein concentration increased between removal of lobe 1 and lobe 2 (see text)	88, 81	84.5

The two upper lobes were rapidly tied off at 15-min intervals. Vascular volumes in the lobes were determined with the use of ^{125}I-labelled albumin as a plasma tracer. The lobes were weighed in the wet condition and after complete drying. The tissue wet weight/tissue dry weight ratios were then calculated, and the ratio for each No. 2 lobe is expressed as a percentage of that in the corresponding No. 1 lobe.

[a] The difference between groups 2 and 3 is significant at the 5% level with the Wilcoxon two-sample test.

weight at a rate of more than 0.2 g/min when the No. 2 lobe was removed, the ratios of the No. 2 lobes were 134, 113, 118, 100 and 117% of the ratios for the corresponding No. 1 lobes. When tested with the Wilcoxon two-sample test (one-sided), there was a significant difference ($P < 0.05$) between groups 2 and 3.

In the two preparations where the perfusate protein concentration was increased (from 23 mg/ml to 50 mg/ml and from 31 mg/ml to 53 mg/ml) between the removal of lobe 1 and lobe 2, the tissue wet weight/tissue dry weight ratio fell. When expressed in relation to the ratios of the No. 1 lobes, the ratios of the No. 2 lobes were 88 and 81%, respectively.

We could thus hardly detect any definite increase in extravascular lung water content in preparations where lung capillary pressure had been increased suddenly but to such a moderate extent that the preparation achieved a new stable weight. The amount of transvascularly filtered fluid in this situation is apparently very small but it is sufficient for a new transvascular equilibrium to be reached. This new equilibrium must stem from filtration-caused changes in some interstitial compartment near the exchange vessels. As long as oedema is not developing, that is as long as capillary pressure has not been raised above a level that produces oedema, this interstitial compartment apparently does not expand by more than a very modest degree. The total increase in extra-vascular fluid in these circumstances must have been less than 10 %. Somewhat larger increments in extravascular fluid were observed in preparations where filtration goes on in such a way that oedema would eventually have developed. Much larger values for extravascular water were found in lobes where atelectasis or oedema were present.

Some further information on pulmonary transvascular fluid exchange and on the interstitial compartment involved may be deduced from experiments by Bø et al. (1974). These workers used isolated perfused lungs placed within a Perspex casing, whereby alveolar pressure, 'pleural' pressure and thus also transpulmonary pressure could be changed at will. Bø et al. were able to arrange their experiments in such a way that with a satisfactory perfusion there was only a small pressure fall (1–2 mmHg) from the arterial to the left atrial side of the pulmonary vascular bed. Thereby they knew fairly accurately what capillary pressure level prevailed in their preparation. When pulmonary arterial pressure and left atrial pressure were raised high enough from initially low values, a steady weight gain could be achieved, indicating a continuous outward transvascular filtration of fluid. When alveolar and 'pleural' pressure were increased to the same extent in such a preparation, then transvascular filtration of fluid fell markedly or even stopped completely, as judged from the preparation weight. In another type of experiment, Bø, Hauge and Nicolaysen (unpublished work) also had outward transvascular filtration of fluid going on at a high capillary pressure. When they increased left atrial pressure, alveolar pressure and 'pleural' pressure to the same extent, the rate of transvascular filtration of fluid remained the same. These results must mean that the in-creased alveolar pressure 'reaches' the wall of filtrating vessels, where it reduces or offsets the filtrating effect of the increased capillary pressure. This again indicates that vessels near the alveoli are largely responsible for the pressure-induced transvascular shift of fluid in our isolated lung preparations.

What sort of changes are occurring in the interstitial fluid compartment close to the capillaries during transvascular shifts of fluid? One would assume from all available information that this compartment is initially a very small one (that is, small as compared to capillary blood volume, for example). A moderate expansion or reduction in volume must efficiently change either the protein concentration (with the colloid osmotic pressure) or the hydrostatic pressure within this compartment, or both. We favour the view that changes in protein concentration are important in this connection. Since the protein content of lung lymph is fairly high, we find it reasonable to assume that there is normally also a high protein concentration in the interstitial fluid of the lung. If the small amount of fluid in the relevant interstitial space has a high protein concentration when capillary pressure is low, this fluid would be rapidly and efficiently diluted by small amounts of a transvascularly-added filtrate. The addition of small amounts of protein-poor ultrafiltrate would thus efficiently reduce the high colloid osmotic pressure of the interstitial fluid. Such a reduction in the extravascular colloid osmotic pressure would represent an efficient and rapidly adjusting counter-force in conditions where filtration is induced by an increase in capillary hydrostatic pressure. With such a mechanism, changes in the transcapillary fluid balance in the lung could be efficiently and rapidly readjusted, as a result of very small transvascular shifts of fluid. In addition, interstitial hydrostatic pressure may of course also change, adding to the tendency for transvascular filtration and reabsorption of fluid in the lungs to be a self-limiting process.

References

Bø, G., NICOLAYSEN, G. & HAUGE, A. (1974) Effects of positive alveolar pressure on pulmonary transvascular fluid filtration, in *Proc. Int. Union Physiol. Sci. 11*, 55, New Delhi
Bø, G., HAUGE, A. & WAALER, B. A. (1975) *J. Appl. Physiol. 38*, 608-614
LUNDE, P. K. M. & WAALER, B. A. (1969) *J. Physiol. (Lond.), 205*, 1-18
NICOLAYSEN, G. (1971) *Acta Physiol. Scand. 82*, 417-432
STARLING, E. H. (1896) *J. Physiol. (Lond.), 19*, 312-326

Discussion

Crosbie: Were the rabbit and cat lungs inflated by negative pressure?

Waaler: No, we used positive pressure ventilation.

Dickinson: Clinically, a good way of driving liquid out of the alveoli is to put a patient on positive pressure ventilation. Your method seems to drive fluid out of the interstitial spaces back into the bloodstream when alveolar pressure is increased, Dr Waaler.

Waaler: In the preparation described, increased alveolar pressure tends to reduce the rate of outward transvascular filtration of fluid.

Staub: Did you mean that you *know* that liquid can be driven out of the lungs by positive pressure, Dr Dickinson?

Dickinson: I have personally held a bag and had to squeeze hard to push the liquid back again. Unfortunately, when you let go it all reaccumulates unless you have done something meantime to cure the patient. It is quite a good way of getting rid of pulmonary oedema clinically.

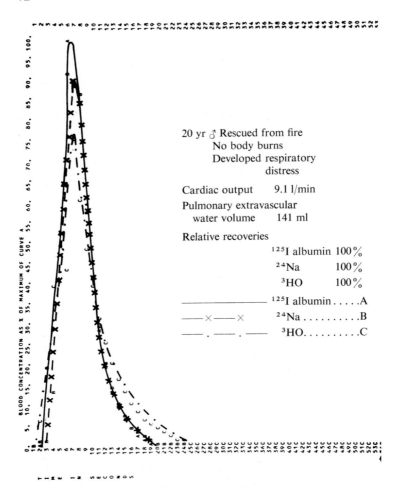

FIG. 1. (Crosbie) Multiple indicator dilution curves obtained from a patient with acute respiratory distress syndrome produced by toxic smoke inhalation. He is being ventilated by intermittent positive pressure with added peak-end expired pressure.
FI_{O_2} 20.93; Pa_{O_2} 49 mmHg (6.5 kPa); Pa_{CO_2} 38 mmHg (5.05 kPa); pH 7.43; Sa_{O_2} 86%; cardiac output 9.1 l/min; chest X-ray within normal limits. Note the reduced amount of water (normal pulmonary extravascular water volume, 200 ml) in the lung capillary bed and the close fit of the labelled sodium to the albumin, indicating normal capillary permeability.

Staub: I have often heard radiologists and clinicians make this statement, but I have never seen any data to prove it.

Crosbie: We measured the pulmonary extravascular water volume in a young man who developed the acute respiratory distress syndrome after inhalation of smoke. We found that the lung water was about 50% of the normal value. He was being ventilated by positive pressure with added peak-end expired pressure at the time. Fig. 1 (Crosbie) shows the actual multiple indicator dilution traces we obtained. He was hypoxaemic, with a high cardiac output and normal chest X-ray. Chinard (1966) showed similar effects in isolated perfused dog lung preparations when the alveolar pressure was raised.

Strang: Dr Waaler's point is that he can limit the rate of accumulation of fluid, not that he can drive it out of the lung.

Hughes: When airway pressure is increased in patients, the cardiac output may be reduced temporarily and capillary pressure lowered relative to alveolar pressure, so that the hydraulic driving force is changed. That is one explanation of why oedema goes away and yet comes back again when pulmonary blood flow readjusts to its original level.

Dickinson: If the liquid is prevented from accumulating in alveoli then it would eventually get swept up by the lymphatics.

Waaler: The main point of doing these experiments in *isolated* lungs is of course that we can then control the vascular pressures completely. If 'pleural' pressure, alveolar pressure and left atrial pressure were raised to the same extent, the rate of transvascular filtration of fluid remained the same.

Michel: Since you could calculate pulmonary vascular resistance in your experiments, have you estimated whether the area of the capillary bed available for filtration was constant or changing when left atrial pressure was varied?

Waaler: We feel fairly confident that the area remained constant in these experiments. When, in well-perfused preparations, we increased the left atrial pressure in steps of 5 mmHg (0.66 kPa), we obtained increments in the amount of fluid filtered out which were proportional to the increase in left atrial pressure. We wouldn't expect this if the surface had also increased.

Michel: When you change the alveolar pressure are you also sure that you are not changing the filtration area, which of course could be an alternative explanation for the changes of filtration rate?

Waaler: Yes, under the conditions of these experiments we believe that we are not changing the filtration area.

Staub: What is the maximum increase in left atrial pressure that will allow a new stable condition to be reached, Dr Waaler? You showed continuous weight gain at 10 mmHg (1.33 kPa). Is that the same in all animals or does it vary from lung to lung?

Waaler: This varies from lung to lung. The bottom part of the lung is positioned about 7 cm below the left atrial cannula, so when stable weight is no longer obtained the first place where continuous outward transvascular filtration of fluid occurs will be at the bottom of the preparation, where there is an additional 5 mmHg in capillary pressure. Rabbit plasma also has a lower protein concentration than dog or human plasma, but usually in these preparations we can raise the left atrial pressure by 5–10 mmHg from 1 mmHg or 2 mmHg and still get a new stable weight. If we perfuse the preparation with blood, it looks as if the left atrial pressure can be raised a bit more before oedema develops.

Staub: How long does it take to reach a new stable weight?

Waaler: About two or three minutes.

Staub: In the unanaesthetized sheep it takes about two hours to reach a new steady state of transvascular fluid balance as measured by lymph flow when left atrial pressure is increased. I wonder why it is so much quicker in the isolated lung?

Waaler: If we are right that there is a small extravascular space which is relevant in this connection, then one would expect this new stable weight to be reached fairly soon, when the first few microlitres of fluid have been pushed out of the vessels. If fluid filtration continues at a high capillary pressure then the interstitial space will soon become 'over-expanded'.

Strang: Presumably when he is measuring lymph flow Dr Staub is unable to follow such rapid changes in net filtration.

Staub: In the sheep, a rise of even 5 cmH$_2$O (0.5 kPa) in left atrial pressure means that about an hour is needed before a new steady state lymph flow is achieved. I am asking why the isolated lung behaves differently.

Waaler: If transvascular fluid filtration is still going on in our preparation after 4 or 5 min, it will usually continue until definite oedema appears.

Dickinson: Does the lymph come out rather faster at that (later) stage or is it still not flowing much?

Waaler: Surprisingly little lymph comes from these preparations.

Staub: That is reasonable, because the lymphatics are dead in the isolated lobes!

Guyton: We also had similar findings in isolated lungs; even after several hours there was practically no lymphatic flow. Dr Staub is right—the lymphatics do not function significantly in such a preparation.

Dr Waaler, did enough fluid actually transfer across the capillary membrane to change the colloid osmotic pressure of the interstitial fluid by an amount sufficient to give the balance that you were looking for?

Waaler: The trouble is that we don't know how big the relevant interstitial space is initially. The total increase in extravascular water content is less than 10% in a new stable-weight situation, but the volume of the interstitial space around the capillaries would then have increased relatively more. I would guess that the volume of this space has at least been doubled.

Lee: Is there a regional distribution of wet weight/dry weight changes? Do they become uniform right through?

Waaler: We tried to cut some of the removed upper lobes in slices 1 cm thick. We could then detect some effect of gravity down those slices, with a slight increase in the wet weight/dry weight ratio from top to bottom.

Strang: You assumed that the concentration of protein in the interstitial fluid was quite high—several grams/100 ml. There is certainly quite a lot of evidence that interstitial fluid in the body generally has quite a substantial albumin concentration, similar to that in lymph. Some of this evidence comes from injecting labelled albumin into the circulation and estimating the size of the extravascular albumin pool (Sterling 1951; Myant 1951). There are also direct measurements of interstitial protein concentration in muscle, which in general agree (Creese *et al.* 1962).

Michel: In organs such as the lungs, where the rate of filtration is low, one might expect the pericapillary protein concentration to be high. It is determined by the flux of protein across the capillary wall divided by the filtration rate, and where the filtration rate is low obviously the concentration will be relatively high.

This leads on to a technical difference between the isolated lung and the intact lung. In the intact lung, with the lymphatics working efficiently there is some means of keeping the pericapillary protein concentrations at a lower level. In the isolated lung there is only diffusion to distribute the protein in the interstitial space. If the protein concentration is high to start with and a little water is filtered into the interstitial space, only diffusion can lower that concentration. Perhaps the phenomenon which Dr Waaler has talked about, and which I suspect is a genuine phenomenon, is applicable to a different extent in the intact animal because the degree of washout of the interstitial space is different.

Staub: Were the lungs ventilated, Dr Waaler?

Waaler: Yes, and they were apparently well maintained. On electron micrographs made during the first hours of perfusion these preparations don't look different from fresh lungs.

Olver: Where is the anatomical site of the protein pool in the lung? If it is in the basement membrane there might not be much convection.

Waaler: We don't know really, but the basement membrane has the right sort of dimensions and it might well represent the interstitial space in question.

References

CHINARD, F. P. (1966) The permeability characteristics of the pulmonary blood-gas barrier, in *Advances in Respiratory Physiology* (Caro, C. G., ed.), Edward Arnold, London

CREESE, R., D'SILVA, J. L. & SHAW, D. M. (1962) Interfibre fluid from guinea-pig muscle. *J. Physiol. (Lond.) 162*, 44-53

MYANT, N. B. (1951) Observations on the metabolism of human gamma globulin labelled by radioactive iodine. *Clin. Sci. 11*, 191-201

STERLING, K. (1951) The turnover rate of serum albumen in man as measured by I^{131} tagged albumen. *J. Clin. Invest. 30*, 1228-1237

Dynamics of subatmospheric pressure in the pulmonary interstitial fluid

ARTHUR C. GUYTON, AUBREY E. TAYLOR, ROBERT E. DRAKE
and JAMES C. PARKER

Department of Physiology and Biophysics, University of Mississippi School of Medicine, Jackson, Mississippi

Abstract Systems analyses are presented for several aspects of pulmonary fluid dynamics, especially those related to (1) transport of fluid between the pulmonary interstitial spaces and the alveoli, (2) the possibility of a mechanism for concentrating protein in the lymph vessels, and (3) the effects of very high resistance to fluid flow in the alveolar septal wall. The analysis of fluid transport between the interstitial space and the alveoli, assuming that there is no active secretory or active absorptive process, shows that the interstitial fluid pressure in the normal lung cannot be more positive than the fluid pressure in the alveoli. Since the surface tension of this fluid causes it to have a subatmospheric pressure, the calculated maximum pressure for interstitial fluid in the normal lung is about −2 mmHg (−0.266 kPa). At any pressure more positive than this the alveoli will fill with fluid.

The systems analyses for concentrating protein in the pulmonary lymphatics and for the effects of high resistance to fluid flow in the alveolar septal wall offer possible explanations for very negative pressures of pulmonary interstitial fluid, even though calculations of the interstitial fluid pressure based on the assumption that the colloid osmotic pressure of pulmonary interstitial fluid is equal to the osmotic pressure of pulmonary lymph give estimated pressures of pulmonary interstitial fluid approaching 0 mmHg.

In previous studies we have suggested that pressure in pulmonary interstitial fluid is normally subatmospheric, with values probably at least as low as −5mmHg (−0.66 kPa) and possibly as low as −16 mmHg (−2.13 kPa) (Guyton & Lindsey 1959; Meyer *et al.* 1968). Though there are many reasons for believing in this concept of a subatmospheric pressure in pulmonary interstitial fluid, there are also other findings that must be explained before it can be accepted with assurance. Therefore, the purpose of the present paper is to explore further this concept and its physiological basis.

REASONS FOR BELIEVING THE SUBATMOSPHERIC PRESSURE CONCEPT

The safety factor against oedema

One of the most important reasons for postulating a subatmospheric pressure in pulmonary interstitial fluid is that the lungs have a large safety factor against oedema. Ordinarily oedema will not occur in the dog's lung until the left atrial pressure rises above 23 to 25 mmHg (3.06–3.33 kPa) or until the plasma colloid osmotic pressure falls below about 10 mmHg (1.33 kPa) (Guyton & Lindsey 1959). From these data one can calculate that the lungs normally have a safety factor against oedema of about 20 mmHg (2.66 kPa). One interpretation of this is that the absorptive pressures tending to move fluid from the interstitial spaces into the pulmonary capillary blood are about 20 mmHg greater than the pressures tending to filter fluid out of the capillaries into the interstitial spaces. If this were true, then the interstitial fluid pressure could be as low as −20 mmHg. This interpretation is probably far from being entirely true, yet even if it is partially true the pressure would still be in the negative range—somewhere between 0 and −20 mmHg.

Measurements of subatmospheric pressure in perforated capsules implanted in the lung

Using the implanted perforated capsule technique that has been used in many studies of peripheral interstitial fluid pressure, Meyer *et al.* (1968) investigated the pulmonary interstitial fluid pressure. In 34 dogs in which we succeeded in implanting the capsules in lungs without causing serious inflammation, the pressures in the capsules averaged −5.8 mmHg (−0.77 kPa) but in a few capsules the pressures were as low as −16 mmHg (−2.13 kPa). Furthermore, the less the degree of inflammation and the less the degree of fibrosis around the capsules, the more negative were the measured pressures. Because it was impossible ever to implant a capsule without at least some degree of inflammation, it was our impression that the values measured in the capsules with the least inflammation, values between −10 and −16 mmHg, probably more nearly represented the true pulmonary interstitial fluid pressure.

Negative pressure in the fluid lining the alveoli

Another very compelling reason for believing that the pulmonary interstitial fluid pressure is substantially subatmospheric is that there is a strong negative pressure in the fluid that lines the alveoli. This can be understood best by

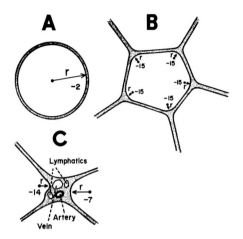

FIG. 1. Negative fluid pressures (mmHg) generated by the surface tension (ST)(dyn/cm) of the fluid in the alveoli. P = (0.15 × ST)/r(cm). (A) Pressure in a spherical alveolus. (B) Pressures at alveolar angles. (C) Pressures adjacent to a perivascular space.

referring to Fig. 1. Fig. 1A illustrates a hypothetical spherical alveolus with a radius of 75 μm. Many studies have demonstrated that the fluid on the inner surface of an alveolus of this size has enough surface tension to cause the fluid to pull away from the alveolar epithelium with a pressure at least as negative as −2 to −3 mmHg (Clements & Gierney 1965). This is based on the following formula for pressure (P) versus surface tension (ST):

$$- \, P \, (mmHg) = \frac{0.0015 \times ST \, (dyn/cm)}{r \, (cm)}$$

If the surface tension is 10 dynes/centimetre (10×10^{-5} N/cm) (a very low value) the pressure of the fluid of a spherical alveolus 75 μm in diameter would be −2 mmHg (−0.27 kPa). However, the shape of the alveolar walls is more like that of Fig. 1B than Fig. 1A; this figure shows acute angles where the septal walls bifurcate. If we assume the radii of curvature of these angles to be about 10 μm the negative pressure of the fluid in these angles comes to −15 mmHg (−2 kPa). Fig. 1C illustrates schematically a perivascular space, with calculated negative fluid pressures in the adjacent alveolar angles of −14 and −7 mmHg (−1.86 and −0.93 kPa); these negative pressures try to expand the perivascular spaces as well as pull fluid through the alveolar membrane.

The question must now be asked: if the pressure of the fluid in the alveoli is subatmospheric, what prevents this from pulling fluid outwards through the septal walls into the alveoli, thereby causing the alveoli to fill with fluid? Indeed, as more fluid enters an alveolus, the radius of the alveolar bubble becomes smaller, and the negative pressure of the alveolar fluid becomes even more negative. Therefore, once started, the process of alveolar flooding should be self-accelerating.

This filling of the alveoli with fluid could be prevented by two mechanisms. (1) There could be an active transport mechanism that causes fluid to be absorbed from the alveoli into the interstitial spaces. Or (2) there could be a more negative pressure in the pulmonary interstitial fluid than in the alveolar fluid. The first of these possibilities is very doubtful because the active transport that has been observed has been in the wrong direction, causing secretion of fluid from the interstitial space into the alveoli (Olver *et al.* 1972). Furthermore, measurements of diffusion through the alveolar membrane of both water and dissolved substances have shown the alveolar epithelium to be exceedingly leaky (Taylor *et al.* 1965), probably much too leaky ever to prevent transudation of fluid from the interstitial spaces into the alveoli if the pressure of the alveolar fluid is more negative than that of the interstitial fluid.

A systems analysis of alveolar fluid dynamics

To illustrate the significance of the negative pressure in the alveolar fluid and its tendency to cause flooding of the alveoli, we have developed the simple systems analysis of Fig. 2, which is self-evident for those who are familiar with systems analysis notation. Briefly, Blocks 1 through 6 calculate the volume of fluid in the alveoli and the average radius of the fluid in the alveoli. Blocks 7, 8, and 9 calculate the radius of the fluid in the angles of the alveoli. The pressure of the fluid in the alveoli (output of Block 1) is determined by whichever is less, the radius of the fluid in the angles or the average radius. The only significant assumption made in this systems analysis is that there is no active transport through the pulmonary epithelial membrane.

Fig. 3 illustrates computer readouts for the time-courses of the alveolar fluid volume and the least radius of the alveolar fluid under the following conditions: initially, the average radius of the alveolus was 76 μm, the radius of the fluid in the angles 15 μm, and the pulmonary interstitial fluid pressure −10 mmHg. Under these conditions the volume of fluid and the least radius remained constant. Then suddenly the pulmonary interstitial fluid pressure was raised to some higher value—to −5 mmHg, to −3 mmHg, −1.5 mmHg, 0 mmHg, or +2 mmHg. Note that so long as the pulmonary interstitial fluid pressure remained less than −2 mmHg the volume of fluid increased up to a new steady-state value but did not continue increasing until the alveolus filled.

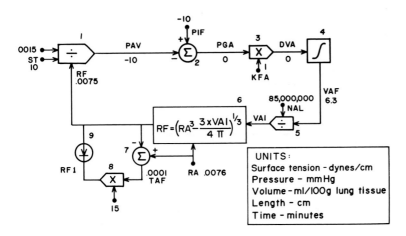

Fig. 2. Systems analysis of alveolar fluid dynamics. DVA – rate of change of alveolar fluid volume; KFA – filtration coefficient for fluid through the alveolar membrane; NAL – number of alveoli in 100 g lung tissue; PAV – pressure of alveolar fluid; PGA – pressure difference between pulmonary interstitial fluid and pulmonary alveolar fluid; PIF – interstitial fluid pressure; RA – average radius of the alveolus; RF – average radius of the inner surface of the fluid lining of the alveolus; RFl – radius of the fluid surfaces in the angles of the alveoli; ST – surface tension; TAF – thickness of the alveolar fluid lining; VAF – volume of alveolar fluid in 100 g lung; VA1 – volume of alveolar fluid in 1 alveolus. (Values on lines = steady-state values. Italicized numbers = block numbers.)

The radius of the fluid in the angles of the alveoli rose from the initial value of 15 μm to a higher value as the angles increased their fluid. When the pulmonary interstitial fluid was raised to a pressure greater than −2 mmHg, the angles of the alveoli filled completely, and the fluid bubble of the alveolus became spherical at a maximum radius of about 72 μm. Thereafter, further filling of the alveolus decreased this spherical radius of curvature, the pressure of the fluid in the alveolus became progressively more negative, and fluid was pulled into the alveoli at an accelerating pace until the alveoli became completely filled.

Computer readouts for final steady-state levels of filling and least radii of the fluid in the alveoli are shown in Fig. 4 for three different sizes of alveoli, with average radii of 76, 38 and 21 μm. Note that a pulmonary interstitial fluid pressure at least as negative as −10 mmHg is required to prevent filling of the 21 μm alveoli. For the 38 μm alveoli, complete filling of the alveolus occurs at −4.2 mmHg (−0.56 kPa). For 76 μm, complete filling occurs when the pulmonary interstitial fluid pressure rises above −2.2 mmHg (−0.29 kPa).

Thus, if we assume that there is no active transport from the alveoli into the pulmonary interstitial spaces, it is clear that a very negative pulmonary inter-

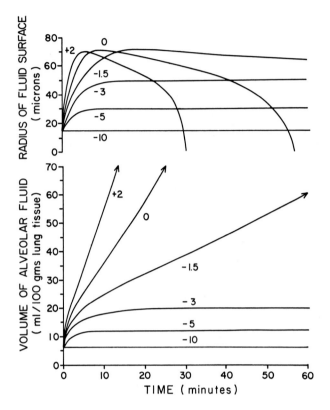

FIG. 3. Computer readout for the time course of changes in volume of alveolar fluid and least radius of the fluid in the alveolar angles. Initial conditions: pulmonary interstitial fluid pressure, – 10 mmHg; radius of the fluid in the septal angles, 15 μm; volume of alveolar fluid, 6.3 ml/100 g lung tissue. The numbers on the curves represent values to which the pulmonary interstitial fluid pressure was suddenly raised.

stitial fluid pressure is required to prevent flooding of the normal alveoli—and investigators have so far failed to find any such active transport.

THE DIFFICULTY MANY PEOPLE HAVE IN UNDERSTANDING THE TISSUE MECHANICS OF SUBATMOSPHERIC PRESSURE

At this point we need to detour for a moment and speak of the most overwhelming argument that we have had to meet time and time again in convincing others that there is truly a subatmospheric pressure in interstitial fluid, whether in the lungs or in the peripheral tissues. That argument is the following: 'It simply can't be'. That is, many investigators have come to the conclusion that

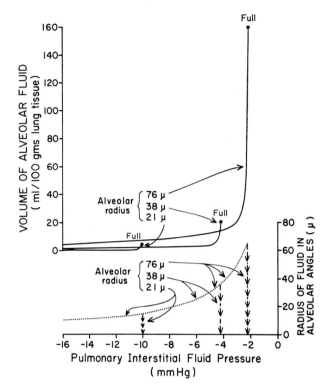

FIG. 4. Computer readout of the steady-state volume of alveolar fluid and radius of the fluid in the alveolar angles at different pulmonary interstitial fluid pressures and for alveoli of different average radii.

subatmospheric pressure cannot exist in the fluids of the body, for the simple reason that atmospheric pressure is acting against the soft tissues from outside the body, and therefore the pressures on the inside cannot be less than the atmospheric pressure. In fact, this argument was used by McDonald (1968) in a recent review of circulatory dynamics. Also, Staub (1974) inferred this possibility in relation to his belief that the interstitial fluid pressure of the alveolar septa is probably near to or equal to atmospheric pressure.

However, on studying the structure of the alveolar septal wall, one can readily understand how a subatmospheric pressure can exist in the fluid within the septal sandwich. The septum has two epithelial cell surfaces plus, between the epithelial cell layers, a dense segment composed of basement membranes and a small amount of connective tissue. Remembering that a basement membrane itself has a porous mucopolysaccharide structure, generally with space diameters of 12 nm upwards, one can understand that these spaces are at least 30 times as large as the diameter of the water molecule and more often 100 or more times as large. Therefore, the interstitial 'space' is not a single large space at all, but instead is the interstices of a 'sponge'. Critical studies of the hydraulic forces required to remove fluid from tissue mucopolysaccharide have demonstrated that −7 to −12 mmHg (−0.93 to −1.6 kPa) pressure is required to compact tissues to the degree of compaction normally found in the body (Granger 1975).

Therefore, it is probably time to put to rest the idea that it is impossible to have subatmospheric pressures in the interstitial fluids. Instead, measurements on tissue mucopolysaccharides indicate that the degree of compaction normally found in tissues could not exist without subatmospheric pressures.

A POSSIBLE MECHANISM FOR CONCENTRATING PULMONARY LYMPH AND ITS SIGNIFICANCE FOR THE CONCEPT OF A SUBATMOSPHERIC PRESSURE IN INTERSTITIAL FLUID

An argument against the concept of a subatmospheric pressure in pulmonary interstitial fluid that has often been put forward is the following: several investigators have attempted to calculate the pulmonary interstitial fluid pressure using a modified Starling equation for equilibration of pressures at the capillary membrane:

$$P_{isf} = P_c - \pi_c + \pi_{isf} - F_l/K_{fc}$$

in which P_{isf} is the interstitial fluid pressure, P_c is the capillary pressure, π_c is the plasma colloid osmotic pressure, π_{isf} is the interstitial fluid colloid osmotic pressure, F_l is lymph flow, and K_{fc} is the capillary membrane filtration coefficient. After the values of this equation have been filled in as best one can, the pulmonary interstitial fluid pressure works out to be nearly equal to 0 mmHg or only slightly negative. However, there are many opportunities for error in this type of calculation. For instance, it has not been possible to measure the colloid osmotic pressure of interstitial fluid. Therefore, investigators have had to assume the value of this to be equal to the colloid osmotic pressure of the lymph flowing from the lungs. Furthermore, none of the other values in the equation are known with certainty, with the possible exception of the plasma colloid osmotic pressure. Therefore, the values used for calculation could have been in error. Indeed, from reported average values, we have also calculated by this same equation interstitial fluid pressures of the order of −6 mmHg (−0.8 kPa) (Guyton et al. 1975).

However, even if we assume that the 0 mmHg calculation is completely correct, there are still several plausible ways in which a subatmospheric pressure

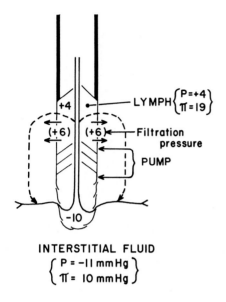

FIG. 5. A lymph vessel mechanism for concentrating lymph protein. Values given in mmHg. π = colloid osmotic pressure.

in pulmonary interstitial fluid is compatible with these calculations. Two of these are (1) the likelihood that the colloid osmotic pressure of pulmonary lymph does not represent the colloid osmotic pressure of the pulmonary interstitial fluid because the lymph vessels have a concentrating mechanism for the lymph protein, and (2) the possibility of restricted movement of fluid in the alveolar septal walls, which would cause in normal lungs an 'effective' pulmonary capillary filtration coefficient of very low value, thereby making the last term of the capillary equilibrium equation quantitatively very important and giving a very negative pulmonary interstitial fluid pressure (Taylor & Gibson 1975).

Lymph vessel mechanics for concentrating protein

Fig. 5 illustrates a simple mechanism by which protein could become concentrated in lymph. This mechanism is based on recent work by Zweifach & Prather (1975) and Hargens & Zweifach (1975) showing that the lymphatics of the mesentery develop considerable positive pressure even in the very small collecting lymphatics, and that this causes filtration of fluid out of the lymphatics into the surrounding tissue spaces, thus concentrating the lymph protein. Note in Fig. 5 that fluid enters the terminal lymphatics, and the pressure increases as

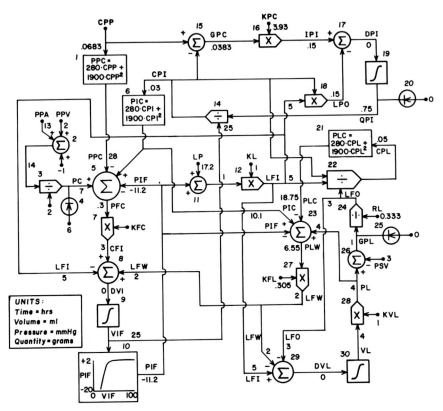

FIG. 6. A systems analysis of the interstitial fluid system of the lung, depicting especially a postulated concentrating mechanism for lymph protein. CFI – rate of filtration of fluid through the pulmonary capillaries into the interstitial spaces; CPI – concentration of protein in the interstitial fluid; CPL – concentration of protein in the lymph; CPP – concentration of plasma proteins; DPI – rate of change of protein quantity in the interstitial fluid; DVI – rate of change of interstitial fluid volume; DVL – rate of change of volume of fluid in the lymphatics; GPC – difference between protein concentration in the plasma and in the interstitial fluid; GPL – difference between the pressure in the lymphatics and the pressure at the outflow point; IPI – rate of leakage of protein from pulmonary capillaries into the interstitial fluid; KFC – filtration coefficient for the pulmonary capillaries; KL – constant for converting LP + PIF into fluid flow into the lymphatics; KPC – coefficient for protein leakage from the pulmonary capillaries into the interstitial spaces; KVL – constant for converting volume of fluid in the lymphatics to pressure in the lymphatics; LFI – flow of fluid from interstitial spaces into the lymphatics; LFO – flow of fluid out of the pulmonary lymphatics; LFW – filtration of fluid out of the lymphatics into the interstitial spaces; LP – increase in pressure caused by lymphatic pump; LPO – rate of flow of protein out of the interstitial fluid into the lymphatics; PC – pulmonary capillary pressure; PFC – filtration pressure across the pulmonary capillary membrane; PIC – colloid osmotic pressure of the pulmonary interstitial fluid; PIF – pressure of the interstitial fluid of the lung; PL – fluid pressure in the lymphatics; PLC – colloid osmotic pressure in the lymph; PPA – pulmonary arterial pressure; PPC – colloid osmotic pressure of the plasma protein; PLW – pressure difference across the lymphatic wall; PPV – pulmonary venous pressure; PSV – outflow pressure at the end of the lymphatics; QPI – quantity of protein in the interstitial fluids; RL – resistance of the lymphatics; VIF – interstitial fluid volume; VL – volume of fluid in the lymphatics. (Values on lines = steady-state values per 100 g lung. Italicized numbers = block numbers.)

the lymph flows upwards beyond the successive valves. In this figure the pressure is shown to rise from an interstitial fluid pressure value of −11 mmHg (−1.46 kPa) up to a lymphatic vessel pressure as high as +4 mmHg (0.53 kPa). This +4 value is chosen because this is approximately the pressure required to cause the lymph to flow out of the chest into the positive pressure region of the neck veins. With an interstitial fluid pressure of −11 mmHg, an interstitial fluid colloid osmotic pressure of 10 mmHg, a lymphatic pressure of +4 mmHg, and an intralymphatic colloid osmotic pressure of 19 mmHg (2.53 kPa), one calculates a filtration pressure across the walls of the lymphatic vessels of 6 mmHg (0.8 kPa). Therefore, fluid continues to filter out of the lymph vessel back into the interstitial fluid, which keeps the interstitial fluid dilute, while a much more concentrated lymph flows from the exit of the lymph vessel.

Another embodiment of a lymph-concentrating mechanism would be for the fluid of the lymph to filter out of the larger lymphatics and be absorbed into the surrounding capillaries. However, the filtration coefficient of the smaller lymphatics is probably far greater than that of the larger lymphatics, so that it is more likely that lymph concentration would occur in the collecting lymphatics that exist in the perivascular spaces rather than in the larger lymphatics. Indeed, it is the collecting lymphatics of the mesentery where protein concentration has been observed to occur.

A systems analysis of pulmonary interstitial fluid dynamics and lymphatic concentration of protein

Fig. 6 illustrates a systems analysis of pulmonary interstitial fluid dynamics, with a possible lymph-concentrating mechanism included. It has three major components: (1) analysis of fluid and protein filtration through the walls of the pulmonary capillaries, (2) analysis of the dynamics of the interstitial fluid compartment itself, and (3) analysis of lymph flow, lymphatic pumping, and filtration of fluid out of the lymph vessels back into the fluid compartment. The analysis allows one to predict the effects of various changes in physiological conditions on such factors as pulmonary interstitial fluid pressure, interstitial fluid volume, interstitial fluid protein concentration, interstitial fluid colloid osmotic pressure, lymph flow, lymph protein concentration, rate of filtration of fluid through the lymph vessel walls, and a number of other factors. Using this analysis we have been able to make some surprising predictions about the efficacy of a lymph-concentrating mechanism, as will be discussed in the following sections.

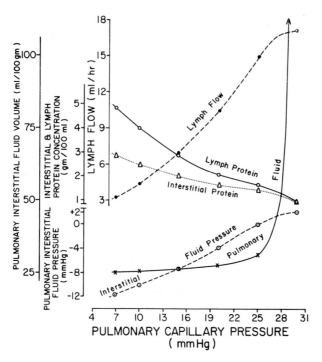

FIG. 7. Computer readout of steady-state values for different lung fluid variables at different pulmonary capillary pressures (as predicted from the systems analysis of Fig. 6). Note the greater protein concentration in the lymph than in the interstitial fluid and also the sudden development of oedema at a pulmonary capillary pressure above 28 mmHg.

Analysis of the lymph-concentrating mechanism at different levels of increased pulmonary capillary pressure

Fig. 7 shows a computer readout for changes in the steady-state values of several variables—changes produced by different pulmonary capillary pressures as predicted by the systems analysis of Fig. 6. Note the progressive increases in both the interstitial fluid pressure and the lymph flow as the pulmonary capillary pressure rises from the normal value of 7 mmHg up to 30 mmHg (0.93–4 kPa). Note also that the pulmonary interstitial fluid volume remains almost normal until the capillary pressure rises above 25 to 28 mmHg (3.32–3.72 kPa), at which level the pulmonary interstitial fluid pressure rises from the subatmospheric pressure range into the supra-atmospheric pressure range; then there is a dramatic increase in pulmonary interstitial fluid volume (assuming that the fluid that floods the alveoli is part of the interstitial fluid). This is exactly what is found in animal experiments (Drake & Taylor 1975).

Note also the predicted values for the concentrations of interstitial fluid protein and lymph protein. In the normal state, the predicted concentration of the lymph protein is about 75% greater than the concentration of interstitial fluid protein. However, as the lymph flow increases, the lymph remains in the lymph vessels for shorter periods, so less filtration occurs. Also, the pressure gradient across the lymphatic wall becomes less favourable for filtration. Therefore, the analysis predicts that lymph protein concentration will approach interstitial fluid protein concentration as the lungs approach the oedematous state.

The important feature of the analysis in Fig. 6 is that it was made with the assumption that the filtration coefficient of all the lymphatics in the lungs is only 1/33rd of the filtration coefficient of the pulmonary capillaries. Though the filtration coefficient for a lymphatic bed has never been measured, anatomical studies of the lymphatics in certain tissues, particularly in the omentum, indicate that the lymphatic filtration coefficient in some tissues can be as great as the filtration coefficient of the blood capillaries, and perhaps even several times as great. Therefore, a filtration coefficient of the pulmonary lymphatics equal to only 1/33rd of the pulmonary capillary filtration coefficient is very small, even though the lungs probably have much less lymphatic surface area than blood capillary surface area.

The reason why so much concentration of the proteins can be achieved in a lymphatic bed with such a low filtration coefficient is simply that the flow of lymph along the lymphatic vessels is so slow that a long time is available for filtration to occur. Thus, Fig. 7 demonstrates that protein can be concentrated markedly in pulmonary lymph even with a minimal lymphatic filtration coefficient.

Effect of different levels of lymphatic filtration coefficient

Fig. 8 illustrates effects of changes in the lymphatic wall filtration coefficient. Zero filtration coefficient means no fluid whatsoever filters out of the lymphatics. Therefore, at zero coefficient the lymph protein concentration is equal to the interstitial fluid protein concentration. However, as the lymphatic filtration coefficient increases, lymph outflow falls, while lymph protein concentration rises progressively higher. On the other hand, this has almost no effect on the interstitial fluid protein concentration, as shown in the figure.

In the upper part of Fig. 8 are shown (1) the true interstitial fluid pressure, and (2) the interstitial fluid pressure that would be calculated from the Starling equilibrium equation given earlier (p. 84) if the interstitial fluid protein concentration is assumed to equal the measured lymph protein concentration.

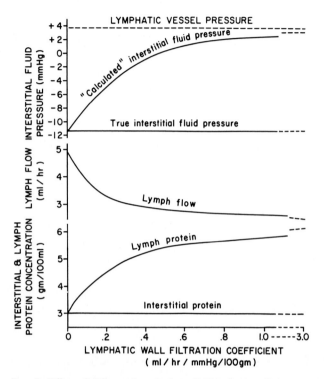

FIG. 8. Effect of different lymphatic wall filtration coefficients on interstitial fluid and lymph variables, showing (top) the hazard of calculating interstitial fluid pressure by assuming that protein concentration in interstitial fluid equals protein concentration in lymph.

Since the true interstitial fluid protein concentration is lower than the lymph protein concentration, the calculated interstitial fluid pressure would always be considerably greater than the true interstitial fluid pressure. Indeed, the analysis shows that, at a lymphatic wall filtration coefficient of 0.46 ml h⁻¹ mmHg⁻¹, the calculated interstitial fluid pressure would be equal to zero even though the true interstitial fluid pressure should be -11.3 mmHg (-1.50 kPa). This filtration coefficient is approximately 20 to 25 times less than that of the pulmonary capillaries.

Another important feature of Fig. 8 is that once the lymphatic filtration coefficient rises above a certain minimal value, a further increase in lymphatic wall filtration coefficient does not cause much additional concentration of the lymph protein. The reason for this is that as the lymph protein concentration rises to a progressively higher value, the high colloid osmotic pressure of the protein itself prevents further filtration of fluid out of the lymphatic and therefore prevents further concentration of the lymph.

A corollary to the above principle is that once the lymphatic wall filtration coefficient has risen above this same minimal level, the calculated interstitial fluid pressure—when the Starling equilibrium equation is used and it is assumed that the lymph protein concentration equals the interstitial protein concentration—will always approach the pressure level in the lymphatic vessel and not the pressure level in the interstitial fluid spaces. This is illustrated by the top curve of Fig. 8 which shows a lymphatic vessel pressure between 3 and 4 mmHg and a calculated interstitial fluid pressure that approaches this value rather than the actual value of the interstitial fluid pressure itself.

Thus, one can see that even with minimal filtration of fluid through the lymphatic walls, the practice of calculating interstitial fluid pressure by assuming that interstitial fluid protein concentration equals lymph flow concentration becomes a fruitless exercise because it gives a value almost equal to the lymphatic pressure level and not to the interstitial fluid pressure level.

A final thought concerning the lymph-concentrating mechanism is the following: on the basis of what we know today about the physical structure and function of lymphatic vessels, there is really no reason to argue whether lymph is concentrated or not, because it is impossible to believe that fluid will not filter out of the very flimsy lymphatic vessels in the face of the well-demonstrated lymphatic pressures that are now known to be reached. Instead, the argument should be about the degree to which lymph is concentrated. We would like to suggest that the degree of concentration might be very significant.

POSSIBILITY OF A VERY LOW 'EFFECTIVE' PULMONARY CAPILLARY FILTRATION COEFFICIENT

Another explanation for the very high concentrations of protein in lymph and yet the likelihood of a very negative interstitial fluid pressure would be the following combination of conditions:

(1) A very low pulmonary capillary filtration coefficient for water.
(2) A very high pulmonary capillary leakage coefficient for protein.
(3) A very strong lymphatic pump.

Unfortunately, the filtration coefficients measured for water have been much too high to support such a simple explanation. However, there is an alternative explanation by which the filtration coefficient for water could 'effectively' be very low and could have the same effects on interstitial fluid pressure as a truly low coefficient. This explanation is the following:

Much of the filtration in the lungs probably goes from the capillaries into the alveolar septal wall. Then the fluid must flow through the narrow interstitial spaces of these walls before finally reaching the interstices at the angles

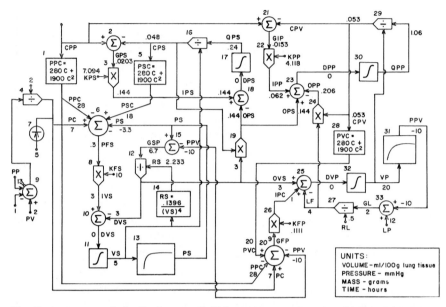

Fig. 9. A systems analysis of pulmonary fluid dynamics, assuming a very high septal resistance for flow of fluid into the perivascular spaces. CPP – concentration of plasma protein; CPS – concentration of protein in the septum; CPV – concentration of protein in the perivascular spaces; DPP – rate of change of protein quantity in the perivascular spaces; DPS – rate of change of quantity of protein in septal fluid; DVP – rate of change of the volume in the perivascular spaces; DVS – rate of change of the volume of the septal interstitial fluid; GFP – pressure differences across the capillary membranes of the perivascular spaces; GL – difference between pumping pressure of the lymphatic pump and pressure in the perivascular spaces; GPP – difference between concentrations of protein in plasma and in perivascular spaces; GPS – difference between concentrations of the protein in the plasma and in the septal fluid; GSP – pressure difference between the septal fluid and the perivascular fluid; IPC – rate of filtration of fluid through the capillaries of the perivascular spaces; IPP – rate of leakage of protein from the capillaries into the perivascular spaces; IPS – rate of leak of protein through the pulmonary capillaries into the septal fluid; IVS – rate of fluid filtration from the pulmonary capillaries into the interstitial fluid of the septum; KFP – filtration coefficient for fluid through the capillaries of the perivascular spaces; KFS – filtration coefficient for the septal capillaries; KPP – coefficient for leakage of protein from the capillaries into the perivascular spaces; KPS – coefficient for leakage of protein through the pulmonary capillaries into the septal fluid; LF – lymph flow; LP – pumping pressure caused by lymphatic pump; OPP – rate of flow of protein in the lymph from the perivascular spaces; OPS – rate of flow of protein from septal fluid into the perivascular spaces; OVS – rate of flow of fluid from the interstitial fluid of the septa into the interstitial fluid of the perivascular spaces; PA – arterial pressure; PC – pulmonary capillary pressure; PFS – pressure across the capillaries in the septum; PPC – colloid osmotic pressure of the plasma; PPV – pressure of fluid in the perivascular spaces; PS – pressure of the interstitial fluid in the septum; PSC – colloid osmotic pressure in the interstitial fluid of the septum; PV – venous pressure; PVC – colloid osmotic pressure of the fluid in the perivascular spaces; QPP – quantity of protein in the perivascular spaces; QPS – quantity of protein in septal fluid; RL – resistance to lymph flow; RS – resistance to flow of fluid from the septal spaces to the perivascular spaces; VP – volume of fluid in perivascular spaces; VS – volume of septal interstitial fluid. (Values on lines = steady-state values/100 g lung. Italicized numbers = block numbers.)

of the alveoli, and thence the perivascular spaces. If there is great resistance to this flow, the following effects would be expected:

(1) A prolonged transit time for fluid flow through the alveolar septal wall so that the protein concentration in this fluid would rise very high.

(2) A very low pressure in the perivascular spaces of the lungs because of the lymphatic pump.

(3) A high pressure gradient between the interstitial spaces of the alveolar septal wall and the perivascular space.

(4) A progressive increase in the thickness of the septal wall as the interstitial fluid pressure rises towards zero; this would automatically decrease the septal wall resistance, thus preventing the pressure in the septal space from rising far above zero and therefore also preventing rupture of the alveolar septal epithelium.

Systems analysis of a septal flow resistance mechanism

Fig. 9 provides a self-explanatory systems analysis involving the above principles. From this analysis one can predict for different physiological conditions the values of many different variables, among which are the following: interstitial fluid pressure of the alveolar septum, interstitial fluid pressure in the perivascular spaces, colloid osmotic pressure in the alveolar septum, colloid osmotic pressure in the perivascular spaces, lymph flow, lymph protein concentration, and so forth.

Predicted effects of increases in pulmonary capillary pressure

Fig. 10 gives computer predictions of the effects of increases in pulmonary capillary pressure. Note especially that the perivascular pressure rises rapidly in comparison with the rise in alveolar septal interstitial fluid pressure. This is because, as the septal interstitial fluid pressure rises towards zero, the septal volume increases. And this decreases resistance to flow from the septum to the perivascular space, therefore also decreasing the pressure gradient between these two areas.

Because of high flow resistance in the septal wall of the simulated lung, fluid is predicted to flow slowly to the perivascular spaces. Therefore, from the point of view of fluid movement from the septal capillaries all the way to the perivascular spaces, the overall effect can be expressed as a very low 'effective' pulmonary capillary filtration coefficient, though this low value is caused mostly by septal resistance rather than capillary pore resistance. This concept could explain the low filtration coefficient that Staub (1974) has measured in non-

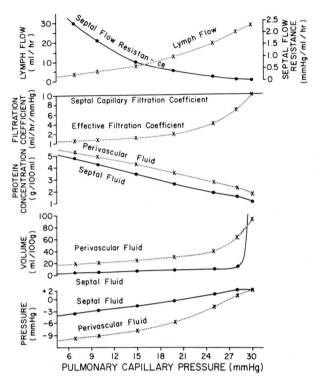

FIG. 10. Computer readout of steady-state values for different pulmonary fluid variables at progressively raised pulmonary capillary pressures. Note the flooding of the alveoli at a pulmonary capillary pressure greater than 28 mmHg. Note also that at normal pulmonary capillary pressures the 'effective' filtration coefficient is very low, but as the oedematous state of the lung is approached at high pulmonary capillary pressures, the 'effective' filtration coefficient becomes very high and approaches the true capillary filtration coefficient.

oedematous lungs even though we (Guyton & Lindsey 1959), Mellins *et al.* (1969) and Taylor & Gaar (1969) have measured much higher filtration coefficients during the development of oedema. Note also in Fig. 10 that the true filtration coefficient remains constant in both the normal lung and the oedematous lung. This is in contrast to the 'effective' filtration coefficient which is very low in the normal lung and yet very high in the oedematous lung.

SUMMARY AND CONCLUSIONS

Our previous studies, and those of others, have produced many reasons for believing that the pulmonary interstitial fluid pressure is normally sub-atmospheric and that this pressure is supra-atmospheric only in the state of pulmonary oedema. Indeed, the analysis of alveolar fluid dynamics presented here shows that the surface tension of the fluid in the alveolus produces a persistent subatmospheric pressure in this alveolar fluid. Furthermore, if we assume that there is no active transport of substances from the alveoli into the interstitial spaces, the maximum pulmonary interstitial fluid pressure that is compatible with non-flooded alveoli is a pressure no more positive than the pressure of the fluid in the alveoli. For a normal-sized alveolus of 75 μm radius, this means an interstitial fluid pressure at least as negative as −2 mmHg. For an alveolus with a radius of 21 μm, the pressure must be at least as negative as −10 mmHg.

Yet the interstitial fluid pressure as calculated from Starling's equation for equilibrium at the pulmonary capillary membrane, in the hands of some investigators, has not been consistently subatmospheric even for the normal lung. However, these investigators have assumed that the protein concentration in interstitial fluid is equal to the protein concentration in pulmonary lymph. The likelihood that this assumption is in error has been explored in this paper by a systems analysis of a possible lymph-concentrating mechanism. This analysis shows that even the smallest amount of pulmonary lymphatic filtration would play havoc with any calculation of pulmonary interstitial fluid pressure in which the protein concentration in pulmonary interstitial fluid was assumed to equal the concentration of protein in lymph. The analysis shows that with even minimal pulmonary lymphatic filtration, the calculated interstitial fluid pressure would be nearly equal to the intralymph vessel pressure and not equal to the true interstitial fluid pressure.

Another analysis demonstrated that high resistance to fluid flow in the alveolar septal walls could cause an extremely low 'effective' filtration coefficient for transfer of fluid from the pulmonary capillaries to the perivascular spaces. A mechanism of this type, coupled with a strong lymphatic pump, could also give very negative pulmonary interstitial fluid pressures while at the same time giving a high lymph protein concentration.

It is possible—indeed likely—that all of these mechanisms are normally functioning in the lungs.

ACKNOWLEDGEMENT

This work was supported by US Public Health Service Grants-in-Aid HL 11678 and HL 11477.

References

CLEMENTS, J. A. & GIERNEY, D. F. (1965) Alveolar instability associated with altered surface tension, in *Handb. Physiol.* Section 3: *Respiration*, vol. 2 (Fenn, W. O. & Rahn, H., eds.), pp. 1565-1584, American Physiological Society, Washington, D.C.

DRAKE, R. E. & TAYLOR, A. E. (1975) Calculation of the edema safety factor in isolated dog lung. *Fed. Proc. 34*, 400

GRANGER, H. J. (1975) Transcapillary exchanges and their regulation, in *Systems Analysis of Biomedical Transport* (Reneau, D. D., ed.), Dekker, New York

GUYTON, A. C. & LINDSEY, A. W. (1959) Effect of elevated left atrial pressure and decreased plasma protein concentration on the development of pulmonary edema. *Circ. Res. 7*, 649-657

GUYTON, A. C., TAYLOR, A. E. & GRANGER, H. J. (1975) *Circulatory Physiology, II; Dynamics of the Body Fluids*, Saunders, Philadelphia

HARGENS, A. R. & ZWEIFACH, B. W. (1975) Exchange between blood, tissue and peripheral lymph in mesentery. *Fed. Proc. 34*, 400 (abstr. 1024)

McDONALD, D. A. (1968) Hemodynamics. *Annu. Rev. Physiol. 30*, 525-556

MELLINS, R. B., LEVINE, O. R., SKALAK, R. & FISHMAN, A. P. (1969) Interstitial pressure in the lungs. *Circ. Res. 24*, 197-212

MEYER, B. J., MEYER, A. & GUYTON, A. C. (1968) Interstitial fluid pressure. V. Negative pressure in the lung. *Circ. Res. 22*, 263-271

OLVER, R. E., REYNOLDS, E. O. R. & STRANG, L. B. (1972) Foetal lung liquid, in *Foetal and Neonatal Physiology* (Cross, K. W., ed.), pp. 186-207, Cambridge University Press, London

STAUB, N. C. (1974) Pulmonary edema. *Physiol. Rev. 54*, 678-811

TAYLOR, A. E. & GAAR, K. A. (1969) Calculation of equivalent pore radii of the pulmonary capillary and alveolar membranes. *Rev. Argent. Angiol. 111*, 25-40

TAYLOR, A. E. & GIBSON, W. H. (1975) Concentrating ability of the lymphatic vessels. *Lymphology*, in press

TAYLOR, A. E., GUYTON, A. C. & BISHOP, V. S. (1965) Permeability of the alveolar membranes to solutes. *Circ. Res. 16*, 353-362

ZWEIFACH, B. W. & PRATHER, J. (1975) Micromanipulation of pressure in terminal lymphatics in the mesentery. *Am. J. Physiol. 228*, 1326-1335

Discussion

Dickinson: I take it that with these calculations you get substantially the same order of figures for interstitial pressure negativity as you got in capsule experiments?

Guyton: If one assumes the protein concentration in interstitial fluid to be the same as the protein concentration in pulmonary lymph, and if reasonable values for plasma colloid osmotic pressure and pulmonary capillary pressure are assumed, one can use the Starling equation for capillary equilibrium to calculate the interstitial pressure. Such data gathered from different laboratories give a calculation for interstitial fluid pressure of somewhere between −6 mmHg (−0.8 kPa) and +1 mmHg (+0.133 kPa). In our paper, we have described some of the ways in which these calculations and the concept of a considerably negative interstitial fluid pressure can be reconciled. The first analysis that we presented relating alveolar fluid to interstitial fluid pressure simply calculates the maximum interstitial fluid pressure that one could predict if there is no active mechanism for transporting fluid out of the alveolus and back into the septal space.

Olver: What is known about the permeability of lymphatic walls to small solutes? If we accept that interstitial fluid has the same electrolyte composition as plasma, and since we know that the ionic composition of the collected lymph is the same as that of the plasma, presumably ions must be leaving the lymphatics along with water?

Guyton: I would postulate that the lymphatic wall is at least as leaky as the blood capillary membrane. Its structure is even more flimsy than that of the blood capillary, and it does not have much basement membrane. It looks as if it is more permeable than the blood capillary, which should give full equilibrium of ions.

Adamson: Did you include the effect of pulmonary surfactant in your first model? In other words, would a change in radius be associated with a constant surface tension or not?

Guyton: We used integrated curves during the respiratory cycle, as published by Clements & Gierney (1965). From these, 15 mmHg (2 kPa) would be about the average for the surface tension. At maximum alveolar size this rises to about 30 mmHg (4 kPa), while at minimum alveolar size it falls near to zero. After determining the average value of 15 mmHg we reduced this to 10 mmHg (1.33 kPa) to be on the safe side and used the value of 10 mmHg in the model. This gave less negative interstitial fluid pressures than we would have calculated if we had used the actual average value.

Staub: Since a hydrostatic pressure of 19 mmHg (2.53 kPa) is equivalent to 1 mosmol, if the alveolar epithelial cells were able to increase their electrolyte composition by 1 mosmol, it would account for the interstitial pressure difference being negative.

Guyton: This is true, but the known active epithelial transport is backwards to the mechanism that you postulate—that is, transport is towards the alveolus rather than out of it.

Staub: We have recently completed a study by quantitative autoradiography of radioactively labelled serum albumin in the lung lymphatics of normal mice. From the very smallest lymphatics (less than 10 μm diameter) to the largest at the lung hilum (about 40 μm diameter) we found no evidence for a change in concentration of the tracer proteins (Nicolaysen *et al.* 1975).

Of course, there is no way of knowing what happens in the interstitial tissue of the lung. We are talking only about your model that includes concentration of protein within the lymphatics, Dr Guyton. Inside the lymphatics there is no evidence of protein concentration in the normal animal.

Guyton: Are you sure that you are not beyond the first few lymphatic valves?

Staub: The smallest lymph vessels we measured were of the size expected for lymph capillaries.

Guyton: I agree that that is a small lymphatic, but you cannot be sure that you are not beyond the first few valves.

Staub: If you mean is there a smaller lymphatic that we could not see, I know of no way to answer that question. We measured every lymph vessel that we could detect.

Guyton: Let's go back to the concept that concentration of protein could occur within the first few segments of the lymphatics. Zweifach (1972) in studies in the mesentery found that the lymphatic pressure had already risen by about 3 mmHg (0.4 kPa) by the time the lymph had flowed past the first two valves. After it had flowed beyond the first six or seven valves, which is not a long distance, the pressure had risen to 6 or 7 mmHg (0.8–0.93 kPa). If the lymphatic membrane is extremely permeable, one would expect fluid to filter out of the lymphatics from the very beginning. I am only proposing this as one possible version of what could happen, not as a law. Hargens & Zweifach (1975) have indeed demonstrated marked concentration of protein in the lymphatics. Therefore, I would be very suspicious of assuming that the interstitial fluid protein concentration in the lungs is equal to the pulmonary lymph protein concentration.

Fishman: As vessels coalesce they increase in calibre. In determining the concentration of radioactive tracers in these three-dimensional structures from counts made in a single plane, how is the thickness of the vessel taken into account? How accurate are estimates of concentration or dilution of a tracer in a vessel that is changing calibre along its course?

Staub: You are talking now about whether the diameter can be measured accurately. In a cylinder the smallest diameter is always the true one.

Robin: Evans' blue dye instilled into the water-filled lung becomes enormously concentrated in pulmonary lymph, with lymph: plasma ratios of about 15:1, so clearly a large molecule can somehow become concentrated in the lymph. The other fact is that in the water-filled lung, concentrations of lymphatic sodium decrease by about 30%, while protein concentrations remain unchanged (Acevedo & Robin 1972). One interpetation, of course, is that protein is concentrated in the lymphatic fluid even though water is being absorbed into the lymphatics,

Hughes: Gil & Weibel (1969) showed that the surfactant layer was thicker in the corners of alveoli and also in crypts and crevices.

Guyton: That is the way it should be. The question is, what is the radius of curvature of the surfactant layer in the crypts? If it is very small, the pressure of the fluid underneath that surfactant layer, the fluid between the fluid surface and the epithelial wall, should be quite negative.

Dejours: What kind of surface tension coefficient did you use, Dr Guyton?

Guyton: We used the surface tension between the fluid and the air in the alveolus.

Strang: The most uncertain part of the argument is the value of surface tension you use at the interface. It could be very much lower than 15 or even 10 dynes/cm (15 or 10 $\times$ 10^{-5}N/cm), even down to 1 or 2 dynes/cm (10^{-5}N/cm or 2 $\times$ 10^{-5}N/cm).

Guyton: Even at 1 or 2 dynes/cm the calculated fluid pressure would still be a negative value. This would make a quantitative difference but not a conceptual difference.

Staub: That value of 10 dynes/cm is reasonable for the average surface tension during the respiratory cycle.

Strang: Yes, but now we are referring to a situation in which one part of the air–liquid interface is contracting. If the usually accepted theory relating to surfactant films is correct, the surface tension value should fall rapidly. Hence the relationships become complicated, because the pressure is not determined by a constant coefficient.

Dickinson: Are you seriously challenging the inescapable theoretical analysis that surface tension must create a negative pressure, even if it is only minutely negative?

Strang: No.

Guyton: You are talking about dynamic coefficients, Dr Strang. Our analysis is for the steady-state condition, not for the dynamic state. Once the alveolus is in the steady-state condition, presumably the surface tension also returns to its steady-state value.

Strang: I don't understand the analysis well enough to know exactly. Nevertheless, your curves reach an end-point when the air space would fill up with liquid. At that point, when the equilibrium for that air space is breaking down as the space begins to fill up, the value of surface tension will tend to change in a direction which will upset the equilibrium in favour of stabilization of the air space.

Guyton: In the steady-state analysis there is infinite time for equilibrium to occur, and at infinite time the rate of change is infinitesimal. Consequently the average surface tension, and not the dynamic surface tension, is the one that would apply in our analysis.

Waaler: You envisage concentration building up along the lymphatic vessels over very short distances on both sides of the valves, and you also think that this has consequences for fluid movements across the lymphatic walls. But what about the valves? Would you not have filtration and diffusion across the valves as well?

Guyton: Yes.

Waaler: Is that included in the analysis?

Guyton: I don't think it has to be included. We simply calculated what happens once a certain pressure is reached. We don't know how many valves the lymph must pass to get up to that pressure. But let's get this clear: we are not saying that concentration of protein in the lymphatics is a proved mechanism. We are simply saying that we have to be very suspicious of using protein values from lymph as the values for protein in the interstitial space.

Farhi: If the liquid tends to accumulate initially in the crypts, wouldn't that reduce the tension where it has the highest value?

Guyton: It is not the surface tension in the crypts that determines the critical point for alveolar collapse. Instead, it is the average surface tension that is important. If we define 'surface tension pressure' as the average pressure underneath the surface of the alveolar fluid, then when the surface tension pressure in the alveolus is less than the interstitial fluid pressure there will be flow of fluid from the interstitial space outwards into the alveolus, assuming that there is no active transport mechanism to make it do otherwise.

Olver: There is evidence that some parts of the respiratory epithelium can actively transport ions.

Guyton: But even your own evidence shows that that transport is in the wrong direction (Olver *et al.* 1972).

References

Acevedo, J. C. & Robin, E. D. (1972) Effect of intrapulmonary water instillation on pulmonary lymph flow and composition. *Am. J. Physiol. 223*, 1433-1437

Clements, J. A. & Gierney, D. F. (1965) Alveolar instability associated with altered surface tension, in *Handb. Physiol.* Section 3: *Respiration*, vol. 2 (Fenn, W. O. & Rahn, H., eds.), pp. 1565-1584, American Physiological Society, Washington, D.C.

Gil, J. & Weibel, E. R. (1969) Improvements in demonstration of lining layer of lung alveoli by electron microscopy. *Respir. Physiol. 8*, 13-36

Hargens, A. R. & Zweifach, B. W. (1957) Exchange between blood, tissue and peripheral lymph in mesentery. *Fed. Proc. 34*, 400

Nicolaysen, G., Nicolaysen, A. & Staub, N. C. (1975) *Microvasc. Res. 10*, 138-152

Olver, R. E., Reynolds, E. O. R. & Strang, L. B. (1972) Foetal lung liquid, in *Foetal and Neonatal Physiology* (Cross, K. W., ed.), pp. 186-207, Cambridge University Press, London

Zweifach, B. W. (1972) Physiology of terminal lymphatics in the mesentery. *Pflügers Archiv. Gesamte Physiol. Menschen Tiere 336*, 565-569

Effect of lung inflation on alveolar permeability to solutes

EDMUND A. EGAN, II

Department of Pediatrics, University of Florida College of Medicine, Gainesville, Florida

Abstract   The alveolar epithelium separates gas and liquid phases in the lung. Osmotic forces available for separating these phases will be determined by the solute permeability of the epithelium. The relative rates of diffusion of several simultaneously studied solutes of known molecular size have been used for measuring the equivalent pore radius across the alveolar epithelium *in vivo* in the perinatal period and in adult animals. In perinatal sheep, the equivalent pore radius increases from 0.5 nm in the fetal state to 1.5–4.5 nm during the first minutes of spontaneous ventilation. Postnatal animals, 12–60 hours of age, have pore radii of 0.7–1.4 nm. Static inflation of the lungs, in fetal lambs, produced pressure-dependent increases in pore radii. In adult sheep and rabbits the measured radius of equivalent pores across the epithelium *in vivo* was positively correlated with the degree of inflation of the lungs ($P < 0.005$). Measurements varied from 0.5 nm at low levels of inflation to large leaks at high levels. These experiments indicate that solute permeability across the alveolar epithelium is a dynamic function of the inflation of the lung, rather than a static feature.

The alveolar epithelium is a barrier which allows diffusion of respiratory gases while it separates the gas in the alveoli and the liquid in the vascular and interstitial spaces of the lung. This barrier function between the two phases in the lung is maintained despite the high permeability of the alveolar epithelium to water. Indeed, large volumes of water rapidly cross the alveolar epithelium in either direction in fresh water and salt water drowning experiments (Swann & Spafford 1951). Two forces are potentially available which can act across this epithelial barrier to sustain the phase separation: a hydrostatic pressure gradient, and an osmotic pressure gradient due to the ability of the epithelium to restrict solute diffusion. Several measurements of lung epithelial permeability to solutes have been reported. In fetal sheep, Normand *et al.* (1971) document an alveolar epithelium only slightly permeable to solutes, equivalent to a barrier in which water and solutes can diffuse only through cylindrical pores 0.5 nm in radius. However, similar studies in postnatal animals report measurements varying from an equivalent pore radius of 0.6–1.0 nm (Taylor & Gaar 1970) to transfer by 'leaks' (Wangensteen *et al.* 1969). The studies reported here were initiated because of the variability, in postnatal experiments, of alveolar epithelial permeability to solutes, and because it was calculated that fetal alveolar permeability to solutes was not consistent with the observed time for absorption of fetal lung liquid at the onset of ventilation. If the fetal permeability persisted, many hours would be needed for the Na^+ and Cl^- ions to diffuse into the interstitium; and absorption of fetal lung liquid would take much longer than the four hours observed (Humphreys *et al.* 1967).

METHODS

The relative rates of diffusion of water-soluble, lipid-insoluble, non-electrolyte solutes of different molecular sizes can define the passive permeability across the alveolar epithelium. The details of the methods have been published previously (Normand *et al.* 1971; Egan *et al.* 1975), and are briefly reviewed here. Trace amounts of radioactively labelled non-electrolyte solutes of known molecular size were mixed with naturally occurring fetal lung liquid or with a normal saline solution. Among these solutes was at least one large molecule, the size of albumin or larger, which we presumed would not cross the alveolar epithelium and whose change in concentration would reflect only the change in volume of the liquid in the air spaces. After this liquid was infused into the atelectatic air spaces, the area to be studied was inflated with an absorbable gas, oxygen or nitrous oxide, and held inflated by application of positive pressure. In fetal animals, the placental circulation remained intact and the entire lung could be studied. In postnatal experiments, only part of the lung was isolated for study and the remainder was ventilated to sustain the animal. After a period of inflation lasting about 15 min the lung was deflated, enabling the alveolar liquid to be sampled. Several inflation periods were used in each animal.

The samples of alveolar liquid were passed through appropriate Sephadex gel filtration columns to separate solutes of different sizes but with similar or interfering radioactive labels. The concentration of each solute in each sample was determined by appropriate beta scintillation or gamma counting.

The findings were analysed using a two-compartment model for diffusion, because solute diffusion through the capillary endothelium is not much restricted compared to that through the alveolar epithelium. Since diffusion follows first-order kinetics, the log concentration for each solute was plotted versus time. The calculated slope for each test molecule was corrected for changes in concentration produced by changes in volume of the alveolar liquid by sub-tracting the slope of the impermeant test molecule. The adjusted slope is the rate constant for diffusion for each solute. The rate constant of a solute for diffusion out of the alveolar space, K_o, is related to the equivalent pore size by Equation 4 of Normand $et\ al.$ (1971)

$$K_o = \frac{A/dx}{V} \times D_T \times F\ (a/r) \tag{1}$$

where $\dfrac{A/dx}{V}$ is total pore area per unit pore length divided by alveolar liquid

volume, D_T is the free diffusion coefficient for the particular solute at the experimental temperature, and $F(a/r)$ is the function relating restriction to diffusion of a molecule of radius a by a cylindrical pore of radius r, as given in Equation 8 of Solomon (1968).

Since in each experiment the term $\dfrac{A/dx}{V}$ is common for each solute, the best

r value was found by trial and error which fits all the experimental K_o values in the relationship:

$$K_o/D_T = F\ (a/r)$$

RESULTS

Dr Richard Olver and I collaborated on the first set of experiments on adult rabbits. The right lung was isolated surgically and ventilated; the left lung remained available for study. Fig. 1 presents the experimental results from one of these animals. In the left-hand panel, the log concentration for five solutes is plotted against time. The concentration of the albumin increases, indicating that alveolar liquid is absorbed, and the rate of change of the con-centration of the other solutes differs from the slope of albumin in inverse relationship to their molecular size. On the right-hand panel, the solid line is the theoretical relationship between K_o and molecular size for a 4 nm pore. The line is constructed to pass through the experimental urea point as a way of arbitrarily defining the unmeasured area term in Equation 1. The points are the experimental K_o values obtained from the left-hand panel. The broken line is the theoretical relationship expected between K_o and molecular size if diffusion occurred through sites of no limiting pore radius, and this line is again constructed to pass through the experimental urea K_o. As can be seen, in this animal the diffusion rates of solute molecules of different sizes approximate the theoretical relationship expected for diffusion limited to definite water-filled

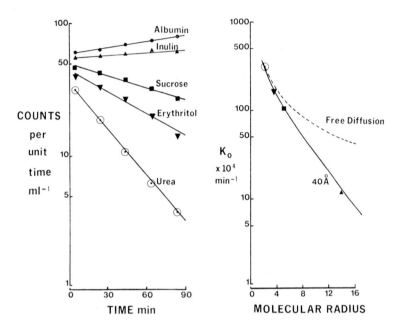

FIG. 1. Adult rabbit. Tracers are ^{131}I-labelled albumin, [14C]inulin, [3H]sucrose, [14C]-erythritol and [14C]urea, infused into the left lung of the animal, which was then inflated with oxygen for 20-minute periods.

Left panel. Ordinate: count rates per unit volume of the labelled markers. Abscissa: experimental time. The slope is calculated by least squares method.

Right panel. Ordinate: values of K_o (rate constant) calculated from the slopes in the left-hand panel. Abscissa: molecular radius. The solid line is the theoretical relationship expected between K_o and molecular radius for a 4.0 nm pore radius; the broken line is the expected relationship for diffusion unrestricted to pores. Points are the experimental K_o values from the left-hand panel. Both lines constructed to pass through the urea point.

channels 4 nm in radius much more accurately than the relationship predicted by free diffusion through large 'leaks'.

Although albumin was never detected in the arterial blood when injected into the alveolar space, the large volume of distribution of the vascular system makes such a technique relatively insensitive. To test the assumption that albumin was an accurate volume marker, large amounts of ^{131}I-labelled albumin were injected intravenously into two animals several hours before saline was infused into the alveoli. Permeability to albumin was measured by the rate of appearance of albumin in the alveolar liquid, as seen in Fig. 2. The alveolar epithelium is not completely impermeable to albumin but the rate of appearance is slow, the half-time for equilibration in this animal being several days. Two conclusions were drawn from this information. First, as our

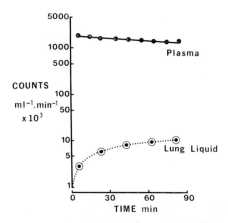

FIG. 2. Adult rabbit in which ^{131}I-labelled albumin was injected intravenously before time 0. The isolated left lung was infused with a normal saline solution and inflated. The counts per unit volume of ^{131}I-labelled albumin in blood and its appearance in lung liquid are plotted against time. Half-time (T $^1/_2$) for equilibration is 70 hours.

experiments lasted less than two hours more than 99 % of the albumin remained in the alveoli, so albumin was a satisfactory volume marker for our purpose. Second, a calculated equivalent pore size is a convention for quantifying permeability, but here some larger sites of transfer constituted a small fraction of the total.

The experiments on adult rabbits produced an average equivalent pore radius across the alveolar epithelium of 2.6 nm, with a range of between 2.0 and 4.0 nm. These results showed a much greater variability than did the determinations of Normand et al. (1971) in fetal sheep. Further, the radii were much larger than the pore radii determined by Taylor & Gaar (1970) but were still too small to account for significant diffusion of macromolecules.

The next set of experiments (done with Drs Strang and Olver) was generated by the fact that each mammal at birth must absorb a significant amount of fetal alveolar liquid, which is close to normal saline in composition. Calculations of the restriction to Na^+ and Cl^- diffusion that is imposed by the equivalent pore radii of 0.5 nm observed in fetal sheep showed that this absorption could not take place in the time observed unless either the pore radii or the total pore area increased greatly. In confirmation of this hypothesis, a very slow rate of lung liquid absorption was reported by Olver & Strang (1974) after secretion of fetal lung liquid had been inhibited with cyanide.

In mature fetal lambs exteriorized at Caesarean section equivalent pore radii across the alveolar epithelium were determined in the fetal state and during the first minutes of spontaneous ventilation; the radii were also determined in

TABLE 1

Calculated radii of equivalent pores across the alveolar epithelium of fetal, natal and post-natal lambs

| Status | N | Pore radius (nm) | |
		Average	Range
Fetal	14	0.55	0.5-0.6
At birth	7	4.00	1.5-5.6
12–60 hours of age	4	1.1	0.7-1.4

N: no. of animals

newborn lambs 12–60 hours after spontaneous vaginal delivery. In the fetal animals, the natural lung liquid was used and the molecular probes were mixed with it. The animals studied in the fetal state were then induced to breathe by application of cold water to the snout. Placental circulation was left intact during the entire time so that we could deflate the lungs of the ventilating fetus merely by closing the tracheal cannula and still sustain the animal from the placenta while we took samples. The newborn lambs were studied in the same manner as the adult rabbits, except that previously collected fetal lung liquid was used as the liquid vehicle for the radioactive tracers infused into the alveoli.

Table 1 summarizes the results of these experiments. The fetal equivalent pore radius was confirmed as 0.5 nm, but at the onset of ventilation the equivalent pore size increased markedly, to between 1.5 and 5.6 nm. However, by 12 hours after birth the equivalent pore size was much closer to the fetal values than those seen during the liquid absorption phase, although in every case pore radius remained larger than fetal values. The equivalent pore radii measured during the phase of absorption of lung liquid are in the range which minimally restricts the diffusion of small solutes, such as Na^+ and Cl^-, yet almost totally restricts the diffusion of large solutes, such as proteins. This will aid absorption of lung liquid by allowing rapid diffusion of Na^+ and Cl^- out of the alveoli while the oncotic pressure difference between the lung liquid and the interstitial fluid that is produced by the low protein content of fetal lung liquid is maintained.

In another group of fetal experiments, an attempt was made to define factors which might be important in producing the changes in alveolar epithelial permeability that we had observed during the change from fetal to postnatal life. Exteriorized mature fetal lambs, with intact placental circulation, were inflated statically with nitrous oxide, oxygen or normal saline after our trace molecules had been mixed into the fetal lung liquid. The results were independent of the gas used, so the results are grouped.

TABLE 2

Calculated radii of equivalent pores across the alveolar epithelium of statically inflated lungs of fetal sheep

Experiment	N	Pore radius (nm)	
		Average	Range
Low pressure gas (25–35 cmH$_2$O [2.45–3.43 kPa])	6	0.8	0.6-1.2
High pressure gas (41–45 cmH$_2$O [4.02–4.41 kPa])	8	–	>7.5
Liquid saline	5	0.9*	0.6-1.1

*Excludes one animal with large pores after two infusions of saline.
N: no. of animals

Table 2 details the results of these static inflation experiments. Low pressure inflation (that pressure necessary to initiate inflation of fetal lungs) produced a small increase in pore radius across the alveolar epithelium, but only to the size range seen in the postnatal lambs, not to values observed in the perinatal, spontaneously ventilating animals. High pressure inflation, a pressure fully expanding the lungs, produced large pores or leaks across the alveolar epithelium. We were unable to duplicate the range of pore radii which we had observed in the spontaneously ventilating fetal lambs and which markedly increased permeability to small solutes yet restricted protein diffusion. In the saline-inflated animals pore radius increased slightly—the same pattern as seen with low pressure gas inflation. However, in one animal, massive infusion of saline produced leaks, as seen in the high pressure gas inflation.

At this point we had two different results in postnatal experiments: newborn lambs with pores of 0.6–1.2 nm, and adult rabbits with pores of 2.0–4.0 nm. In retrospect, it appeared that the rabbits had been studied at high lung volumes, and the newborn lambs at much less than total lung volume. Thus, another set of experiments was conducted in adult sheep to determine whether the size of the equivalent pore radii across the alveolar epithelium was related to the inflation of the lung. From our perinatal static inflation experiments, it seemed certain that expansion could induce a change from a small equivalent pore size to a leak. We felt it was logical to assume that control of this variable was what had produced the intermediate pore sizes in the adult rabbits and in the fetal lambs we studied at the onset of breathing.

In adult sheep, a catheter with a circumferential balloon was passed through the tracheal cannula and fixed into a bronchus by inflation of the balloon; this

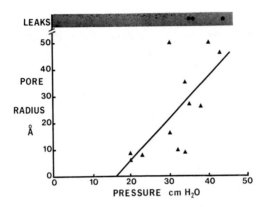

FIG. 3. Experiments on adult sheep. Ordinate: calculated radius of equivalent pores across the alveolar epithelium. Abscissa: the static inflation pressure used to inflate isolated lung segments. Regression line was calculated excluding the three experiments with leaks ($r = 0.685$ [$P < 0.005$]).

isolated one part of a lung. The remainder of the lungs sustained the animal. A normal saline solution with the trace molecules was infused into the atelectatic isolated area, followed by inflation with oxygen to a specific pressure and held inflated by a continuous positive pressure of 18 cmH$_2$O (1.77 kPa). Transpulmonary pressure varied with respiration in this preparation as the thorax had not been open and the animals were breathing spontaneously.

In Fig. 3, the equivalent pore radius is plotted against the inflating pressure. There is a significant correlation between inflation pressure and equivalent pore radius across the alveolar epithelium. Values of less than 1.5 nm, comparable to those seen in the newborn lambs, are seen at the lower inflation pressures, while values between 1.5 and 5.0 nm and leaks are seen at higher inflation pressures.

The variability of the pore size at similar inflation pressures is still significant in these experiments on adult animals. Therefore, a second group of adult sheep were studied in which the residual volume and total capacity of the isolated segment were measured before the experiment, and the total volume in the air space of the segment, liquid and gas, was used as the independent variable. Fig. 4 shows the plot of the 14 experiments studied. The relationship between the volume of gas and liquid in the lung and the equivalent pore size across the alveolar epithelium is similar to that in the pressure-defined experiments ($r = 0.796$ [$P < 0.005$]). At alveolar volumes of less than 50% of total lung capacity the alveolar epithelium has equivalent pore radii of less than 1.5 nm. As total lung capacity is approached, large pores or leaks occur.

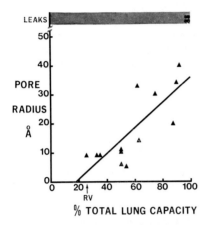

Fig. 4. Experiments on adult sheep. Ordinate: calculated equivalent pore radius across the alveolar epithelium. Abscissa: the total volume of liquid and gas expressed as a percentage of total capacity of the isolated segment. Regression line was calculated excluding animals with 'leaks' ($r = 0.795$ [$P < 0.005$]).

DISCUSSION

This phenomenon of differing pore radii across alveolar epithelium has been described in response to physical stimuli in the renal tubule (Boulpaep 1972) and the frog cornea (Zadunaisky 1971). The dependence of alveolar epithelial permeability on lung inflation helps to explain the variability in previous measurements of permeability to non-electrolyte solutes. The ability of the alveolar epithelium to increase the size of paracellular pathways for solute transport is important in the adaptation to ventilation and the absorption of fetal lung liquid at birth, and may be of importance in other situations in postnatal life.

The leaks produced at high pressures and high inflations in both the fetal and adult investigations are of further interest. If size no longer restricts solute diffusion, then only hydrostatic forces are available to act across the alveolar epithelium to maintain the separation of gas and liquid. It is not yet known whether such leaks are reversible in a short period of time or whether longer-term healing must occur before a less permeable alveolar epithelium is re-established. Therapeutic techniques involving hyperinflation of the lungs for respiratory failure would seem to influence the permeability of the alveolar epithelium, and changes in its permeability might be important in some pulmonary pathological processes.

ACKNOWLEDGEMENTS

Components of these studies were supported by the Medical Research Council, NIH Grant HL 16864-01, and cooperative funds from the Florida Heart Association and its chapters. I wish to acknowledge the scientific assistance of Mr C. M. J. Bright, Miss Valerie Cole and Mr Bruce McIntyre.

References

BOULPAEP, E. L. (1972) Permeability changes of the proximal tubule of Necturus during saline loading. *Am. J. Physiol.* 222, 517-531

EGAN, E. A., OLVER, R. E. & STRANG, L. B. (1975) Changes in the non-electrolyte permeability of alveoli and the absorption of lung liquid at the start of breathing in the lamb. *J. Physiol. (Lond.)* 244, 161-179

HUMPHREYS, P. W., NORMAND, I. C. S., REYNOLDS, E. O. R. & STRANG, L. B. (1967) Pulmonary lymph flow and the uptake of liquid from the lungs of the lamb at the start of breathing. *J. Physiol. (Lond.)* 193, 1-29

NORMAND, I. C. S., OLVER, R. E., REYNOLDS, E. O. R. & STRANG, L. B. (1972) Permeability of lung capillaries and alveoli to non-electrolytes in the foetal lamb. *J. Physiol. (Lond.)* 219, 303-330

OLVER, R. E. & STRANG, L. B. (1974) Ion fluxes across the pulmonary epithelium and the secretion of lung liquid in the foetal lamb. *J. Physiol. (Lond.)* 241, 327-357

SOLOMON, A. K. (1968) Characterization of biological membranes by equivalent pores. *J. Gen. Physiol.* 51, 335-364s

SWANN, H. G. & SPAFFORD, N. R. (1951) Body salt and water changes during fresh and sea water drowning. *Tex. Rep. Biol. Med.* 9, 356-362

TAYLOR, A. E. & GAAR, A. K. (1970) Estimation of equivalent pore radii of pulmonary capillary and alveolar membranes. *Am. J. Physiol.* 218, 1133-1140

WANGENSTEEN, O. D., WITTMERS, L. E. & JOHNSON, J. A. (1969) Permeability of the mammalian blood gas barrier and its components. *Am. J. Physiol.* 216, 719-727

ZADUNAISKY, J. A. (1971) Electrophysiology and transparency of the cornea, in *Electrophysiology of Epithelial Cells* (Giebisch, G., ed.), pp. 225-255, Schattayer, Stuttgart & New York

Discussion

Widdicombe: Was the change in pore radius reversible, and if so, how quickly?

Egan: I can't answer that from a single experiment. Newborn lambs had a pore radius of 1.0 nm by 12 hours of age. It appears that the reversal from the 4.0 nm pore radius to the smaller size occurs within this time span. I have not studied the same lung consecutively at a high inflation and then at a low inflation.

Hughes: When you introduced the substances into the air-filled lung, where were they actually deposited? Could they be deposited at bifurcations of the airway system?

Egan: The liquid and tracers were never introduced into an air-filled lung, but an atelectatic one. Gas was added after the liquid, ensuring that all the liquid was in alveoli.

Gatzy: How do you know that distribution to a different or larger surface area doesn't account for some of these phenomena? When you inflate with gas, for example, do you take redistribution into account in your equations?

Egan: The pore radius is calculated by comparing the relative rates of diffusion of molecules of different sizes. If total pore area alone, and not pore radius varied with inflation, the relative rates of diffusion of the different molecules should remain constant, even if the absolute rates change. The differences in the relative rates of transfer of the experimental tracer molecules with lung inflation meant that pore radius and not just area was variable.

Maetz: If I understand you properly, this is a membrane where hydrostatic pressure can be changed from the inside, the blood side, and produce an increase in pore radius. The hydrostatic pressure can also be changed from the air side with an increase in the pore radius. That is interesting because in experiments on gall bladder or isolated rumen only changes in hydrostatic pressure from the inside actually made the membrane leaky, and not changes from the outside (see discussion of this problem in House 1974).

Dickinson: But are there not two membranes which have been stretched in different directions?

Egan: It may be true that the alveolar epithelial membranes can be stretched from the interstitial fluid side and be disrupted, but I have not seen that documented. We are stretching it only from the air side.

Schneeberger: Did you try to study the distribution of probe molecules in the alveolar space? I know that is difficult with small molecules but you could add, say, Evans' blue dye to the administered material and try to trace its anatomical distribution. How do you know that absorption is actually occurring at the alveolar surface level? Have you any evidence that it might be occurring at the bronchial alveolar junctions, for instance?

Egan: The liquid was infused into the lung, and then the oxygen was added after it. From calculations of the relative volumes of the airway and alveoli all the fluid must be down in the terminal air spaces. The airway contains only gas. All the fluid is in the alveolus and the changes we measure reflect alveolar permeability and not airway permeability. However, this conceivably may not be true in the fetal animal where the fetal fluid is in the airway as well as in the potential air spaces.

Robin: Is the lining epithelium in the fetal lung structurally different from that in the adult lung, and does it become attenuated as the lung becomes more adult?

Egan: Yes, but I think that by the end of gestation, when these animals were studied, there is very little morphological difference between adult and newborn respiratory epithelium. The alveolar lining is so thin that the distance between the air space and the capillary spaces is already down to 0.2 μm in newborn rats (Weibel 1967).

Robin: I wasn't thinking so much of space differences as of differences in the epithelial membrane. Although it is true that the fetal lung is one kind of model for looking at lung transport properties, it doesn't have to be identical in this respect with the adult lung. If the cells acquire new functions, or different functions, they might have different transport properties in addition to diffusion differences or differences in pore size.

Hughes: What is the current theory about this sudden change in pore size at birth?

Egan: In the first phase, when there is still both liquid and gas in the fetal lung, there is probably a high lung volume. Extrapolating from our work on adult lungs I would say that if the alveolus is at a high volume the permeability of the epithelium is markedly increased. As the fluid is absorbed the resting volume of the lung may indeed be less and the alveolar epithelium becomes less permeable to solutes.

Hughes: Is there any evidence that lung volume shrinks in the first few hours after birth?

Egan: Clinically the lung volumes that have been measured have only been gas volumes. Initially both gas and liquid are present and I think that the total volume of the air space is unknown. There is probably between 15 and 30 ml liquid/kg body weight in the air space, at least at the start of breathing.

Normand: There is certainly good evidence that with a mechanically unsound lung, such as an immature lung, the onset of ventilation may disrupt the alveolar wall to a considerable extent. Ordinary light microscopy shows that in the lung of an infant dying of hyaline membrane disease, most of the epithelium has been destroyed (Lauweryns 1965).

When we did some rather crude experiments, ventilating the lungs of immature fetal lambs, we found that macromolecular transfer across the alveolar wall was on the basis of free diffusion and there was no significant barrier, whereas there was evidence of sieving when mature lungs were ventilated (Normand *et al.* 1970).

Adamson: Does pore size alter in fetal lungs that have been distended beyond the functional residual capacity?

Egan: I can't be sure. Our analysis of the fetal data led us on to the adult work and the idea that lung volume is probably the important parameter in determining pore radius. We did not measure the permeability in fetal and perinatal animals as a function of the total volume in the lung.

Olver: Regarding the volume of the lung after birth, the functional residual capacity (FRC) is the same at 10 minutes as it is at two or three days (Klaus *et al.* 1962). One interpretation of this is that the liquid moves out of the potential air spaces of the lung rapidly, say within 10 minutes. Alternatively the FRC could sit on top of the liquid in the alveoli. The lung liquid could then be reabsorbed from that space at a rather slower rate. It takes about six hours for the lungs to reach a steady weight after birth but of course one doesn't know how the liquid is partitioned between the alveoli and the interstitial space in that first six hours.

Hughes: You said that pore size jumped from 0.6 nm in fetal lambs to 4 nm at birth, but when you doubled the volume in the fetal lung with saline the pore size was only 0.9 nm.

Egan: By just adding saline we did not reproduce the large pore radius we observed in the spontaneously ventilating lambs. We have not reproduced the changes at birth by static inflation with gas or saline yet, and we are only speculating that the important factor in changing pore size is the volume.

Strang: Twice the lung volume isn't equal to the air of a full inspiration plus the lung liquid. The amount of lung liquid in the fetus at term is about 30 ml/kg, roughly 1 FRC. When the animal takes its first breath, it probably takes in about 2 FRC of gas, making a peak lung volume of 3 FRC, which is large indeed. If one tries to expand the lung to that degree with saline, the whole preparation begins to fall apart because the lung weighs so much; it pushes the heart to one side and the blood can't get back into the thorax.

Olver: We did this experiment once in the fetal lamb. We tripled the amount of lung liquid present by adding two volumes of saline, on top of what was already there, and that led to unrestricted diffusion.

Durbin: Why not add air to the saline-filled fetal lung, as the animal does with its first breath?

Staub: You get very funny distributions when you do that. The air doesn't fill all parts of the lung equally.

Durbin: Perhaps, but I think the problem is to build up a final pressure which may then distend the pores irreversibly.

Strang: That is what we tried to do. I am not sure why it was so difficult. We stimulated breathing by pouring cold water on the exteriorized fetal lamb, and stopped it by ceasing the cold stimulation. When breathing stopped, we sampled liquid from the lung. We found quite a lot of molecular transfer, indicating fairly big holes in the epithelium, but it was not unrestricted by any means. The estimated pore radius came out between 3.4 nm and 5.6 nm. When we tried to define the degree of lung expansion needed to produce these changes, which we did by adding gas to a given level of inflating pressure, we never seemed to hit it right (Egan *et al.* 1975). We either got a very small pore or a very big one, and I am not sure why that was. It wasn't until Dr Egan got back to Florida that he seemed to be able to find the knack of inflating the lung just the right amount.

References

EGAN, E. A., OLVER, R. E. & STRANG, L. B. (1975) Changes in non-electrolyte permeability of alveoli and the absorption of lung liquid at the start of breathing in the lamb. *J. Physiol. (Lond.)* 244, 161-179

HOUSE, C. R. (1974) *Water Transport in Cells and Tissues*, pp. 333-339, Edward Arnold, London

KLAUS, M., TOOLEY, W. H., WEAVER, K. H. & CLEMENTS, J. A. (1962) Lung volume in the newborn infant. *Pediatrics 30*, 111-116

LAUWERYNS, J. M. (1965) Hyaline membrane disease; a pathological study of 55 infants. *Arch. Dis. Child. 40*, 618-625

NORMAND, I. C. S., REYNOLDS, E. O. R. & STRANG, L. B. (1970) Passage of macromolecules between alveolar and interstitial spaces in foetal and newly ventilated lungs of the lamb. *J. Physiol. (Lond.) 210*, 151-164

WEIBEL, E. R. (1967) Postnatal growth of the lung and pulmonary gas exchange capacity, in *Development of the Lung (Ciba Found. Symp.)*, Churchill, London; Little Brown, Boston

General discussion I

Dickinson: It appears that we are near a consensus that increased pressure opens up pores, at least in one direction, in perhaps two membranes. We have heard a lot about pressure, surface tension and other things. We seem well poised to ask how the fetal lung becomes inflated and how an oedematous lung clears its fluid at birth.

Strang: The fetal lung in the lamb contains about 30 ml liquid/kg body weight, so in the mature fetal lamb there may be 120–150 ml liquid. Some of that liquid may be squeezed out during the delivery process. Karlberg *et al.* (1962) measured the amount of liquid coming out of the human infant's mouth during the passage through the birth canal. Of course there is no way of knowing whether all that fluid came from the lung or whether some was from the stomach; but even if it all came from the lung it would amount to only 30% of the amount in the lung, assuming of course that the human is the same as the lamb in this respect. Quite a lot of fluid may therefore have to be absorbed at the time of birth. Certainly in infants delivered by Caesarean section there is probably plenty of fluid to be absorbed. Anybody who has laryngoscoped a baby to resuscitate it after Caesarean section knows that a lot of fluid comes out between the vocal cords. So the baby is taking its first breath on top of a lot of liquid already in the lung.

It always struck me as very odd that in the fetal lamb there is not much frothing and foaming, and liquid doesn't come through the ventilator tubes as one might expect: which suggests strongly that the fluid is displaced from the fine air spaces into the interstitial parts of the lung. Aherne & Dawkins (1964) obtained histological evidence that the interstitial spaces of the lung become distended with liquid in the hours after delivery. Later we showed (Humphreys *et al.* 1967) that during delivery there was a fourfold or fivefold increase in lymph flow from the lungs during the initiation of positive pressure ventilation;

115

after five or six hours, however, pulmonary lymph flow had returned to below the resting fetal level. So there is plenty of evidence that the fluid is cleared from the fine air spaces and goes through the interstitial space and lymphatics, with some perhaps going directly into the blood. What is not known is whether the fluid is removed in two steps, the first a rapid absorption into the interstitial space, the second a slow uptake from that site; alternatively, it could be absorbed gradually and continuously from the alveolar spaces. My prejudice would be that gas exchange requires the liquid to be absorbed rather rapidly from the alveoli into the interstitial space.

Another point is that the permeability of the fetal pulmonary epithelium, to chloride ions in particular, is so low that a very large pressure would be required to cause the lung liquid to be reabsorbed in a reasonable time. So it looks as though some change is necessary in the epithelium. I imagine that when the lungs are expanded at birth, paracellular pathways open up between epithelial cells, with a large consequential increase in hydraulic conductivity. As Dr Michel mentioned earlier in connection with capillaries, when it comes to pores of molecular dimensions a small increase in size makes a big difference to hydraulic conductivity. Such a change would allow the liquid to be absorbed down the pressure gradients established by the first breath. There is, between lung liquid and interstitial fluid, a gradient of protein osmotic pressure which would also favour absorption.

We are encouraged in this view by some elegant experiments by a number of epithelial physiologists. When the osmotic pressure is increased on one side of corneal epithelium or toad bladder, paracellular pathways have been shown to open up (Zadunaisky 1971; Wade *et al.* 1973).

Maetz: Do surfactants already exist in fetal lung liquids or do they only appear after birth?

Strang: If by 'appear' you mean 'appear on the alveolar surface', two stages are identifiable: storage, and secretion into the lumen. Secretion into the lumen in the human probably happens at between 30 and 35 weeks of gestation. In the lamb it is probably at about 130 days (term = 147 days; Reynolds *et al.* 1965). In the rabbit it is on the 28th day of a 31-day gestation (Humphreys & Strang 1967).

Dickinson: Dr Guyton, you can get the air barrier quite nicely down to the alveoli and open up paths for liquid to escape, but it seems that there are great mechanical difficulties, especially of course if there is any lack of surfactant. Have you any suggestions about that?

Guyton: First I would like to ask what the surface tension of the lung liquid is in the fetal lamb?

Strang: When the surface tension of the fluid is measured in a Langmuir trough during compression of the surface film it goes down to very low values, 5 dynes/cm (5×10^{-5}N/cm) or less (Humphreys *et al.* 1967, Fig. 2).

Guyton: What is it during expansion or during the steady state?

Strang: The usually quoted value for a surface film during dynamic expansion is 40–55 dynes/cm, the equilibrium value 25–30 dynes/cm. The lung liquid of the fetal lamb behaves in the manner described for suspensions of surface-active lipoprotein.

Guyton: When air is first pulled into the alveolus the applicable radius is the radius of the ostium; so what is the radius of the ostium? This radius and the surface tension are the two factors that determine the minimal inspiratory pressure required to displace the liquid from the alveolus during the filling process.

Strang: The smallest radius is probably 0.003 cm.

Normand: Dr Lynne Reid's studies show that the alveolus really is not fully developed at this time but the radius of the effective ostium of the terminal air space is about the same as the radius of a mature alveolus or a bit bigger (Reid 1967).

Guyton: What about at the radii of the ends of the respiratory bronchioles?

Strang: In the lungs at birth the respiratory bronchioles are smooth-walled and don't contain out-pouchings recognizable as alveoli. The bronchioles open into a primitive acinus consisting of smooth-walled alveolar sacs.

Guyton: The first breath requires a pressure of about -40 mmHg (-5.3 kPa).

Olver: Pressures of -70 to -80 mmHg (-9.31 to -10.6 kPa) have been recorded (Karlberg *et al.* 1962). They are transient pressures and we don't know what proportion is exerted across the epithelium.

Guyton: Presumably the septal interstitial spaces between the alveoli must also be subjected to at least as negative a pressure. Fluid movement from the alveoli into the septal spaces caused by this negative pressure could account for the swelling of the interstitial spaces.

Dr Strang, how much of the fluid goes into the blood and how much of it goes into the lymph?

Strang: Between a third and a half goes to the lymphatics and the rest to the blood (Humphreys & Strang 1967).

Guyton: One would therefore expect dilution of the interstitial fluid.

Strang: That is observed and reflected in the lymph.

Guyton: One would also expect a great deal of absorption of liquid into the blood because of that dilution.

Strang: A lot of the initial inflating pressure that has been recorded during the first breath may be taken up in accelerating the liquid in the airways. There is a large flow resistance, because lung liquid is about 1000 times more viscous than air, and there is also a substantial inertial component in accelerating the liquid fast enough during the first breath (Howatt *et al.* 1965).

Olver: At the second breath there may still be a substantial pressure gradient across the lung (Karlberg *et al.* 1962). It isn't just the first breath. Large transpulmonary pressures may be generated after air has reached the alveoli and may be important in opening up the intercellular junctions and allowing the lung liquid to be absorbed. From the low chloride permeability of the alveolar epithelium we originally thought that, whatever the forces available, liquid couldn't be reabsorbed rapidly. As water moved down the pressure gradient, the increased osmotic pressure produced inside the alveoli by the restricted permeability to solutes would counterbalance that movement.

Guyton: Unless you open up large peri-epithelial pores.

Olver: Yes; that would markedly increase hydraulic conductivity.

Guyton: Could expansion of the interstitial spaces open these junctions between the epithelial cells? In other words, have you measured epithelial permeability after creating lung oedema?

Egan: We have started such experiments, but it is too soon to talk about them. If the interstitial space is filled with fluid the small airways tend to close early, and the hyperexpansion of distal airways in interstitial pulmonary oedema shown by Milic-Emili & Ruff (1971) would tend to produce high lung inflation, which I assume could change epithelial permeability.

Guyton: That would be one explanation. Another explanation would be that mechanical stretching of the interstitial spaces by interstitial oedema fluid could in some way open the pores.

Olver: The nearest thing we did to that in the fetus was to increase left atrial pressure to about 7 cmH$_2$O (0.68 kPa)—enough to more than double pulmonary lymph flow. That didn't make any difference to the rate of lung liquid secretion. For that reason we thought that hydrostatic pressures up to that level were not terribly important. Presumably one could reach a stage at which they become important.

Dickinson: The problem of clearing water from the lungs is not exclusive to neonatology. When someone has been rescued from the sea the saline fluid is rapidly absorbed. Surgeons in intensive care units sometimes pour isotonic saline down the lungs to wash out asthmatic secretions. This completely fills up lungs which may have very little nitrogen in them. The alveoli are flooded but clear quite rapidly. Do you think the same mechanisms are in force there, with high transient negative pressures developing inside the chest, or would other mechanisms be available in an adult lung for clearing isotonic fluid from the alveoli?

Hugh-Jones: I don't know the reference but the Japanese used to use one lung as an artificial kidney and fill it with isotonic saline. Those lungs used to clear quickly.

Robin: Dr Kylstra (1957) also studied the ability of the lung to clear many solutes from the blood.

In humans, pulmonary lavage with isotonic saline takes about six to eight hours as judged by X-ray. On the other hand, residual effects of saline seem to persist for a long time. For example, gas exchange does not really return to its basal state in the average patient for 12 to 24 hours, though that may not have anything to do with the residual liquid. It certainly doesn't clear immediately.

Hugh-Jones: Do you know anything about the clearing of the salt and chloride? If you sample the liquid in the lung is there a change?

Robin: Not with isotonic saline, not to any substantial degree.

Egan: I think that agrees with what we find in the adult sheep. Iso-osmotic saline is absorbed at about 0.1%/min. Full absorption would require a fairly long time. It is a little difficult to sample the liquid. We have to put down at least 25% of the air-space capacity of the isolated segment of lung as isotonic saline to ensure that we get a representative sample down for measuring the concentration of the solutes. A few millilitres are not enough.

Farhi: I would like to come back to the problem of distension of the lung and increased pore size. Obviously one cannot inflate a lung to more than its vital capacity, but there are cases—after surgery, or after atelectasis has occurred—in which the remaining aerated lung is distended to much more than its normal total capacity. Is there any evidence that there is a greater tendency for fluid to leak across the alveolar membrane of these areas?

Egan: Newborn infants may have a syndrome that Avery *et al.* (1966) called transient tachypnoea of the newborn. On radiographs they have hyper-expanded lungs. I don't know whether anybody has specifically measured the volume of the lung but it is impressive on chest X-rays. I would like to think that this initial hyperexpansion of the lung so changes epithelial permeability that protein diffuses from the interstitial space into the lung liquid. This would soon eliminate the normal osmotic pressure produced by a difference in protein concentration, and so would delay the absorption of lung liquid. In fact Dr Avery hypothesized that such a delay was the aetiology of the syndrome.

Guyton: About 15 years ago we saw a phenomenon which we could never explain. Maybe someone here can explain it. We inflated one lung with liquid, the other with air, and studied the effects of different mean pressures in the liquid-filled lung on the fluid in the intrapleural space. When the pressure was above about 15 mmHg (2 kPa) in the alveoli, fluid began to pour into the intrapleural space, and terrific pleural effusion developed. When we lowered the pressure to about 11 mmHg (1.46 kPa) the leaks closed. That is, when the alveolar pressure rose above a critical level, liquid flowed rapidly into the pleural space; when the pressure was slightly lower the openings closed, so this was not simply a case of alveoli being ruptured.

Egan: At 10 cmH$_2$O (0.98 kPa) a lung containing liquid is completely filled.

Agostoni: In the experiment I showed earlier (p. 61), both lungs were filled with saline and the level of saline in the filling system was kept at a different height from the bottom of the lung. In the supine dog we went up to 10 cm above the top of the lung. We saw no pleural effusion under these conditions. When the dog was in the head-up position the level of saline in the filling system was kept to a maximum at the top of the lung, because the lung volume then was 115% of the total lung capacity. If we had needed higher levels we might have reached a point at which there would have been some break in the lung. You said you were more than 10 cm above the top of the lung, Dr Guyton. We didn't have any pleural effusion but our distension of the lung was less than yours.

Dickinson: Could you regard the pleural space as being in any way analogous to the pulmonary interstitial space?

Agostoni: Roughly yes, since both belong to the interstitial space. Some differences, however, should be pointed out. First, we have heard that the protein content of the pulmonary interstitial space may be higher than that of the pleural liquid. Indeed, in the pleural liquid of rabbits and dogs the protein concentration is about 1.3 and 1.8 g/100 ml, respectively, the computed colloid osmotic pressure being 4.8 and 3.2 cmH$_2$O (0.47 and 0.31 kPa), respectively (Agostoni 1972). In this connection, it must be remembered that pleural liquid can be sampled directly, whereas pulmonary interstitial liquid cannot. Finally, on one side pleural liquid is facing the capillaries of the systemic circulation and on the other side those of the pulmonary circulation (even in those species in which the visceral pleura is supplied by the bronchial circulation the capillary blood is drained by the pulmonary veins) (Agostoni 1972), whereas the pulmonary interstitial liquid faces only the capillaries of the pulmonary circulation.

Maetz: We have heard about the mechanical factors of pressure and so on which may intervene. Could an endocrine factor which changes the permeability of the lining of the lung come into the picture?

Strang: Many changes take place in the nervous system and the adrenals at the time of birth. None of these things have been investigated from this point of view, as far as I know.

Widdicombe: Prostaglandins are bound to crop up at any symposium nowadays. J. R. Vane and his colleagues (Palmer *et al.* 1973) have shown that when the lungs are mechanically deformed, prostaglandins are released. What do these do to intercellular spaces?

Fishman: I think that the demonstration of enhanced synthesis and release of prostaglandins during mechanical stimulation of the lung is about as far as recent investigations have gone with respect to the topic of the present meeting.

Crosbie: The bomb-blast lung is another major problem for intensive care units these days. Healthy young people injured in this way respond very well to intermittent positive pressure and often the lung damage is the only injury they have. With the shock-lung syndrome itself it may take up to a month for the alveolar-capillary damage to disappear.

Dickinson: But the lung is capable of eventually getting back complete functional normality even after an injury of this sort. After an acute attack of pulmonary oedema the lung can recover extraordinarily rapidly.

Dejours: Does the fetal lung ever contain amniotic fluid?

Strang: Not usually: not in health.

Dejours: The fetus makes some so-called respiratory movements. Doesn't some amniotic fluid move in and out?

Strang: Very little. If the umbilical cord is occluded the fetal lamb can be made to gasp. It makes massive respiratory movements, generating pleural pressures as low as -70 cmH$_2$O (-6.86 kPa). That pressure is sufficient to shift about 10–15 ml liquid (Howatt *et al.* 1965). The rapid shallow breathing that occurs in the unasphyxiated fetus shifts only 1 or 2 ml (Dawes *et al.*1972).

Some experiments have shown that radio-opaque dyes injected into the amniotic fluid can subsequently be found in the lung when the fetus makes asphyxial gasps. The assumption is that when the fetus has been breathing amniotic fluid for a long time the tracer becomes mixed with lung liquid. It is unlikely that the shallow movements observed in normal intrauterine life will produce any significant mixing of amniotic and lung liquid (Howatt *et al.* 1965; Dawes *et al.* 1972).

Dejours: I asked this question because it has been reported that drugs or amino acids injected into the amniotic fluid could pass into the fetus. Do these enter through the digestive tract?

Olver: Yes. The fetus makes swallowing movements and can swallow appreciable amounts of amniotic fluid. At the simplest level we distinguish between amniotic fluid and lung liquid on the basis of electrolyte composition, which is very different. The difference excludes any appreciable mixing between the two.

Adamson: We have been interested in the effects of fetal breathing movements on the flow of lung liquid (Adamson *et al.* 1975). A tracheal cannula in the form of a loop placed in the lamb fetus *in utero* shows fine oscillations in the liquid-filled loop when the fetus breathes. This appears to be against a closed glottis, as there is little movement of liquid from the oral pharynx back into the lung. Any movement of liquid is generally from the lung into the oral pharynx. This is not a steady flow, but rather like the Manhattan skyline, with short periods of flow and then no flow at all. Retrograde flow is a very unusual event and it is rarely more than 3 or 4 ml.

Fishman: Could I get some clarification? If one lung is filled with fluid, Dr Egan, blood flow will be diverted from that lung and absorption will necessarily be slow.

Egan: In the rabbit we began using a fluid-filled preparation. We used isotopic water to make sure that none of the other solutes were flow-limited in their transfer. The blood flow was so low, in a fluid-filled lung, that we were getting a flow limitation of solute transfer. To study this adequately I think one has to have gas in the lungs. It appears important to have an adequate alveolar Po_2 to keep pulmonary resistance low, so that the solute movement is not flow-limited.

Fishman: Is the idea to raise the oxygen tension of the liquid in the lung in order to promote vasodilation of the pulmonary vessels, thereby neutralizing some of the mechanical compressive forces of gravity?

Egan: Liquid and gas are needed. If the lung is filled with liquid alone I think there will be a very low flow, unless resistance is raised in some other parts of the lung. Conceivably one could study a fluid-filled segment of lung by raising pulmonary resistance in other parts by some other mechanism. When we used a liquid-filled lung we could not study it.

Robin: In an adult lung filled with iso-osmotic saline, pulmonary blood flow decreases sharply. Since the lung is collapsed before being filled with saline, one can show a sharp reduction in Po_2. When the lung is filled with saline, although it is not ventilated, the Po_2 goes up sharply because pulmonary blood flow has been rapidly reduced (Smith *et al.* 1970). On the other hand, sufficient pulmonary flow is retained for endogenous solutes, such as urea, creatinine, glucose, etc., to go through the residual blood flow and appear in the saline in that lung. I don't think anybody has precise estimates of how much the pulmonary blood flow is reduced, but it is reduced substantially. Of course, if you are looking at permeability coefficients of substances that are flow-limited, then there are major problems because you are assuming that there is no flow limitation for your measurement of permeability coefficients.

Egan: Water was included in our first experiments on rabbits, and in every case it was at least 10 times faster than urea, which is the small solute used in the experiments described in my paper. If water moves in the same channels as solutes, then we really should not have flow limitation for the solutes that I showed.

Staub: We used radioactive microspheres to measure blood flow before and after fluid-filling of the left lower lobe in the dog. Even though airway pressure of the fluid-filled lobe was well below the main pulmonary artery pressure, we found that blood flow decreased almost 75% after fluid filling. Nevertheless, the rate at which tritiated water was removed from the fluid-filled lung lobe was still so fast that it could barely be measured. Even with the markedly reduced blood flow the removal of the tritiated water was not flow-limited.

Hughes: I would like to return to the point Dr Farhi raised about the mechanical effect of stretching the lung and making the epithelial pores bigger. There is no reason why it shouldn't make the endothelial pores bigger as well, and over-expanded lungs are in danger of pulmonary oedema.

Dickinson: Earlier somebody said that stretching in one direction appears to increase the permeability of epithelial pores, but the point was made by analogy with gastric mucosa so that wouldn't necessarily apply to the alveolar epithelium.

Hughes: Expansion of the lung is fairly isotropic; however the structures are arranged they are going to be stretched axially as well as radially. So endothelial intercellular junctions could get a similar stretch at high lung volumes to the alveolar epithelial junctions.

Dickinson: If there was significant axial stretching I would agree.

Egan: In the adult sheep in which the gas and the liquid volume reached total lung capacity a leak occurred. In some such experiments, instead of the saline being absorbed, it began to be diluted by addition of a net flux of water from the interstitial space into the lung space. I don't know whether that is pulmonary oedema, nor have I any idea what the effect is on the capillaries.

Hughes: The best human experiment is acute asthma, where the lung volume goes up to 150% of the total lung capacity and in a matter of a week it can return to 50% of total lung capacity. That is a huge change in lung distension. Apart from measurements of the volumes and pressures, this hasn't been studied from the point of view of liquid exchanges across any of the membranes.

Hugh-Jones: There is no evidence of any increased movement of liquid in acute asthma, is there?

Hughes: There is generally not overt oedema but no one has used more sensitive techniques to test that point.

Lee: In people dying from acute asthma what is the wet weight/dry weight ratio of the lung? Most respiratory physicians think that the bronchi constrict in asthma, but it could well be that the small bronchi appear to constrict because of peribronchial cuffing by oedema fluid when something happens to capillary permeability.

Dickinson: Few clinicians would think that was a matter of functional constriction. At necropsy the airways are manifestly blocked.

Lee: They are blocked with proteinous exudate. Not many people ask where this comes from.

References

ADAMSON, T. M., BRODECKY, V., LAMBERT, T. F., MALONEY, J. E., RITCHIE, B. C. & WALKER, A. M. (1975) Lung liquid production and composition in the 'in utero' foetal lambs. *Aust. J. Exp. Biol. Med. Sci. 53*, 65-75

AGOSTONI, E. (1972) Mechanics of the pleural space. *Physiol. Rev. 52*, 57-128

AHERNE, W. & DAWKINS, M. J. R. (1964) The removal of fluid from the pulmonary airways after birth and the effect on this of prematurity and prenatal asphyxia. *Biol. Neonatorum 7*, 214-229

AVERY, M. E., GATEWOOD, O. B. & BRUMLEY, G. (1966) Transient tachypnea of the newborn. *Am. J. Dis. Child. 111*, 380-385

DAWES, G. S., FOX, M. E., LEDUEK, B. M., LIGGINS, G. C. & RICHARDS, R. T. (1972) Respiratory movements and rapid eye movement sleep in the foetal lamb. *J. Physiol. (Lond.) 220*, 119-143

HOWATT, W. F., AVERY, M. E., HUMPHREYS, P. W., NORMAND, I. C. S., REID, L. & STRANG, L. B. (1965) Factors affecting pulmonary surface properties in the foetal lamb. *Clin. Sci. 29*, 239-248

HUMPHREYS, P. W. & STRANG, L. B. (1967) Effects of gestation and prenatal asphyxia on pulmonary surface properties of the foetal rabbit. *J. Physiol. (Lond.) 192*, 53

HUMPHREYS, P. W., NORMAND, I. C. S., REYNOLDS, E. O. R. & STRANG, L. B. (1967) Pulmonary lymph flow and the uptake of liquid from the lungs of the lamb at the start of breathing. *J. Physiol. (Lond.) 193*, 1-29

KARLBERG, P., CHERRY, R. B., ESCARDO, F. E. & KOCH, G. (1962) Respiratory studies in newborn infants. II. Pulmonary ventilation and mechanics of breathing in the first few minutes of life, including the onset of respiration. *Acta Paediatr. 51*, 121-136

KYLSTRA, J. A. (1957) Lavage of the lung. *Acta Physiol. Pharmacol. Neerl. 7*, 163-221

MILIC-EMILI, J. & RUFF, F. (1971) Effects of pulmonary congestion edema on the small airways. *Bull. Physio-pathol. Resp. 7*, 1181-1196

PALMER, M. A., PIPER, P. J. & VANE, J. R. (1973) Release of rabbit aorta contracting substance (RCS) and prostaglandins induced by chemical or mechanical stimulation of guinea-pig lungs. *Br. J. Pharmacol. 49*, 226-242

REID, L. (1967) The embryology of the lung, in *Development of the Lung (Ciba Found. Symp.)*, Churchill, London

REYNOLDS, E. O. R., JACOBSON, H. N., MOTOYAMA, E. K., KIKKAWA, Y., CRAIG, J. M., ORZALESI, M. M. & COOK, C. D. (1965) The effect of immaturity and prenatal asphyxia on the lungs and pulmonary function of newborn lambs: the experimental reproduction of respiratory distress. *Pediatrics 35*, 382

SMITH, J. D., MILLEN, J. E., SAFAR, P. & ROBIN, E. D. (1970) Intrathoracic pressure, pulmonary vascular pressures and gas exchange during pulmonary lavage. *Anesthesiology 33*, 401-405

WADE, J. B., REVEL, J. P. & DiSCALA, V. A. (1973) Effect of osmotic gradients on intracellular junctions of the toad bladder. *Am. J. Physiol. 224*, 407-415

ZADUNAISKY, J. A. (1971) Electrophysiology and transparency of the cornea, in *Electrophysiology of Epithelial Cells* (Giebisch, G., ed.), pp. 225-255, Schattayer, Stuttgart, New York

Comparative aspects of salt and water transport across lung

R. D. KEYNES

Physiological Laboratory, University of Cambridge

Abstract   Calculation suggests that the outward flux of water from the surface of the lung into the expired air could be driven by a relatively small standing osmotic gradient. The structure of this alveolar epithelium does not appear to possess the characteristics of a typical secretory epithelium. These considerations argue against the occurrence of active transport in the alveoli of the adult mammalian lung.

I have been asked to consider the question of transport across the lung from the comparative standpoint. In attempting to comply, I can at least claim that my approach will be characterized by lack of prejudice, if I may equate a reprehensible ignorance of lung physiology with open-mindedness on the subject!

The lung of the mammal, unlike that of its water-breathing ancestors, is not needed to play a direct role in regulating the salt balance of the organism. This is not necessarily true of the fetus, where the possibility clearly exists that there may be an active or passive flux of ions across the alveolar epithelium. But other speakers will be dealing with the mammalian fetus, and with adult fish and amphibia, and I will not trespass on their territory. In trying to think about transport across the alveolar epithelium it did, however, occur to me that the lung of the air-breathing vertebrate could be regarded as responsible for more than an exchange of gases, since there is in fact a continuous flux of pure water flowing outwards from the surface of the alveoli and of the pulmonary air passages. I therefore thought that it might prove instructive to calculate the approximate magnitude of this water flux, both for comparative purposes, and to see whether it was likely to raise any obvious transport problems.

Suppose that we take the water content of air expired at 37 °C as 0.05 g/l and the resting minute volume of a normal man as 6 l. The total rate of loss of water via the lungs will be 5×10^{-3} g/s. Assuming for the purpose of my argument that this all takes place across the alveoli themselves, whose area is said to be 75×10^4 cm^2, the water flux per unit area is 6.7×10^{-9} g cm^{-2} s^{-1}. To set this figure in some sort of perspective, the rate of loss of water from the surface of various insects is around 20 mg cm^{-2} h^{-1}, or 6×10^{-6} g cm^{-2} s^{-1} (Prosser & Brown 1961). For another comparison, the flux of labelled water across the gill epithelium of fresh water teleosts was determined by Motais et al. (1969) as about 100 μl cm^{-2} h^{-1}, or 3×10^{-5} g cm^{-2} s^{-1}. By these standards, the flux calculated above for the alveolar epithelium is a rather small one. Even so, it may be worth enquiring whether there is any difficulty in providing the necessary driving force. Suppose the hydraulic permeability coefficient, L_p, is taken as 3.5×10^{-6} g cm^{-2} s^{-1} osmol^{-1}, as in toad skin (Bentley 1961), the observed flux could be produced by an osmotic pressure difference of $6.7 \times 10^{-9}/3.5 \times 10^{-6} = 1.9 \times 10^{-3}$ osmol. Hence a very mild steady-state hypertonicity of the intra-alveolar fluid could bring about the water movement, and no active transport mechanism need be invoked to account for evaporation from the lung.

This comforting conclusion does not, all the same, provide a solution for the problem that arises if there is an appreciable leakage of fluid into the alveoli from the capillaries, as there may be if the mean value of hydrostatic pressure minus air pressure acting outwards exceeds the colloid osmotic pressure acting inwards. It appears to be generally held that the normal route for removal of such exuded fluid is via the lymphatics (Greene 1965), but the possibility exists that the alveolar lining might be organized as a secretory epithelium capable of transporting sodium chloride back into the blood stream accompanied by water. If such a mechanism existed in the lung, one would expect (Keynes 1969) the alveolar epithelium to display certain characteristic features, such as the asymmetrically positioned junctional complexes of Farquhar & Palade (1963), the extensive intercellular canaliculi involved in fluid coupling, and an abundance of mitochondria. From the ultrastructural studies of Schneeberger-Keeley & Karnovsky (1968), in which they investigated the distribution of horseradish peroxidase (EC 1.11.1.7) in the lungs of mice after intravenous injection, it seems that although the peroxidase molecules were able to penetrate the endothelial junctions into the basement membranes, they were stopped from entering the alveolar space by the presence of zonulae occludentes between the epithelial cells. Although these impenetrable zones were in the right location, at the air side of the epithelial cells, to function as the 'tight' junctions of a secretory epithelium transporting ions away from this side, they did not have the typical appearance described by Farquhar & Palade (1963) and, despite the pitfalls in arguing from histology to function, they may be considered as unlikely to serve the same purpose. In other respects, too, the alveolar epithelium does not look as if it were specialized for secretion and, fervent advocate though I am of the ubiquity and importance of secretory epithelia, I hesitate to add the lining of the alveoli to their ranks.

Since this brings to a rather premature end all that I can usefully say that is directly relevant to the lung, I would like to take this opportunity of mentioning briefly some studies by Dr A. E. Hill (1975) on the general question of the mechanism of coupling between water and solute fluxes in secretory epithelia, which throw considerable doubt on the validity of Diamond's standing-gradient osmotic flow theory. The argument is basically that a strictly isotonic secretion cannot be achieved in any known tissue with the observed geometry and passive water permeability of the intercellular canals. Calculations based on Segel's (1970) analytical solution for the standing gradient system indicate that for the secreted fluid to be isotonic with the bathing medium to within 3%, it is necessary either that the value of L_p for the walls of the intercellular canals should be several orders of magnitude greater than in any known type of membrane, or that the canals should be very much longer and thinner than they appear to be in any electron micrograph. Diamond & Bossert's (1967) contrary conclusion rested on quite unrealistic assumptions about the length and diameter of the canals in gall bladder epithelium. I recommend to anyone interested in this field a close study of Hill's (1975) paper.

References

BENTLEY, P. J. (1961) Directional differences in the permeability to water of the isolated urinary bladder of the toad, *Bufo marinus. J. Endocrinol.* 22, 95-100

DIAMOND, J. M. & BOSSERT, W. H. (1967) Standing-gradient osmotic flow. A mechanism for coupling of water and solute transport in epithelia. *J. Gen. Physiol.* 50, 2061-2083

FARQUHAR, M. G. & PALADE, G. E. (1963) Junctional complexes in various epithelia. *J. Cell Biol.* 17, 375-412

GREENE, D. G. (1965) Pulmonary oedema, in *Handb. Physiol. Section 3: Respiration*, vol. 2 (Fenn, W.O. & Rahn, H., eds.) ch. 70, American Physiological Society, Washington, D.C.

HILL, A. E. (1975) Solute-solvent coupling in epithelia: a critical examination of the standing-gradient osmotic flow theory. *Proc. R. Soc. Lond. B Biol. Sci. 190*, 99-114

KEYNES, R. D. (1969) From frog skin to sheep rumen: a survey of transport of salts and water across multicellular structures. *Q. Rev. Biophys.* 2, 177-281

MOTAIS, R., ISAIA, J., RANKIN, J. C., & MAETZ, J. (1969) Adaptive changes of the water permeability of the teleostean gill epithelium in relation to external salinity. *J. Exp. Biol.* 51, 529-546

PROSSER, C. L. & BROWN, F. A. (1961) *Comparative Animal Physiology*, 2nd edn, Saunders, Philadelphia

SCHNEEBERGER-KEELEY, E. E. & KARNOVSKY, M. J. (1968) The ultrastructural basis of alveolar-capillary membrane permeability to peroxidase used as a tracer. *J. Cell Biol.* 37, 781-793

SEGEL, L. A. (1970) Standing-gradient flows driven by active solute transport. *J. Theor. Biol.* 29, 233-250

Discussion

Dickinson: Dr Schneeberger, in relation to the epithelial membrane, are the tight junctions usually nearer the alveolar surface or nearer the interstitial surface? Compared with the other membranes, are there abundant mitochondria in lung epithelium? And do you see any intercellular canaliculae such as are seen in frog skin?

Schneeberger: As I mentioned earlier (pp. 3–21), in mouse alveolar epithelium the junction involved is a so-called tight junction rather than a desmosome. The tight junctions are usually in the distal portion of the intercellular cleft. Mitochondria are quite numerous in type II pneumocytes but not particularly abundant in type I pneumocytes. A thick glycocalyx is particularly prominent in type II pneumocytes. Intercellular junctions of alveolar epithelium are fairly straight, except perhaps for those between type I and type II pneumocytes. These characteristics do not fit the criteria that Dr Keynes listed for secretory epithelia. Of the two types of cell, type II pneumocytes are the more likely candidates for being secretory cells. They are fewer in number than type I pneumocytes.

Adamson: We have been interested in trying to identify a cell in the fetal lung which would be a secreting cell. There are cells with microvilli which appear to have tight junctions. Mitochondria are not often seen, but these cells contain a lot of glycogen, which could be another source of energy. In the lung of the fetal lamb at 100 days, such cells are seen in the main bronchi, and as the lamb becomes more mature, these cells (bronchiolar cells) are seen perhaps more peripherally in the bronchi. These cells appear to be absent in the adult sheep lung. It would therefore seem best to consider the fetal lung as a separate entity from the adult lung when we are looking at cells involved in secretion.

Schneeberger: When I described these alveolar lining cells I was referring to the adult lung. I agree that lung liquid has a unique ion composition. We have to explain that and try to establish which cells are the secretory ones.

Maetz: The 'chloride cells' in fish gills are often thought to be mitochondria-rich cells but in 2 μm thick sections under a high-powered electron microscope, and with a special coloration specific to the membranes, very few mitochondria are seen. They are very long and branched and wavy, so that when they are cut in thin sections it looks as if there are a lot, but really we have just cut the 'sausage' in many smaller slices (M. Pisam, personal communication). Many cells, including hepatocytes, are now considered to have only one or two mitochondria, and the chloride cell is one of these types. The mitochondria occupy a large volume of cell content, however.

Keynes: It is reasonable to say that in the tissues with a lot of mitochondria, the mitochondria produce ATP and ATP drives the sodium pump. But if this is a secretory epithelium with relatively little potassium adenosine triphosphatase (ATPase, EC 3.6.1.3), it might instead have active chloride transport, and we have no idea how this active chloride transport is actually coupled to metabolism. There is apparently no chloride-activated ATPase in any animal cell, though Dr Durbin has reported that there is thiocyanate-sensitive ATPase.

Durbin: I think the evidence is quite good now that acid secretion in the stomach is dependent on ATP as an energy source. This conclusion is based primarily on two recent observations. Stimulation of respiration by cyclic AMP in isolated oxyntic cells is inhibited by oligomycin, which is an effective inhibitor of oxidation coupled to phosphorylation (F. Michelangeli, unpublished work, 1975). Also Lee *et al.* (1974) have shown that ATP will support proton movement in gastric microsomes. Undoubtedly the lung transports at a lower rate than the stomach, and it would be interesting to know the relative volumes of mitochondrial space in the two organs.

Keynes: Insect tissues also have an ubiquitous electrogenic potassium-transporting system, but nobody has been able to find any potassium-activated ATPase. In insect Malpighian tubules, organs where a great deal of active transport goes on, there are plenty of mitochondria, but apparently no ATPase.

Olver: The number of cells as a proportion of the total is also perhaps not entirely relevant. After all, in the amphibian stomach the oxyntic cells make up only a minority of the total number of cells in the epithelium, yet of course this is the site of active hydrogen ion transport.

Durbin: In fact they make up about 25–30% of the total number in epithelium (Helander *et al.* 1972).

Robin: Two lines of evidence support your conclusions, Dr Keynes. One concerns the energetics of lung tissue. S. L. Young *et al.* (1973, unpublished) did a series of studies on the metabolic pathways in the isolated perfused rat lung. They showed clearly that the lung contains a large population of cells, which by extrapolation are alveolar epithelial type I cells, which have a high rate of aerobic glycolysis. Most ATP generation then comes about through glycolysis, which is relatively inefficient in terms of moles of ATP provided per mole of substrate consumed. This itself is an interesting paradox, since one of the tissues that has an overabundance of molecular oxygen has 'decided' that it will generate ATP largely through glycolysis. The second line of evidence is that rates of bidirectional sodium transport are not affected by the addition of ouabain to the saline-filled dog lung, which suggests at least that sodium–potassium-activated ATP is not involved in sodium transport.

Durbin: But the fetal lung actively transports solute which is coupled to water movement, doesn't it?

Olver: Yes. It is also true that there is active ion transport in the adult mammalian trachea and we could probably extrapolate that right down through the tracheobronchial system. I am not quite sure what those studies that you referred to actually mean, Dr Robin. It is important to know where the ouabain was put and what effect was being looked for.

Robin: I find it hard to believe that if tracheal mucosa, for instance, has active transport of sodium, type I alveolar epithelial cells must also have it.

Olver: I didn't say that.

Strang: There are a lot of different epithelial cells in the lung and we ought to be careful before we base any conclusions on the appearance of one type of epithelial cells. Type II cells, as Dr Schneeberger has said, have quite a lot of the relevant structural features for active ion transport, and they are fairly numerous. Although they occupy only about 10% of the area of the lung surface they contribute about half the total number of cells (Thurlbeck & Wang 1974).

Keynes: I entirely agree about the danger of looking at an electron micrograph and concluding what the function of a cell is. Dr Schneeberger, you said that in lung epithelium there are desmosomes rather than tight junctions. But is not the whole of the nomenclature rather misleading? It turns out that in gall bladder epithelium the main characteristic of the so-called tight junctions is that they have an extremely low electrical resistance. In other words, in the electrical sense they are very loose junctions. Was I right in concluding that in the lung you don't see the characteristic staining of a line down the middle? These lines which Farquhar & Palade (1963) described seem to be characteristic of secretory epithelia.

Schneeberger: I was speaking about the alveolar epithelium, not about upper airway epithelium which I have not looked at in detail. What we see in the alveolar epithelium is not a desmosome-like structure but a tight junction. Freeze-fracture images show that they are composed of a complex network of strands. At the alveolar level then, there are no desmosome-like structures. The transepithelial resistance across the adult alveolar epithelium has not been established, and all we have at the moment is the freeze–fracture image of the junction.

Gatzy: Isn't it true that horseradish peroxidase will penetrate beyond the desmosomes up to the tight junctions? I don't think the desmosomes are part of the junctional complex. The tight junction is generally regarded as the site of the paracellular electrical resistance.

Keynes: Is there a desmosome-type junction between the other cells in fish gills?

Maetz: In the gill epithelium there seem to be tight junctions essentially everywhere. Preliminary results of recent freeze–fracture studies by C. Sardet in Paris suggest that rather complex junctional processes occur. I think that it is a typical feature of the gill to be a tight membrane. Fish gill has an osmotic permeability about 10 times less than frog skin or frog bladder, even in the absence of neurohypophysial hormones (see Maetz, this volume).

Donald: As far as I can remember R. V. Christie and others demonstrated in the 1930s that inspired air was saturated with water vapour at an early stage in the upper respiratory passages. Are there later views on this subject?

Dickinson: That would support Dr Keynes' point even more strongly.

Staub: Older studies indicated that incoming fresh air was saturated with water vapour before it reached the carina of the trachea. Therefore, no water is lost from the alveolar surfaces. Furthermore, the fluid flux up the tracheo-bronchial tree in 24 hours is small. There really isn't much net exchange of fluid from the respiratory portions of the lung in the adult compared to the fetus.

Dejours: Regarding the saturation of the ingoing air, mammals and birds may be subjected to an enormous loss of water during muscular exercise or in thermal polypnoea. So what happens to the reabsorption of salt in these situations?

Keynes: One needs better figures, but it is not clear to me that there is a transport problem in explaining the evaporation of water. My sums showed that a difference of 2 mosmol was enough for the water to be sucked through passively. If saturation with water vapour occurs much earlier and through a much smaller area of tracheal epithelium, then one only has to use rather larger osmotic permeability coefficients. I chose the smaller values deliberately and I still ended up finding that a difference of only a few milliosmoles in tonicity across the membrane would be enough to provide a driving force for the water.

Olver: Since the area across which this evaporative water loss is taking place may be two or three orders of magnitude less than you suggested, a much larger driving force than that calculated may be necessary. Mélon (1968) reported that there is active sodium transport across the nasal mucosa towards the lumen which might be important in that respect.

References

FARQUHAR, M. G. & PALADE, G. E. (1963) Junctional complexes in various epithelia. *J. Cell Biol.* *17*, 375-412

HELANDER, H. F., SANDERS, S. S., REHM, W. S. & HIRSHOWITZ, B. I. (1972) Quantitative aspects of gastric morphology, in *Gastric Secretion* (Sachs, G., Heinz, E. & Ullrich, K. J., eds.), Academic Press, New York

LEE, J., SIMPSON, G. & SCHOLES, P. (1974) An ATPase from dog gastric mucosa: changes of outer pH in suspensions of membrane vesicles accompanying ATP hydrolysis. *Biochem. Biophys. Res. Commun. 60*, 825-832

MÉLON, J. (1968) Activité sécrétoire de la muqeuse nasale. *Acta Oto Rhino Laryngol. Belg. 22*, 11-244

SCOTT, W. N., SAPIRSTEIN, V. S. & YODER, M. J. (1974) Partition of functions in epithelia: localization of enzymes in 'mitochondria-rich' cells of toad urinary bladder. *Science (Wash. D.C.) 184*, 797-800

STEINMETZ, P. R. (1974) Cellular mechanisms of urinary acidification. *Physiol. Rev. 54*, 890-956

THURLBECK, W. M. & WANG, N. S. (1974) The structure of the lungs, in *MTP Int. Rev. Sci. Physiol. Series One*, vol. 2, *Respiratory Physiology* (Guyton, A. C. & Widdicombe, J. G., eds.), Butterworths, London

Transport of ions and water across the epithelium of fish gills

J. MAETZ

*Groupe de Biologie Marine du Département de Biologie du Commissariat à l'Energie Atomique,
Station Zoologique, Villefranche-sur-mer*

Abstract The teleostean gill is characterized by an exceptionally low permeability
to water. Water moves along the osmotic gradient across the gill, being gained
in fresh water and lost in sea water. Coupling of water movement to solute
movement has not been reported.

In fresh water, the gill is the site of independent active uptake of sodium and
chloride. Na^+ uptake is coupled to H^+ or NH_4^+ excretion, Cl^- uptake to HCO_3^-
excretion. Amiloride blocks sodium transport and thiocyanate inhibits the
chloride pump.

In sea water, sodium and chloride exchanges across the gill are about 100
times faster than in fresh water, up to 100% of the internal sodium or chloride
being exchanged per hour. Chloride is actively excreted, while sodium movement
may well be passive. The chloride pump is associated with a mechanism for
Na/K exchange; both pump and Na/K exchange are blocked by thiocyanate and
possibly by ouabain.

Three enzymes are involved in the ionic pumps: carbonate dehydratase
(EC 4.2.1.1; carbonic anhydrase), sodium/potassium-stimulated adenosinetriphosphatase (EC 3.6.1.3, ATPase) and anion-stimulated ATPase. Specialized
cells ('chloride cells') are presumably the site of the active transport.

At the beginning of this century, Fredericq (1901) discovered that the osmotic
pressure of the body fluids of bony fishes (teleosts), whether living in fresh
water or in sea water or migrating from one medium to the other, is relatively
constant, being at a level similar to that found in higher vertebrates and equivalent to about one third of the osmotic pressure of sea water.

What was known 50 years ago of the contrasting ways in which sea water
and fresh water teleosts maintain their osmotic and mineral balance is summarized by the classical models proposed by Homer Smith (1930) and August
Krogh (1939). In fresh water, water enters osmotically through the gills and
the kidney has the task of clearing this water by excreting abundant and dilute
urine. The renal loss of sodium and chloride, as well as the passive losses of
these electrolytes across the gill, are compensated by an 'active' uptake of ions

133

by the gills against a considerable concentration gradient. The gut is believed to play a negligible role in fresh water fish. In sea water, water is lost osmotically across the gills and the gut is the site of the compensatory mechanism, permitting water balance to be maintained. The fish drinks the external medium and water is absorbed by the gut along with the ingested salts. The entry of sodium and chloride is compensated by branchial excretion of monovalent ions against the chemical gradient. Kidney function is characterized by the reduction of free-water clearance and excretion of the bivalent ions absorbed by the gut.

The purpose of this review is to discuss the functional differences characterizing the gill in fresh water and sea water fish.

Until recently studies on fish gills were made on whole animals, the investigator having access only to the external medium. Pioneer work in the field of membrane physiology was only possible on cellular or epithelial membranes which lend themselves to investigations *in vitro*. Only in the last 15 years has our understanding of the branchial ion transport mechanism made any progress. Perhaps the most significant advance was the discovery of the bioelectric potential generated by the branchial epithelium. This allowed for a better assessment of the driving forces which govern ion movements across the gill. The equation put forward by Goldman (1943) to describe passive ion movement in relation to the electrochemical gradient allowed the passive and active components of ion transfer to be expressed quantitatively. The introduction of radioactive tracers permitted the influx (J_{in}) and efflux (J_{out}) of ions across the gill to be measured without the mineral balance of the animal under study being disturbed. The *net* flux, i.e. the difference between these unidirectional fluxes, may in fact be modified by changes in either influx or efflux. Ussing's criterion (Ussing 1960), which relates unidirectional fluxes and electrochemical gradients, made possible a different approach to the definition of passive transport across the gill.

In this review, I shall attempt to clarify the passive and active ion transfer mechanisms which allow the gill to exhibit, alternately, two pumping activities oriented either towards the outside in sea water or towards the inside in fresh water. I shall also characterize the gill with respect to its permeability to water. Many reviews have recently covered this subject (Motais 1967; Kirschner 1970; Maetz 1971, 1974*a*; Potts 1968, 1972; Motais & Garcia-Romeu 1972).

MECHANISMS OF ION TRANSPORT IN FRESH WATER GILLS

Fig. 1 compares the values of the unidirectional sodium fluxes across the gill of the euryhaline eel (*Anguilla anguilla*) in fresh water and in sea water. In

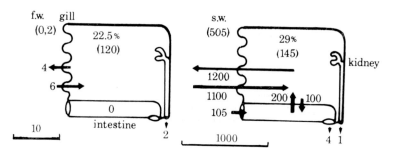

FIG. 1. Comparison of Na$^+$ exchanges in freshwater (f.w.) and sea water (s.w.) eel. External and internal sodium concentrations in µequiv./ml are given in brackets. Internal sodium space, in % body weight. Fluxes (arrow) in µequiv. h^{-1} 100 g^{-1}. Note different scales. (From Maetz 1971).

fresh water the fluxes are relatively slow, representing less than 0.1 % of the exchangeable sodium per hour. The efflux being about two-thirds of the influx, there is a net absorption rate which compensates for loss of sodium in the urine.

Sodium and chloride fluxes across the gill as a function of external concentration

In the goldfish (*Carassius auratus*), sodium and chloride influxes have been shown to vary with external sodium and chloride concentrations. Fig. 2*a* reveals that the two curves display saturation kinetics. They fit the well-known Michaelis-Menten equation:

$$J_{in} = J_{max} (C_{ext})/K_m + C_{ext} \qquad (1)$$

where J_{max} is the maximal rate of influx, J_{in}, in µequiv./(h 100 g) and K_m the Michaelis constant corresponding to C_{ext} in µequiv./l when $J_{in} = 0.5\ J_{max}$. Similar curves were described for the rainbow trout (*Salmo gairdneri*) by Kerstetter *et al.* (1970) and Kerstetter & Kirschner (1972). In some fish, for example the flounder (*Platichthys flesus*) and the eel (Motais 1967), chloride transport is much slower than sodium transport.

Fig. 2*b* shows the sodium and chloride influx curves in goldfish which had been selectively depleted of internal sodium or chloride by being kept in dilute sodium sulphate or choline chloride solutions for several weeks. It is obvious that the maximum rate of transport and the K_m are modified according to the needs of the organism. These functional variations have been interpreted as showing an increase in the number of pumping sites and in the affinity of these sites for sodium or chloride. Conversely, when the fish is salt-loaded, the number of pumping sites and the affinity of the carrier are reduced (Maetz 1974*a*).

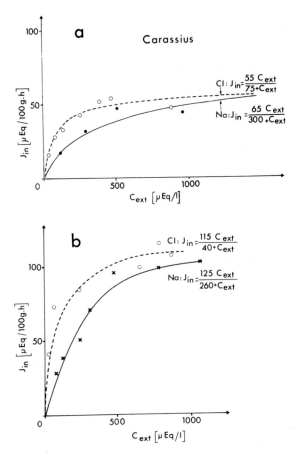

Fig. 2. Sodium and chloride influxes in goldfish (*Carassius*) as a function of external sodium or chloride concentrations. J_{in} in μequiv. h^{-1} 100 g^{-1}; C_{ext} in μequiv./l.
(*a*) Control fish studied in fresh water with added NaCl.
(*b*) Selectively Na⁺- or Cl⁻-depleted fish studied in Na_2SO_4 or choline chloride solutions (no Ca^{2+}).
The Michaelis-Menten equations are given. (Maetz 1972, 1973*a*; De Renzis & Maetz 1973.)

Fig. 3 illustrates the relationship between gill potential and external sodium and chloride concentrations in the goldfish studied in solutions of Ca^{2+}-free sodium sulphate or sodium chloride. Fish studied in choline chloride solutions yielded rather similar curves. In the lowest range of concentrations (0 to 1 mmol/l) the gill potential varied between 55 and 30 mV (negative inside). Ussing's criterion, taking into account the unidirectional fluxes measured in fish kept in this range of concentration, gives a passive equilibrium potential of

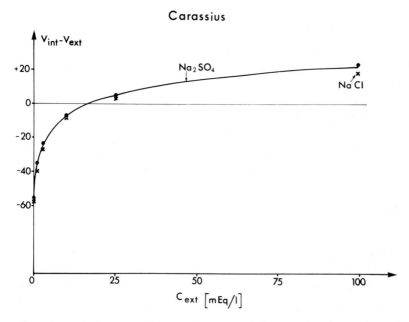

Fig. 3. Gill potential as a function of external sodium concentration in the goldfish (Maetz, unpublished). Potential ($V_{int} - V_{ext}$) in mV; Concentrations in μequiv./l. Na_2SO_4 or NaCl solutions with no Ca^{2+}.

about 190 mV, negative inside for Na^+ and positive inside for Cl^-. Thus active transport of both Na^+ and Cl^- prevails in the goldfish gill.

In the goldfish, sodium and chloride effluxes also vary with external sodium or chloride according to a Michaelis-Menten function, the flux observed in sodium-free or chloride-free media being about three to five times less than in solutions of 1 mmol/l. The change in gill potential observed with increasing sodium or chloride concentrations accounts only partially for the increase in sodium efflux and not at all for the increase in chloride efflux. At least part of these effluxes may result from a coupling between sodium influx and efflux and chloride influx and efflux (Maetz 1972; De Renzis & Maetz 1973; Kerstetter et al. 1970). When there is no external Ca^{2+}, both Na^+ and Cl^- effluxes are stimulated, the action on Cl^- being more discrete. These effects are reversed after addition of Ca^{2+} (Maetz 1974b; Eddy 1975). I have suggested that Ca^{2+} modulates the relative permeabilities of the gill to Na^+ and Cl^- and proposed (Maetz 1974b) that the gill potential is chiefly a Na^+ and Cl^- diffusion potential.

$$V_{int} - V_{ext} = \frac{RT}{F} \ln \frac{P_{Na}(Na_{ext}) + P_{Cl}(Cl_{int})}{P_{Na}(Na_{int}) + P_{Cl}(Cl_{ext})} \qquad (2)$$

where $V_{int} - V_{ext}$ is the potential in mV, R, T, F are the usual thermodynamic constants ($RT/F = 25$ mV at 17 °C), P_{Na} and P_{Cl} are the branchial permeability constants for sodium and chloride expressed in μequiv. h^{-1} 100 g^{-1}/μequiv. l^{-1}, and (Na or Cl_{ext} or $_{int}$) are the external or internal sodium or chloride concentrations in μequiv./l.

$P_{Na}/P_{Cl} = 8$ when there is no Ca^{2+} and about 1 in fresh water or in deionized water with 1.5 mmol Ca^{2+}/l. This change in the relative permeabilities of the gill to sodium and chloride explains why potentials measured in fresh water or in Ca^{2+}-enriched external media are much smaller than those reported in Fig. 3.

Independence of sodium and chloride absorptions: occurrence of separate ionic exchange processes

The curves illustrated in Fig. 2b were obtained from fish studied in either sodium sulphate or choline chloride solutions. Garcia-Romeu & Maetz (1964) showed that sulphate and choline are impermeant ions. Thus Na^+ or Cl^- may be taken up without being accompanied by a permeant co-ion. This independence of Na^+ and Cl^- uptake had already been noted by Krogh (1939). He also observed that when fish selectively depleted of sodium or chloride are returned to a NaCl solution they absorb one ion species and exclude the other.

Absorption of an ion without an accompanying *co-ion* suggests that the ion is taken up in exchange for a *counter-ion*. Krogh (1939) suggested that NH_4^+ and HCO_3^- are the endogenous ions excreted against Na^+ and Cl^- respectively. This would explain why in fish the gill and not the kidney is the major site of ammonia excretion and why most aquatic animals excrete their nitrogenous wastes in the form of ammonia. Maetz & Garcia-Romeu (1964) confirmed Krogh's theory. They showed that addition of ammonium ions to the external medium depressed Na^+ uptake in the goldfish, while injection of ammonium ions stimulated it. Parallel experiments with HCO_3^- confirmed the HCO_3^-/Cl exchange.

A more direct demonstration of this latter exchange was obtained in the goldfish (De Renzis & Maetz 1973). Applying the titration techniques developed for the frog by Garcia-Romeu *et al.* (1969), we showed that there is a direct correlation between base excretion and Cl^- uptake (Fig. 4). A correlation between ammonia excretion and Na^+ uptake has only been demonstrated recently. De Vooys (1968) observed that carp (*Cyprinus carpio*) kept in deionized water where no Na^+ absorption can occur still excrete ammonia. This was confirmed in the trout (Kerstetter *et al.* 1970) and in the goldfish (Maetz 1973a). Kirschner (1970) made the interesting suggestion that H^+ ions rather

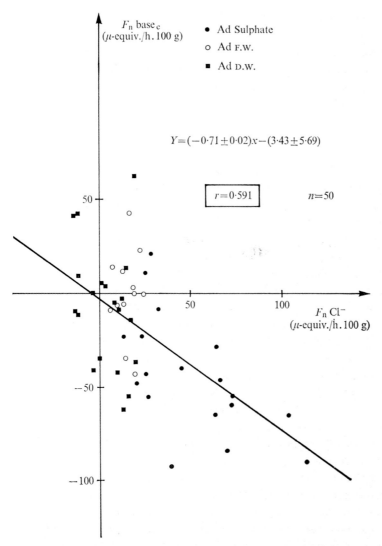

FIG. 4. Correlation between the net flux of base (presumably HCO_3^-) and Cl^- uptake from a choline chloride solution (goldfish, adapted to sodium sulphate solution, fresh [F.W.] or deionized water [D.W.]). Base excretion corrected from ammonia excretion (see De Renzis & Maetz 1973). Net fluxes in μequiv. h^{-1} 100 g^{-1}.

than NH_4^+ may serve as counter-ions for Na^+ uptake. Garcia-Romeu et al. (1969) had demonstrated that H^+ was the counter-ion exchanged against Na^+ in frogs, which are uricotelic and lose small quantities of ammonia through their skin. In our recent review of these controversial aspects of Na^+ and Cl^-

uptake in fresh water fish (Maetz *et al.* 1975), we report that in the goldfish, *in vivo* H^+ ion excretion matches Na^+ net uptake, while in the perfused head of trout (technique in Payan & Matty 1975), a direct correlation between Na^+ influx and ammonia excretion rate is observed. We suggest that H^+ as well as NH_4^+ participate in the exchange and that in some situations fish excrete NH_3 in the un-ionized form.

Inhibitors of Na^+ and Cl^- uptake in fresh water fish

The teleostean gill has long been known to have a high activity of carbonate dehydratase (EC 4.2.1.1; carbonic anhydrase) (Leiner 1938; Maetz 1956a). Interest attaches to this enzyme because it catalyses the hydration of carbon dioxide, making available HCO_3^- and H^+, the counter-ions discussed in the preceding paragraph. If this enzyme plays a key role in the ion absorption mechanism, injection of acetazolamide should inhibit uptake of both Na^+ and Cl^-. Such an effect has indeed been demonstrated in the goldfish (Maetz 1956b; Maetz & Garcia-Romeu 1964). In the trout, Kerstetter *et al.* (1970) confirm that Na^+ uptake was inhibited by acetazolamide. The fact that ammonia excretion remained undisturbed by this inhibitor suggested that there was no linkage between Na^+ absorption and ammonia excretion. However, using the perfused head preparation, P. Payan (unpublished work) has recently found that inhibition of carbonate dehydratase simultaneously blocks Na^+ influx and ammonia loss. Kerstetter & Kirschner (1972) also failed to observe any effect of acetazolamide on Cl^- uptake. This is being reinvestigated on the perfused head preparation.

The two other inhibitors used are more specific in that they block Na^+ and Cl^- uptake independently. One of these is amiloride, a potassium-sparing diuretic compound which is known to cause a rapid and reversible inhibition of sodium transport in frog skin (Ehrlich & Crabbé 1968). While Cuthbert & Maetz (1972) found this drug to be rather ineffective in the goldfish, Kirschner *et al.* (1973) showed that it inhibits Na^+ influx by about 80%, Na^+ efflux and Cl^- exchange remaining undisturbed in the trout. Excretion of the counter-ions was found to be depressed—H^+ excretion by 50% and ammonia excretion by 30%. This suggests that both endogenous ions intervene in the exchange. The second inhibitor, thiocyanate (SCN^-), is an ion found in the lyotropic series of Cl^-. Krogh (1949) discovered that after addition of SCN^- to the external medium, Cl^- loss replaces Cl^- uptake in many fresh water animals. Epstein *et al.* (1973) confirmed, in the goldfish, that low concentrations of SCN^- inhibit Cl^- influx while Na^+ absorption continues unchanged. More recently, similar results were published for the trout (Kerstetter & Kirschner

1974). De Renzis (1974) demonstrated that the goldfish gill is impermeant to thiocyanate and that chloride influx and efflux were both depressed simultaneously, as would be expected from a coupling between chloride influx and efflux. Furthermore, De Renzis observed that when, under the influence of thiocyanate, chloride loss replaces chloride uptake, excretion of the counter-ion HCO_3^- is replaced by its absorption from the external medium. Thus the Cl^-/HCO_3^- exchange seems obligatory and functions in both directions.

Significance of these exchange mechanisms in relation to the maintenance of acid-base balance and respiratory gas exchanges

Dejours (1969) had already indicated an obligatory HCO_3^-/Cl^- exchange. He observed that when the external medium of the goldfish was suddenly changed from a solution of NaCl to one of Na_2SO_4 there was a sharp reduction of the CO_2 output. In some animals, CO_2 was even absorbed from the external medium for as long as 24 h. When these animals were returned to a NaCl solution, CO_2 excretion was resumed and was considerably enhanced.

As oxygen has a relatively low solubility in water, the fish has to maintain a high rate of flow over the gills in order to meet its oxygen demand. From recent work on fish respiration, it emerges that fish cannot jeopardize oxygen uptake in order to regulate the Pco_2 and pH of the blood, as mammals would do, by varying their ventilation rates. It is plasma HCO_3^- rather than Pco_2 which is adjusted because it can be modulated independently of ventilation volume and oxygen transfer rates. These adjustments are effected by way of the branchial HCO_3^-/Cl^- exchange mechanism. Experiments on the effects of an increase in ambient CO_2 or O_2 or of acclimation to various temperatures all point to the importance of this exchange in the maintenance of the acid–base balance of the body fluids (Lloyd & White 1967; Cameron & Randall 1972; Randall & Cameron 1973; P. Dejours, personal communication). Conversely, readjustment of the mineral balance may likewise be associated with changes in the acid–base balance. De Renzis & Maetz (1973) reported that attempts to deplete the goldfish selectively of internal sodium or chloride (see Fig. 2) are accompanied by considerable changes in plasma pH. Sodium depletion leads to acidosis and NH_4^+ accumulation, while chloride depletion is accompanied by alkalosis and HCO_3^- accumulation.

As I pointed out in 1971, 'the fish gill is a multi-purpose organ, specialized for respiratory gas exchanges, the clearance of waste products of nitrogenous metabolism and the maintenance of acid-base and mineral balance... Most of these various and apparently unrelated functions may be in fact intimately linked'.

MECHANISMS OF BRANCHIAL ION TRANSPORT IN SEA WATER

The first attempt to use radioactive tracers in the study of teleostean osmoregulation was made by Mullins (1950). He found that the rate of Na^+
exchange was very slow in the fresh water stickleback (*Gasterosteus aculeatus*)
and rather rapid in salt water. For the salt water fish, he interpreted his results
in terms of the Homer Smith model (Smith 1930). The total influx of Na^+ was
thought to be accounted for by drinking, while the efflux was assumed to occur
across the gill. Mullins' work was not followed up until 10 to 15 years later
when Motais (1961) showed that in the euryhaline flounder the Na^+ turnover
rate involves 25% of the internal Na^+ per hour in sea water, while in fresh
water it accounts for less than 1%. Measuring simultaneously the drinking
and Na^+ exchange rates in this fish, Motais & Maetz (1965) discovered that
the sodium swallowed represents only one-fifth of the sodium influx, the
remainder occurring through the gill. Urinary Na^+ loss accounts for less than
0.1% of the Na^+ efflux. Thus practically all the Na^+ efflux passes across the
gill. These observations on the relative importance of the various sites of ionic
exchange have since been extended to many sea water teleosts. We have
found that Cl^- is exchanged at rates rather similar to those of Na^+.

The first attempt to measure the electric potential across the gill was made
by House (1963). He found that the body fluids of the sea water blenny,
Blennius pholis, were positive to the external medium, and concluded that Cl^-
excretion by the gill was active, being against both electrical and chemical
gradients. For Na^+, however, the chemical gradient is in part or totally
compensated by the electrical gradient. All the subsequent observations of
this kind confirmed House's initial discovery. Whether there is an active
component of sodium excretion or not remains a matter of dispute. Maetz &
Campanini (1966) were the first to observe that transfer of the sea water eel,
Anguilla anguilla, from sea water to fresh water was followed by a reversal of
the gill potential from $+20$ to -50 mV (with reference to the inside milieu),
while in the fresh-water-adapted fish the potential is only -20 mV. Motais
(1961) had shown several years before that transfer from sea water to fresh
water induced instantaneous changes in the Na^+ efflux of the flounder. It is
only recently that the simultaneous potential and flux adjustments in relation
to external salinity changes have been fully understood.

*Sodium influx and efflux readjustments and potential changes in relation to
external salinity*

Motais (1967) measured sodium influx in the sea-water-adapted flounder,
Platichthys flesus, as a function of rapid changes in external salinity. As in

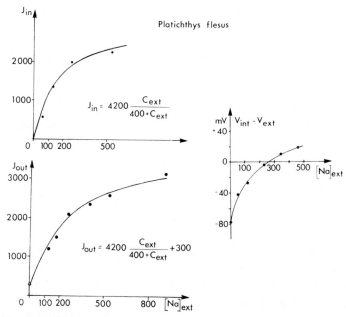

FIG. 5. Sodium influx and efflux (Motais 1967) and gill potential (Potts & Eddy 1973) as a function of external sodium concentration in the sea water flounder, *Platichthys flesus*. Fluxes in μequiv. h^{-1} 100 g^{-1} and $V_{int} - V_{ext}$ in mV. Concentrations in mequiv./l. The Michaelis-Menten equations are given.

fresh water teleosts, sodium influx varies according to a curvilinear function which was interpreted in terms of Michaelis-Menten kinetics (see Fig. 5). The maximal flux is however 4000 μequiv. instead of 35 μequiv. h^{-1} 100 g^{-1}, while the K_m (400 mequiv./l) is 500 times higher. Motais suggested that there was a carrier with a poor affinity for Na$^+$ in the gill. When he studied the changes in sodium efflux in relation to external salinity, he found that the major part of the sodium efflux likewise varied according to a curvilinear function almost identical with that describing Na$^+$ influx. A small part of the Na$^+$ efflux (about a fifth of the total flux) seemed to be independent of external sodium. Motais proposed that the sodium influx and most of the sodium efflux were both effected by a carrier responsible for a coupling between these fluxes, an 'exchange–diffusion' carrier. The small sodium efflux component that was independent of external sodium was thought to represent the sodium pump. If the fish were kept for a longer time in fresh water, this small residual sodium efflux declined slowly, as if the pump were progressively shut off. Similar observations were made on numerous stenohaline and euryhaline teleosts. Differences were seen in the relative importance of the sodium-dependent and independent sodium efflux components: for example, in the euryhaline killifish (*Fundulus heteroclitus*) and in the stenohaline sea perch (*Serranus cabrilla*), the latter component attained about 60 to 70% of the total Na efflux. In the euryhaline fish, the residual efflux observed after transfer to fresh water was, however, subjected to a powerful secondary regulation which checked sodium loss. In the stenohaline species, sodium loss continued unheeded and the fish died.

The model proposed by Motais (1967) was soon criticized by Smith (1969) on the grounds that it ignores the gill potential. The flux-force relationship prevailing across the gill of the sea water fish does not clearly point to the existence of a sodium pump. Potts & Eddy (1973) reinvestigated the pattern of readjustment of sodium in the flounder in relation to changes in external salinity and simultaneously measured the gill potential. They confirmed that the potential switches from +20 to −70 mV (with reference to the body fluids) on transfer from sea water to fresh water, while in intermediate salinities it follows a curvilinear function not unlike that observed for the unidirectional fluxes (see Fig. 5). They discovered that Na^+ and not Cl^- was the ion responsible for the potential pattern. For instance, after the fish was transferred into Cl^--free sea water made up with impermeant monovalent anions, the gill potential remained the same as in sea water. After the fish was transferred into Na^+-free sea water, however, the potential reversed just as it did in fresh water. Potts & Eddy (1973) proposed that the potential was chiefly a diffusion potential described by the equation (2) proposed for the goldfish (p. 137). They calculated that the P_{Na}/P_{Cl} ratio was about 30, and they also suggested that if the gill potential is a sodium diffusion potential, the sodium exchanges across the gill must occur independently and by free diffusion. Moreover, they demonstrated that the changes in sodium efflux in relation to external salinity were satisfactorily explained by the Goldman (1943) equation which takes into account the changes in potential. Almost simultaneously Kirschner *et al.* (1974), from their study of the sodium efflux changes and potential adjustments in the trout, likewise conclude that the exchange–diffusion theory is untenable. More recent investigations on the sea water mullet (*Mugil capito*) in our laboratory suggest that, in this species at least, sodium is probably transferred by a combination of both free diffusion and exchange diffusion processes (Maetz & Pic 1974; Pic & Maetz 1975). For instance, when fish were transferred from sea water to isotonic Ringer or to a solution of 50 mM-Na_2SO_4, the potential decreased by 15 mV or even reversed to −20 mV, while the sodium efflux remained practically unchanged. This suggests that a saturation process exists which is independent of potential changes.

Importance of external potassium in sodium efflux and potential readjustments

Epstein *et al.* (1967) and Kamyia & Utida (1968) discovered substantial increases in the Na/K-dependent adenosinetriphosphatase (EC 3.6.1.3; ATPase) activity in homogenates of the gills of *Fundulus heteroclitus* and the Japanese eel (*Anguilla japonica*). This enzyme was thought to be related to the increased salt load incurred by the fish in salt water and excreted by the gill. In 1969 I proposed a model suggesting that sodium extrusion is effected by an exchange of sodium and potassium which is catalysed by ATPase. Sodium efflux in the flounder was found to be stimulated not only by external Na^+ but also by external potassium, a cation which is present in sea water at a concentration of 10–12 mmol/l. Variations of sodium efflux with external potassium also showed saturation kinetics. Moreover potassium at low concentrations was found to be far more effective than sodium in stimulating sodium efflux. Fig. 6*a* illustrates this point. Furthermore, when the potassium influx was measured as a function of external potassium, the relationship between these two variables was similar to that displayed by the potassium-dependent sodium efflux (Maetz 1973*b*); this therefore suggested that there was a carrier with high affinity for external potassium, a carrier which could be a Na/K ATPase localized on the apical membrane of the branchial 'chloride cells'. In sea water, owing to the high concentration of Na^+ (50 times that of K^+), a competition between the two cations for the potassium site of the enzyme was thought to occur, allowing Na^+ to enter in exchange for internal Na^+. Thus sodium exchange–diffusion would stem from the Na/K ATPase exchange mechanism. The hypothesis that a Na/K exchange carrier is related to the Na/K ATPase activity is substantiated by two types of experiments. Transfer of the flounder, the sea perch and the fat sleeper (*Dormitator maculatus*) into potassium-free salt water is followed by a reversible decrease in sodium efflux and a rise in the plasma sodium level (Maetz 1969; Motais & Isaia 1972*b*; Evans *et al.* 1973). In some fish such as *Dormitator* and *Anguilla* the addition of ouabain (an inhibitor of Na/K ATPase) to the external medium produces an inhibition of the sodium efflux and a rise in plasma sodium (Motais & Isaia 1972*b*; Evans *et al.* 1973). Some discordant observations have however been made. In the eel kept in potassium-free salt water, no significant rise in plasma sodium is observed. In the sea perch, flounder or trout, addition of ouabain to the external medium does not change the sodium efflux (Forrest & Epstein 1972; Motais & Isaia 1972*b*; Kirschner 1973).

The Na/K exchange theory has recently been criticized on the same grounds as the sodium exchange–diffusion hypothesis. Potts & Eddy (1973) (flounder), House & Maetz (1974) (eel) and Greenwald *et al.* (1974) (trout) observed that

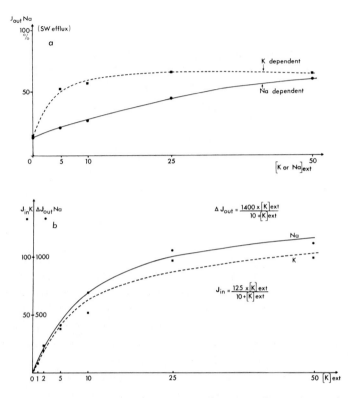

FIG. 6. Sodium- and potassium-dependent sodium efflux and potassium influx in the sea water flounder (Maetz 1969, 1973*b*).
(*a*) Comparison of potassium-dependent and sodium-dependent sodium efflux in % of the sea water efflux.
(*b*) Comparison of potassium influx and potassium-dependent sodium efflux in μequiv. h^{-1} 100 g^{-1}. The Michaelis-Menten equations are given. Concentrations in mequiv./l.

addition of potassium to fresh water depolarizes the gill, which on the basis of the sodium diffusion theory would explain the increase in sodium efflux. Moreover potassium is more potent than sodium in producing these potential changes. This parallels its higher efficiency in 'driving sodium out of the fish'. These observations suggest that potassium participates in the generation of gill potential and that equation (2) (p. 137) should be completed by inclusion of P_K, (K_{ext}) and (K_{int}). All these investigators agree that P_K/P_{Na} is greater than 1 in the various species of fish studied so far. It is evident that at least part, if not all, the Na/K exchanges must be diffusive in nature. Recent quantitative studies by Evans *et al.* (1974) on *Dormitator* and by Maetz & Pic (1974; see also Maetz & Bornancin, 1975) on *Mugil* show, however, that the experimental curve for the changes in Na^+ efflux in relation to external potassium differs widely from that expected from the Goldman (1943) equation for diffusive sodium fluxes in relation to changes in gill potential. For example, transfer of *Mugil* from salt water into a potassium salt solution (20 mM) reverses the potential from $+20$ mV to -10 mV, while the sodium efflux remains unchanged. Thus it seems that Na/K exchanges occur by means of a carrier which is uninfluenced by changes in potential or by free diffusion processes.

Evidence for a chloride pump linked to the Na/K carrier

There is no doubt that Cl^- is excreted actively by the gill. Recent evidence suggests that the chloride pump is responsible for a small part of the gill potential, the major part being the result of sodium and potassium diffusion (Shuttleworth et al. 1974; Pic & Maetz 1975). The electrogenicity of the chloride pump is demonstrated by the significant decrease in the gill potential produced in the flounder and the mullet when thiocyanate is injected into them. SCN has been discovered by Epstein et al. (1973) to be an inhibitor of the chloride pump in the eel.

For technical reasons, the evolution of the chloride influx and efflux as a function of external changes in chloride concentration has not been investigated. Transfer from salt water to fresh water, however, causes a parallel decrease of the sodium and chloride effluxes in many but not all fish (see review by Maetz 1974a). This 'chloride-free effect' is independent of the 'sodium-free effect' seen when the flounder is transferred into sodium-free or chloride-free sea water (Motais 1967). However, Potts & Eddy (1973) have observed that of these two media only sodium-free sea water induces a reversal of the gill potential. Thus the behaviour of the sodium efflux, i.e. no readjustment in chloride-free sea water and instantaneous reduction in sodium-free sea water, is explained in the light of the sodium free-diffusion theory. The chloride efflux behaviour, however, is not explained by these changes in potential: it remains unchanged in sodium-free sea water despite the change in potential and decreases sharply in chloride-free sea water, when there is no change in potential. Moreover, after the fish is transferred to fresh water, the chloride efflux declines, while the reversal of potential would be expected to increase the chloride efflux. Thus the chloride efflux pattern can only be explained by assuming the existence of a chloride pump associated with an exchange–diffusion mechanism uninfluenced by changes in potential.

Epstein et al. (1973) discovered that SCN injected into the intraperitoneal cavity of the eel produces a 60–70% inhibition in the chloride efflux, with the sodium efflux remaining unchanged. SCN produces a rise in both plasma sodium and chloride within a few hours of injection. It may therefore be suggested that extrusion is in some way linked to sodium extrusion. If sodium extrusion is effected by a Na/K exchange mechanism it would be expected that SCN would block the enhancing effect of potassium on the sodium efflux. This is indeed what is observed. Furthermore if chloride extrusion is linked to the Na/K exchange, the addition of potassium to fresh water should enhance not only the sodium efflux but also the chloride efflux. Indeed Epstein *et al.* (1973) observed such a parallel activation. More recently, we have done the same experiments on the mullet (Maetz & Pic 1974; see also Maetz & Bornancin 1975). When we measured gill potential and sodium efflux simultaneously, we noted that the depolarizing effect of potassium remained unchanged after SCN poisoning. Thus the chloride efflux associated with the Na/K exchange process seems to be independent of the gill potential. Furthermore, we showed that the gill was indeed impermeant to SCN, and thus SCN could on no account be excreted by the gill at the expense of Cl^-. Fig. 7 illustrates experiments on the activation effect of potassium on the chloride efflux and the inhibition of that effect by SCN. In the eel, Epstein *et al.* (1973) noted that the chloride efflux observed with SCN inhibition in sea water was more or less identical to the chloride efflux recorded upon transfer to fresh water. They suggested that simultaneous inhibition of the chloride pump entails an inhibition of the chloride exchange–diffusion process.

Importance of Ca^{2+} in gill phenomena

Potts & Fleming (1971) discovered that when *Fundulus kansae* were kept in Ca^{2+}-free or Mg^{2+}-free sea water, the sodium turnover rate was considerably enhanced. Bornancin *et al.* (1972) studied in detail the effects of Ca^{2+} removal on the sea water eel. Fish kept overnight in Ca^{2+}-free sea water showed a raised plasma sodium and sodium space. Sodium influx and efflux across the gill were double those in controls. The effect on sodium influx was annulled within 1 h by the addition of Ca^{2+}, while the effect on efflux was only partially reduced. The sodium leak measured after transfer of the Ca^{2+}-depleted fish to deionized water was found to be increased 3.5-fold, this effect being annulled within 15 h of addition of Ca^{2+}. In Ca^{2+}-depleted fish, the ability of potassium to enhance the sodium efflux was found to be appreciably depressed. Within 15 h of Ca^{2+} being added the Na/K exchange was considerably enhanced. Recently, J. Isaia and A. Masoni (unpublished work) have confirmed these results in eels kept for a much shorter time in Ca^{2+}-free and Mg^{2+}-free salt water. We have extended these observations to the mullet and the flounder (Pic & Maetz 1975; and unpublished work). The mullet proved extremely

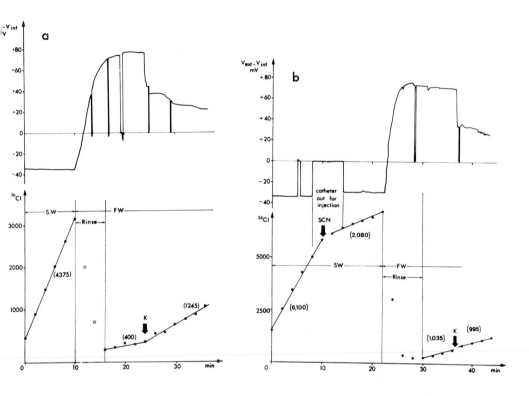

FIG. 7. Chloride efflux and gill potential in the sea water mullet (Maetz & Pic, unpublished).
(*a*) Transfer of control fish from sea water to fresh water; effect of external potassium.
(*b*) Action of SCN injected during the sea water period. Note absence of potassium effect.
Upper trace: $V_{ext} - V_{int}$ in mV.
Lower trace: ^{36}Cl appearance in external bath in c.p.m./ml.
Abscissae: time in min.

sensitive to Ca^{2+} removal. Transfer of this fish from fresh water to deionized water is accompanied by a 2.5-fold increase in the sodium efflux and a smaller increase in the chloride efflux. Addition of Ca^{2+} at the concentration found in sea water, i.e. 10 mmol/l, produced a threefold decrease in the sodium efflux and a twofold decrease in the chloride efflux as well as an instantaneous depolarization of the gill. We suggest (Pic & Maetz 1975) that Ca^{2+} decreases the gill permeability to Na^+, while Cl^- permeability is altered very little. As the gill potential is mainly a diffusion potential dependent on the relative cation: anion permeabilities, the depolarizing effect of Ca^{2+} is thus explained. Similar observations were made on frog and rabbit gall bladders by Diamond and his colleagues (see review by Moreno & Diamond 1975). We have also observed

(Pic & Maetz, unpublished) that after transfer into deionized water, the enhancing effect of potassium on the chloride and sodium effluxes was no longer observed. If, however, the fish were transferred into deionized water with added Ca^{2+} (1 mmol/l), activation of the sodium efflux by potassium was restored without there being an enhancement of chloride efflux by potassium. For this effect to be obtained, HCO_3^- ions (1 mol/l) had to be present in the external medium. Thus, recent observations point to dual Na^+/K^+ and HCO_3/Cl^- exchange mechanisms. The flounder however proved rather unresponsive to Ca^{2+} removal. Motais (1967) had already noted that the sodium efflux was the same whether transferred into fresh or deionized water. After three to four hours of pretreatment in Ca^{2+}-free and Mg^{2+}-free sea water, the sodium efflux observed in sea water increased by 66% while the leak in deionized water was augmented by 100%. The effect of potassium on sodium efflux remained unaltered, however. After only 15–60 min in Ca^{2+}-free and Mg^{2+}-free sea water with added EDTA (1 mmol/l) the sodium efflux is increased by 2.5- to fourfold, while the sodium leak into deionized water is increased by six- to tenfold. Furthermore, the potassium activation effect on sodium efflux is completely abolished, thus confirming the impairment of the sodium extrusion mechanism.

The role of Ca^{2+} in active transport of chloride and its associated Na/K exchange process is currently under investigation in our laboratory.

The inhibitory effects of SCN and the possibility of a HCO_3^-/Cl^- exchange suggest that an anion-sensitive ATPase may be operative in fish gills. Such an enzyme has been discovered in the mitochondrial and microsomal fractions of gill homogenates in the trout (Kerstetter & Kirschner 1974) and in the eel (Maetz & Bornancin 1975). This Mg-ATPase is activated by HCO_3^- and inhibited by SCN. However, the absence of any chloride activation argues against this enzyme having a role in the chloride pump.

CHARACTERISTICS OF BRANCHIAL WATER PERMEABILITY

Both osmotic (P_{os}) and diffusional (P_d) water permeabilities have been measured in fish gills. P_d was estimated by following the radioactive efflux of fish injected with tritiated water (HTO) (Evans 1969; review by Maetz 1974a). Motais et al. (1969) demonstrated that cardiac output was not likely to be a limiting factor for the diffusional HTO efflux. External unstirred layers between branchial secondary lamellae may well be of little importance because the branchial surface is extremely well stirred in vivo. P_d values may however be underestimated because of unstirred layers within the secondary lamellae. Fig. 8 illustrates the comparison of the HTO appearance rates observed in

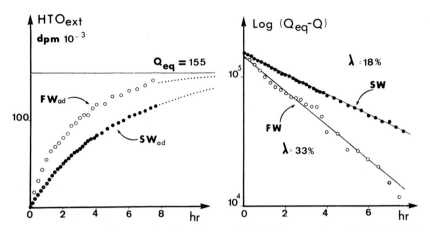

FIG. 8. Rate of appearance of tritiated water (HTO) in sea-water-adapted (SWad) and fresh-water-adapted (FWad) flounders (Motais *et al.* 1969).
Left: HTO appearance in external bath in d.p.m./ml.
Right: $Q_{eq} - Q_t$ (difference between radioactivity attained at equilibrium and radioactivity at time t) on a semi-log plot.
Abscissa: time in min.
Note the turnover rates in %/h (λ).

fresh water and sea water flounders, showing that branchial water permeability is apparently higher in fresh-water-adapted specimens.

Until recently P_{os} was estimated indirectly. In fresh water fish, as urine flow compensates for net inflow of water across the gills and gut, the branchial net flow was taken to be the difference between urine flow and drinking rate. In sea water fish, as the drinking rate is assumed to compensate for urinary and branchial water losses, branchial water loss was taken to be the difference between drinking rate and urine flow. As different groups of fish were used for determining urine flow and drinking rate, and as the water content of the fish used in these experiments was assumed to be in equilibrium, this indirect method is bound to yield unreliable results. More recently, Shuttleworth & Freeman (1974) and J. Isaia & T. Hirano (in preparation) have directly measured water loss and water gain of gills *in vitro* by following the weight changes of gills dipped in either hyperosmotic or hypo-osmotic media. According to Isaia & Hirano the results thus obtained yield P_{os} values in the same range as those obtained indirectly by Motais & Isaia (1972a). Shuttleworth & Freeman (1974), however, find P_{os} values about 10 times smaller than those of Motais & Isaia (1972a). This discrepancy may be explained, at least in part, by the fact that Shuttleworth & Freeman used eels about 20 times heavier than those used by Motais & Isaia.

Motais & Isaia (1972a) found that the P_{os} value for the gill of the fresh water eel, measured in fresh water, was about four times higher than that observed for the gill of the sea water eel measured in sea water, while Shuttleworth & Freeman (1974) recorded no difference whatsoever. Moreover, Isaia & Hirano discovered that the P_{os} measured in the mucosal–serosal direction was significantly different from that in the serosal–mucosal direction, suggesting the phenomenon of 'rectification of flow' already described in other epithelial membranes. Measuring P_{os} in both directions, they discovered that in fact the sea water eel gill is more permeable than the fresh water eel gill when mucosal to serosal P_{os} is considered by measuring the rate of swelling of gills dipped in fresh water. The gill of the fresh water eel is however more permeable than the sea water gill when serosal to mucosal P_{os} is measured by following the rate of shrinkage of gills dipped in sea water. The HTO permeabilities reported above were measured in the serosal to mucosal direction.

Table 1 compares the P_d and P_{os} values for various epithelia. It may be seen that the gill of the teleostean fish is one of the most impermeable membranes whether P_{os} or P_d values are considered. It is also evident that the ratio P_{os}/P_d is very nearly equal to 1, at least in the sea water teleostean gills. This would mean that movement of water across the gill is restricted to very small pores, of the dimensions of the water molecule, thus excluding bulk flow. For calculating P_{os}, however, the gill was assumed to be semi-permeable. This condition may not be fulfilled because the gill in sea water is the site of very fast diffusional flows of ions which may interfere with water movement. This possibility deserves further study. It has been assumed that the fish gill is not the site of water movement caused by solute movement. Such water movements would be in the same direction as osmotically driven water movements (inwards in fresh water and outwards in sea water) and thus would be contrary to the needs of the organism. However, the independence of water and solute movements across the gill has yet to be unequivocally demonstrated.

CONCLUSION

Until recently, few papers about branchial mechanisms were being published. Now, in almost every issue of journals devoted to comparative physiology or experimental biology, several papers appear on this topic. I have often indulged in presenting models of gill functioning. These have rightly been considered as a challenge. It is tempting to generalize on experimental evidence derived from a few species, but one must remember that there are 50 000 species of fish.

Progress in the years to come may be predicted to occur in various directions. Observations on the relation between structure and function in the 'chloride

TABLE 1

Osmotic and diffusional permeabilities of epithelia of organs of various species

Epithelia	P_d ($\mu m/s$)	P_{os} ($\mu m/s$)	P_{os}/P_d	References
Kidney				
Rat proximal tubule	56	2300	41	
Rat distal tubule	16	380	24	
Rabbit collecting duct	3.8	69	18	
Gall bladder				
Dog	1.1	68	62.5	
Fish	0.8	63	76	
Cloaca				
Chicken	0.8	31	36	
Intestine				House 1974
Human ileum	0.2	24	120	
Eel	0.7	47	70	
Gastric mucosa				
Frog	0.5	11	22	
Dog	0.4	6	15	
Urinary bladder				
Frog	1	7.7	7.7	
Skin				
Frog	0.55	5.5	10	
Toad	1.5	23.6	16	
Gills				
Flounder (fresh water)	0.3	0.7	2.6	Motais & Isaia 1972a
Flounder (sea water)	0.17	0.14	0.8	
Goldfish	0.25	1.3	5.2	Motais et al. 1969
Sea perch	0.12	0.16	1.3	
Dogfish (elasmobranch)	0.56	8.1	14.5	Payan & Maetz 1971

cells' which are presumably the sites of ionic transport may prove particularly fruitful, and biochemical investigations of the chloride pump may yield interesting results. One of the most surprising developments in recent years has been the interest that students of respiratory physiology have shown in the fish gill because of the interplay of gaseous and ionic exchanges it shows in relation to acid–base balance. I thought that this interplay was restricted to aquatic animals. This symposium shows that I was wrong.

References

BORNANCIN, M., CUTHBERT, A. W. & MAETZ, J. (1972) *J. Physiol. (Lond.)* 222, 487-496
CAMERON, J. N. & RANDALL, D. J. (1972) *J. Exp. Biol.* 57, 673-680

CUTHBERT, A. W. & MAETZ, J. (1972) *Comp. Biochem. Physiol. 43A*, 227-232
DEJOURS, P. (1969) *J. Physiol. (Lond.) 202*, 113-114P
DE RENZIS, G. (1974) *J. Physiol. (Paris,) 69*, 290A
DE RENZIS, G. & MAETZ, J. (1973) *J. Exp. Biol. 59*, 339-358
DE VOOYS, C. G. N. (1968) *Arch. Int. Physiol. Biochim. 76*, 268-273
EDDY, F. B. (1975) *J. Comp. Physiol. 96*, 131-142
EHRLICH, E. N. & CRABBÉ, J. (1968) *Pflügers Arch. Gesamte Physiol. 302*, 79-96
EPSTEIN, F. H., KATZ, A. E. & PICKFORD, G. E. (1967) *Science (Wash. D.C.) 156*, 1245-1247
EPSTEIN, F. H., MAETZ, J. & DE RENZIS, G. (1973) *Am. J. Physiol. 224*, 1295-1299
EVANS, D. H. (1969) *J. Exp. Biol. 50*, 689-704
EVANS, D. H., MALLERY, C. H. & KRAVITZ, L. (1973) *J. Exp. Biol. 58*, 627-636
EVANS, D. H., CARRIER, J. C. & BOGAN, M. B. (1974) *J. Exp. Biol. 61*, 277-283
FORREST, J. N. & EPSTEIN, F. H. (1972) *Bull. Mt. Desert Isl. Biol. Lab. 12*, 35
FREDERICQ, L. (1901) *Bull. Acad. R. Belg. Cl. Sci. 38*, 428-454
GARCIA-ROMEU, F. & MAETZ, J. (1964) *J. Gen. Physiol. 47*, 1195-1207
GARCIA-ROMEU, F., SALIBIAN, A. & PEZZANI-HERNANDEZ, S. (1969) *J. Gen. Physiol. 53*, 816-835
GOLDMAN, D. E. (1943) *J. Gen. Physiol. 27*, 37-60
GREENWALD, J., KIRSCHNER, L. B. & SANDERS, M. (1974) *J. Gen. Physiol. 64*, 135-147
HOUSE, C. R. (1963) *J. Exp. Biol. 40*, 47-104
HOUSE, C. R. (1974) *Water Transport in Cells and Tissues*, Edward Arnold, London
HOUSE, C. R. & MAETZ, J. (1974) *Comp. Biochem. Physiol. 47A*, 917-924
KAMYIA, M. & UTIDA, S. (1968) *Comp. Biochem. Physiol. 43B*, 611-617
KERSTETTER, T. K. & KIRSCHNER, L. B. (1972) *J. Exp. Biol. 56*, 263-272
KERSTETTER, T. H. & KIRSCHNER, L. B. (1974) *Comp. Biochem. Physiol. 48B*, 581-589
KERSTETTER, T. H. & KIRSCHNER, L. B. & RAFUSE, D. D. (1970) *J. Gen. Physiol. 56*, 342-359
KIRSCHNER, L. B. (1970) *Am. Zool. 10*, 365-376
KIRSCHNER, L. B. (1973) See discussion of paper by Maetz (1973*b*)
KIRSCHNER, L. B., GREENWALD, L. & KERSTETTER, T. H. (1973) *Am. J. Physiol. 224*, 832-837
KIRSCHNER, L. B., GREENWALD, L. & SANDERS, M. (1974) *J. Gen. Physiol. 64*, 148-165
KROGH, A. (1939) *Osmotic Regulation in Aquatic Animals*, Cambridge University Press
LEINER, M. (1938) *Z. Vgl. Physiol. 26*, 416-466
LLOYD, R. & WHITE, W. R. (1967) *Nature (Lond.) 216*, 1341-1342
MAETZ, J. (1956*a*) *Bull. Biol. Fr. Belg.* (suppl.) *40*, 1-129
MAETZ, J. (1956*b*) *J. Physiol. (Paris) 48*, 1085-1099
MAETZ, J. (1969) *Science (Wash. D.C.) 166*, 613-615
MAETZ, J. (1971) *Philos. Trans. R. Soc. Lond. B Biol. Sci. 262*, 209-249
MAETZ, J. (1972) *J. Exp. Biol. 56*, 601-620
MAETZ, J. (1973*a*) *J. Exp. Biol. 58*, 255-275
MAETZ, J. (1973*b*) in *Transport Mechanisms in Epithelia (Alfred Benzon Symp. 5)*, (Ussing, H. H. & Thorn, N. A. eds), pp. 427-441, Munskgaard, Copenhagen
MAETZ, J. (1974*a*) in *Biochemical and Biophysical Perspectives in Marine Biology*, vol. 1 (Malins, D. C. & Sargent, J. R., eds.), pp. 1-167 Academic Press, London
MAETZ, J. (1974*b*) *C. R. Hebd. Séances Acad. Sci. Sér. D Sci. Nat. 279*, 1277-1280
MAETZ, J. & BORNANCIN, M. (1975) *Fortsch. Zool. 23*, 322-362
MAETZ, J. & CAMPANINI, G. (1966) *J. Physiol. (Paris) 58*, 248 (abstr.)
MAETZ, J. & GARCIA-ROMEU, F. (1964) *J. Gen. Physiol. 47*, 1209-1227
MAETZ, J. & PIC, P. (1974) *J. Physiol. (Paris) 69*, 270A
MAETZ, J., PAYAN, P. & DE RENZIS, G. (1975) in *Perspectives in Experimental Biology*, vol. 1: *Zoology* (Davies, P. S., ed.), Pergamon, Oxford
MORENO, J. H. & DIAMOND, J. M. (1975) in *Membranes – A Series of Advances*, vol. 3 (Eisenman, G., ed.), Pergamon, Oxford; Dekker, New York
MOTAIS, R. (1961) *C.R. Hebd. Séances Acad. Sci. Sér. D. Sci. Nat. 253*, 724-726

MOTAIS, R. (1967) *Ann. Inst. Oceanogr. Monaco 45*, 1-84
MOTAIS, R. & GARCIA-ROMEU, F. (1972) *Annu. Rev. Physiol. 34*, 141-176
MOTAIS, R. & ISAIA, J. (1972a) *J. Exp. Biol. 56*, 587-600
MOTAIS, R. & ISAIA, J. (1972b) *J. Exp. Biol. 57*, 367-373
MOTAIS, R. & MAETZ, J. (1965) *C.R.Hebd. Séances Acad. Sci. Sér. D Sci. Nat. 261*, 532
MOTAIS, R., ISAIA, H., RANKIN, J. C. & MAETZ, J. (1969) *J. Exp. Biol. 51*, 529-546
MULLINS, L. J. (1950) *Acta Physiol. Scand. 21*, 301-334
PAYAN, P. & MAETZ, J. (1971) *Gen. Comp. Endocrinol. 16*, 535-554
PAYAN, P. & MATTY, A. J. (1975) *J. Comp. Physiol. 96*, 167-184
PIC, P. & MAETZ, J. (1975) *C.R. Hebd. Séances Acad. Sci. Sér. D. Sci. Nat. 280*, 983-986
POTTS, W. T. W. (1968) *Annu. Rev. Physiol. 30*, 73-104
POTTS, W. T. W. (1972) *Verh. Dtsch. Zool. Ges. 56*, 164-172
POTTS, W. T. W. & EDDY, F. B. (1973) *J. Comp. Physiol. 87*, 29-48
POTTS, W. T W. & FLEMING, W. R. (1971) *J. Exp. Biol. 54*, 63-75
RANDALL, D. J. & CAMERON, J. N. (1973) *Am. J. Physiol. 225*, 997-1002
SHUTTLEWORTH, T. J. & FREEMAN, R. F. H. (1974) *J. Exp. Biol. 60*, 769-781
SHUTTLEWORTH, T. J., POTTS, W. T. W. & HARRIS, J. N. (1974) *J. Comp. Physiol. B 94*,
    321-329
SMITH, H. W. (1930) *Am. J. Physiol. 93*, 480-505
SMITH, P. G. (1969) *J. Exp. Biol. 51*, 739-758
USSING, H. H. (1960) in *Handb. Exp. Pharmakol.* (Eichler, P. & Farah, A., eds.), vol 13,
    1-195, Springer, Berlin

Discussion

Keynes: You said that the chloride transport mechanism reverses when fish move between fresh water and salt water, Dr Maetz, and you also think that outward chloride transport takes place from the chloride cells. Does the reverse transport also take place only with chloride cells? Or is it possible that chloride is extruded from the chloride cells, but that when the fish have to pump chloride inwards this takes place in other cells?

Maetz: There is no definitive proof but there is reason to believe that active transport of ions occurs in the mitochondria-rich cells in both fresh-water-adapted and sea-water-adapted fish gills. For instance carbonate dehydratase, which plays a role in ion transport across the gill, seems to be located in these cells (see review by Maetz 1971). Furthermore, Na^+/K^+-activated ATPase seems also to be located almost exclusively in the mitochondria-rich cells (Sargent *et al.* 1975), and this is an enzyme which plays a crucial role in Na/K exchange across the gill in sea water and in sodium absorption by the gill in fresh water (Maetz 1973; Richards & Fromm 1970). Nevertheless, although it is the same cell-type which performs these transport functions, it is highly probable that different cell populations are functional in both media (Shirai & Utida 1970; Masoni & Isaia 1973).

Keynes: Quite a good precedent for reverse transport taking place in the same cells is provided by intestinal epithelium. Normally there is uptake of sodium and chloride but when the intestine is treated with cholera toxin or other toxins, there is a gigantic reverse transport of chloride, which must happen in the same place. This reverse transport may all be tied up with bicarbonate—just how is quite unclear to me at present, but certainly the same cell is capable of pushing the ions either way.

Olver: Cyclic AMP and aminophylline also reverse ion transport in the intestine, don't they?

Keynes: Cyclic AMP is certainly implicated there.

Maetz: Cyclic AMP is also implicated in fish gill function in relation to the role of adrenaline, a hormone which modulates water permeability and active transport of ions (Cuthbert & Pic 1973; Pic *et al.* 1973). It is not clear, however, whether adenylate cyclase (EC 4.6.1.1) intervenes in the reversal of the chloride pump which takes place during transition between the fresh water and sea water habitat.

Dickinson: We heard earlier that in the fetus there is net secretion of liquid from the lung outwards, but we also heard that isotonic liquids put into the adult air-filled lung are very rapidly absorbed. It seems that the mammalian lung is equally capable of transport in both directions.

Olver: That is perhaps a misinterpretation. Isotonic saline is absorbed rather slowly down the protein osmotic pressure gradient between it and plasma. The fact that there is bulk liquid movement under these circumstances says nothing about active transport.

Strang: Still, some kind of reversal in secretion may take place in the lung at birth.

Dickinson: In the fetus the parts that will become the air passages are electronegative with respect to the body. If the lungs of either the fetus or the adult are filled with hypotonic fluid similar to tap water, do the insides of the air passages become electropositive?

Maetz: What is the origin of the potential? To illustrate my question, in the fish gills in sea water the potential has a dual origin. On the one hand, the main part of the potential is a diffusion potential, the gill behaving as a sodium or potassium electrode (Potts & Eddy 1973; House & Maetz 1974). On the other hand, a small part of the gill potential results from the electrogenicity of the chloride pump (Shuttleworth *et al.* 1974; Pic & Maetz 1975). This pump is knocked out when thiocyanate is injected into the fish and this results in a 5 to 10 mV depolarization of the gill potential.

Gatzy: If the chloride concentration in the lumen of the amphibian lung is lowered, the potential increases. It looks as if this is a diffusion potential that arises from the exit of chloride from the cell to the lumen.

Maetz: It could be a chloride-permeable epithelium rather than a sodium-permeable epithelium.

Gatzy: At least the apical membrane appears to be selectively permeable to chloride.

Hugh-Jones: Is the lung of *Dipnoi* (lungfish) a projection from the foregut, like the mammalian lung? Does it too have an active exchange of electrolytes when the fish is in water?

Maetz: I don't think so; the lung remains filled with air. Some teleosts such as the mud-skippers, however, have adaptive structures which enable them to live for lengthy periods on moist surfaces. They have no lungs but some kind of alveolar air-filled bags in the mouth cavity. The lining of these structures contains numerous chloride cells which I presume are related to acid–base balance. There is now more and more evidence of a tie-up between osmoregulation and acid–base balance in fish, whether fresh water or sea water, in crustacea and even in molluscs (see review by Maetz *et al.* 1975).

Keynes: Do you know anything about the structure of the buccal cavity in electric eels, which are air-breathing fish? The electric eel has no gills; it comes up and gulps air at the surface. It might be worth looking at it.

Maetz: I don't know anything about it.

Durbin: Are there any differences in morphology between euryhaline fish in fresh water and sea water conditions? Does the turnover of chloride cells change?

Maetz: There are considerable morphological changes in the chloride cells during the transition from fresh water to sea water. These changes are characterized not so much by an increase in the relative volume of mitochondria as by a considerable expansion of the smooth reticulum, a tubular system which is an expansion of the basolateral membrane. The augmentation in cell surface is illustrated by the much higher Na^+/K^+-dependent ATPase activity found in the chloride cells of the sea-water-adapted fish and by the considerable increase in ouabain-binding sites observed in the gill in sea water (see review by Maetz & Bornancin 1975). We calculated about 10^8 binding sites per chloride cell in the sea-water-adapted eel! Preliminary freeze–fracture studies by C. Sardet (unpublished) have revealed, in the tubules, beautifully organized arrays looking like crystals which characterize the sea water gill of the mullet whereas fresh water gills do not possess this organization. It is interesting to note that these clusters are seen on the A as well as on the B face of the cell membrane.

Schneeberger: Are these arrays clustered?

Maetz: Yes, beautifully clustered. There is also beautiful crystalline organization in the apex in both fresh water and sea water fish. But obviously the surface of exchange is much bigger in the sea water fish because the tubular system is far more developed.

The number of chloride cells is three to four times higher in sea water fish than in fresh water fish. There is also more ATPase in the sea water fish than in the fresh water fish (Utida *et al.* 1971). Studies with tritiated thymidine show that turnover is three or four times faster in sea water than in fresh water (Conte & Lin 1967). The cells wear out and are replaced by new cells. We also studied cell renewal in relation to osmoregulation by using actinomycin. After one dose of 10 μg actinomycin, a sea water eel dies within five days, with complete failure of osmoregulation. A fresh water fish, on the contrary, survives for weeks. It looks as if cell turnover is critical in the sea water fish but not so critical in the fresh water fish (Maetz *et al.* 1969).

Strang: There are, as far as I know, four different cell types in the epithelium of the peripheral parts of the lung: type I, II and III alveolar cells and the Clara cell. We haven't really discussed the structure of these. Can you tell us anything about the structure of epithelial cells in the gill?

Maetz: There are three types of cells: chloride cells, flat squamous cells on the respiratory leaflets, and mucus cells. Chloride cells have sometimes been claimed to be mucus cells. In fact chloride cells are rich in glycoprotein, which they excrete all the time. They have a conspicuous coat of glycoprotein where chloride and sodium ions are trapped in quantities. This coat may have an important role in controlling access of these ions to the membrane.

Olver: Were you looking at the red or the grey mullet?

Maetz: The grey mullet (*Mugil capito*).

References

Conte, P. F. & Lin, D. H. Y. (1967) Kinetics of cellular morphogenesis in gill epithelium during sea water adaptation of *Oncorhynchus* (Walbaum). *Comp. Biochem. Physiol. 23*, 945-957

Cuthbert, A. W. & Pic, P. (1973) Adrenoceptors and adenylcylclase in gills. *Br. J. Pharmacol. 49*, 134-137

House, C. R. & Maetz, J. (1974) On the electric gradient across the gill of the sea water adapted eel. *Comp. Biochem. Physiol. A Comp. Physiol. 47*, 917-924

Maetz, J. (1971) Fish gills: mechanisms of salt transfer in fresh water and sea water. *Philos. Trans. R. Soc. Lond. B Biol. Sci. 262*, 209-249

Maetz, J. (1973) Transport mechanisms in sea-water adapted fish gills, in *Transport Mechanisms in Epithelia (Alfred Benzon Symp. 5)* (Ussing, H. H. & Thorn, N. A., eds.), pp. 427-441, Munskgaard, Copenhagen

Maetz, J. & Bornancin, M. (1975) Biochemical and biophysical aspects of salt secretion by chloride cells in teleosts. *Fortschr. Zool. 23*, 322-362

Maetz, J., Nibelle, J., Bornancin, M. & Motais, R. (1969). Action sur l'osmorégulation de l'anguille de divers antibiotiques inhibiteurs de la synthèse des protèines ou du renouvellement cellulaire. *Comp. Biochem. Physiol. 30*, 1125-1151

Maetz, J., Payan, P. & De Renzis, G. (1975) Controversial aspects of ionic uptake in freshwater animals, in *Perspectives in Experimental Biology*, vol. 1: *Zoology* (Daviès, P. S., ed.), Pergamon, Oxford

Masoni, A. & Isaia, J. (1973) Influence du mannitol et de la salinité externe sur l'équilibre hydrique et l'aspect morphologique de la branchie d'anguille adaptée à l'eau de mer. *Arch. Anat. Microsc. Morphol. Exp. 62*, 293-306

Pic, P. & Maetz, J. (1975) Différences de potentiel trans-branchial et flux ioniques chez *Mugil capito* adapté à l'eau de mer. Importance de l'ion Ca^{++}. *C.R. Hebd. Séances Acad. Sci. Ser. D Sci. Nat. 280*, 983-986

Pic, P., Mayer-Gostan, N. & Maetz, J. (1973) Seawater teleosts: presence of α and β receptors in the gill regulating salt extrusion and water permeability, in *Comparative Physiology* (Bolis, L., Schmidt-Nielsen, K. & Maddrell, S. H. P., eds.), pp. 293-322, North-Holland, Amsterdam

Potts, W. T. W. & Eddy, F. B. (1973) Gill potentials and sodium fluxes in the flounder, *Platichthys flesus. J. Comp. Physiol. 87*, 29-48

Richards, B. D. & Fromm, P. O. (1970) Sodium uptake by isolated-perfused gills of rainbow trout (*Salmo gairdneri*). *Comp. Biochem. Physiol. 33*, 303-310

Sargent, J. R., Thomson, A. J. & Bornancin, M. (1975) Activities and localization of succinic dehydrogenase and Na$^+$/K$^+$activated ATPase in the gills of fresh water and sea water eels (*Anguilla anguilla*). *Comp. Biochem. Physiol. B Comp. Biochem. 51*, 75-79

Shirai, B. D. & Utida, S. (1970) Development and degeneration of the chloride cells during seawater and freshwater adaptation of the Japanese eel, *Anguilla japonica. Z. Zellforsch. Mikrosk. Anat. 103*, 247-264

Shuttleworth, T. L., Potts, W. T. W. & Harris, J. N. (1974) Bioelectric potentials in the gill of the flounder *Platichthys flesus. J. Comp. Physiol. 94*, 321-329

Utida, S., Kamyia, M. & Shirai, N. (1971) Relationship between the activity of Na$^+$ – K$^+$-activated adenosine triphosphatase and the number of chloride cells in eel gills with special reference to sea water adaptation. *Comp. Biochem. Physiol. A Comp. Physiol. 38*, 443-447

Coupling of water to solute movement in isolated gastric mucosa

R. P. DURBIN

Cardiovascular Research Institute, University of California, San Francisco

Abstract Osmosis is apparently the mechanism responsible for the coupling of water to solute transport in biological membranes. Often a secreted or absorbed fluid is essentially iso-osmotic with the solution of origin, or with plasma, and various models have been constructed by Curran, Diamond and others to account for such observations. More information is needed, however, to test further the predictions of these models and to facilitate correlation with known structural details. This study deals with gastric secretion and the effects of the luminal solution on its composition. Although pure gastric juice collected *in vivo* is virtually iso-osmotic with plasma, Teorell, Öbrink and others found that instillation of a buffer solution (glycine) in the lumen led to a twofold increase in the concentration of gastric acid. This effect is not restricted to buffer solutions: the normality of H^+ secreted into an isotonic (120 mM) NaCl solution bathing the isolated bullfrog gastric mucosa was 276 ± 19 mmol/l (13 experiments). Clearly the luminal solution affects the concentration of gastric secretion, probably by reducing an endogenous osmotic gradient. Thus the sites responsible for transport of H^+ must be accessible from the luminal solution.

The common means by which water flow is driven in the everyday world is by hydrostatic or osmotic pressure, and it seems reasonable to assume that these mechanisms continue to operate down to the cellular level, unless results dictate otherwise. The delicate balance often observed between active ion transport and water flow, which yields a virtually isotonic absorption or secretion, would appear to favour osmosis as the primary driving force. Flow of water then provides an appropriate negative feedback which reduces the differences in osmotic pressure towards zero. Such is the ideal, and sometimes it appears an impossible one when we are confronted with hard experimental fact. These matters have been discussed carefully and elegantly by House (1974).

Paradoxically, we can gain insight into the nature of isotonic fluid movement by focusing attention on procedures which disturb the balance between water and ion flows. A classic example of balance and its perturbation is provided in gastric physiology, and this will be considered in more detail.

Gastric juice collected *in vivo* has an osmolarity which exceeds that of blood by at most a few per cent (Moody & Durbin 1965; Makhlouf *et al.* 1966). This is no longer the case when iso-osmotic glycine solution is instilled in the lumen. Teorell (1940), who introduced the term *primary acidity* for the ratio of measured acid output to net volume flow, found that this was 208 mequiv./l with glycine solutions in the cat *in vivo*. Linde *et al.* (1947) observed comparably high values in the dog *in vivo*; these tended to increase as the rate of secretion diminished. Later it was found that instillation of buffer was unnecessary (Moody & Durbin 1965). The acidity (to be equated with primary acidity) of secretion in dog stomach was 198 ± 5 mM with iso-osmotic mannitol in the lumen but 140 ± 4 mM when iso-osmotic HCl was instilled. Presumably the latter situation represents that encountered *in vivo* with an initially empty lumen.

The acidity of gastric secretion is thus seen to depend on the nature of the solute in the lumen. In all likelihood the source of the effect is a difference in permeability, e.g. between HCl and mannitol. It does not seem possible to fit such results to a model in which water flow is segregated from the lumen, for instance if acid were formed within vesicles which emptied into the lumen by a reverse pinocytosis.

These conclusions would be more secure if the instillate effect could be further verified. In principle the isolated gastric mucosa would be ideal for testing, since both bathing solutions are easily available to the experimenter. Surprisingly little is known about coupling of water and solute flows in this tissue, however. In several studies, little correlation could be demonstrated (Durbin *et al.* 1956; Villegas & Sananes 1968); on the other hand, no systematic attempt was made to vary acid secretion by stimulation or otherwise.

In the present study I used a large area of bullfrog gastric mucosa to maximize water flow, and histamine or thiocyanate (SCN^-) to vary acid secretion. Fig. 1 is a schematic drawing of the chambers. Volume flow was measured gravimetrically by filling the volume chamber from a preweighed syringe, and draining the chamber contents into a preweighed vial at the end of a period.

The mucosa was mounted in early experiments with the secretory (luminal) surface facing the volume chamber. This gave results roughly similar to those to be reported, but opposite in sign. Volume recovery was erratic, however, and this seemed to be due to a variable trapping of fluid by mucus secreted during an experiment. The problem was eliminated by reversing the mucosa, so that the nutrient (serosal) surface faced the volume chamber (see legend to Fig. 1 for further details).

In a preliminary test, Parafilm membranes were mounted between the

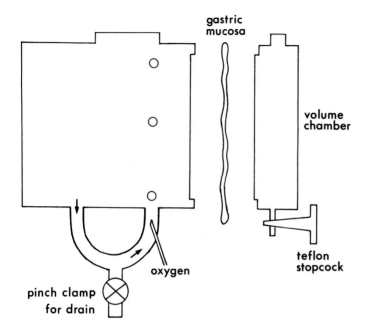

FIG. 1. Schematic diagram of chambers. Area of mucosal window is 11.4 cm², volume of larger chamber to the left about 40 ml and that of volume chamber about 15 ml. Both chambers are open to the atmosphere; volume chamber is neither gassed nor stirred.

chambers and recoveries were determined over the conventional period of 50 min. The evaporation loss in 10 such periods was 23 μl, with a standard deviation of ± 8 μl. The latter is a measure of cumulative errors in weighing, delivery and recovery.

Two different approaches were used to quantitate volume flow associated with acid secretion. In one series of five experiments, mucosae were bathed with solutions containing no added secretagogue for 4 to 6 h. After the initial secretory rate had dropped considerably, acid secretion was stimulated with 10^{-4}M-histamine in the nutrient solution for three consecutive periods. The points (open circles) plotted in Fig. 2 show the means of the last two periods before stimulation, and the means of the second and third periods with histamine (the first period having been considered transitional).

In the second series of eight experiments, mucosae were stimulated from the outset with 10^{-4}M-histamine. After at least three periods in which acid secretion and net flow were measured, the nutrient solution was exchanged for one containing 10mM SCN^- (omitting the equivalent amount of Cl^-) and both rates were followed for another three periods. As before, the last two periods

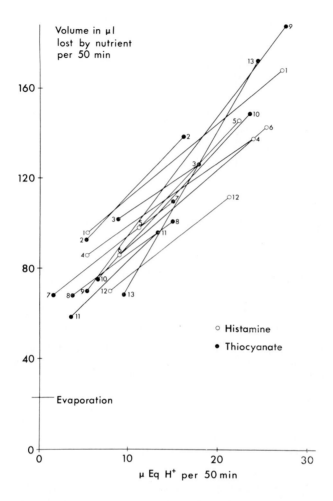

Fig. 2. Comparison of net volume flow (obtained by weighing solution recovered from volume chamber) and acid secretion (obtained by draining large chamber and titrating contents to pH 7.7). Numbers denote individual experiments. For those with open circles, acid secretion and volume flow were stimulated by 10^{-4}M-histamine: closed circles represent experiments in which activity was inhibited by 10^{-2}M-SCN$^-$. Line marked *evaporation* indicates mean loss/50 min with Parafilm membranes.

before addition of SCN$^-$, and the second and third periods with SCN$^-$, were averaged to give the points plotted as filled circles in Fig. 2.

To obtain the effective concentration of the secreted fluid (acidity), the reciprocal slope of each line in Fig. 2 was calculated:

$$\text{acidity} = \frac{\Delta \text{ (acid secretion)}}{\Delta \text{ (volume flow)}} \tag{1}$$

This procedure has the advantage that constant losses due to evaporation or mucus production cancel when the subtraction is performed.

TABLE 1

Acidity of secretion

	$\mu equiv.\ H^+/l$
Histamine (5)	300 ± 20
SCN⁻ (8)	262 ± 28
Combined (13)	276 ± 19

Errors are s.e.m., no. of expts in parentheses. Secretory solution 120mM-NaCl.

Table 1 lists the mean acidity thus calculated. That for histamine stimulation does not differ significantly from that for SCN^- inhibition, and the two have been combined to yield an overall acidity of 276 ± 19 mmol/l. From the projected y-intercepts of Fig. 2, we can calculate a mean y-intercept of 54 ± 6 μl. Consequently the volume flow y in μl/50 min can be written as

$$y = 54 + H^+/0.276 \tag{2}$$

where H^+ is acid secreted in μequiv./50 min. If y and H^+ are expressed in the more conventional units of μl cm^{-2} h^{-1} and μequiv. cm^{-2} h^{-1}, respectively, Eq. 2 takes the form

$$y = 5.7 + 3.6\ H^+ \tag{3}$$

since the chamber area is 11.4 cm^2.

The last two equations apply only to the conditions of the present study. The mean y-intercept in Eq. 2 is rather high in comparison with the evaporation loss with Parafilm (23 μl). The difference could be due to there being better stirring with a mucosa present, hence greater evaporation, or it could be due to a real net flow associated with mucus production or electrogenic Cl^- movement. In an attempt to quantitate the latter, I used solutions in which sodium isethionate, K_2SO_4 and $CaSO_4$ replaced the corresponding Cl^- salts (Durbin et al. 1974). The chambers did not allow measurement of electrical activity other than potential difference; this was observed to reverse in sign when Cl^- was excluded, indicating that electrogenic Cl^- movement had disappeared. The acid secretion and net volume flow in the third period with Cl^--free solutions were 1.3 ± 0.3 μequiv./50 min and 80 ± 10 μl/50 min in six experiments. This volume flow, when corrected for that presumed to be associated with the small acid secretion, does not differ significantly from the value of 54 μl/50 min for the y-intercept found in the presence of Cl⁻: it seems that little or no fluid movement is associated with electrogenic Cl⁻ transport.

The hyperacidity reported here could reflect the relative impermeability of NaCl compared to HCl, or it might be normal for the bullfrog. For this reason experiments were performed in which iso-osmotic sucrose solutions were instilled on the secretory surface. The experiment was begun with 120mM-NaCl as usual for several periods, and continued with 220 mM-sucrose for the rest of the time. Either histamine (10^{-4}M) was added to stimulate further secretion, or SCN⁻ (10 mM) was added to inhibit secretion, as before.

In general, sucrose appeared to reduce fluid movement, with variable effects on acid secretion. As a result, the slope of lines plotted as in Fig. 2 approached zero, and the acidity (reciprocal slope) became meaninglessly large. Another approach can be used, however, on the assumption that the y-intercept does not change when sucrose is substituted for NaCl. The acidity can then be obtained from

$$y = 54 + H^+/(acidity)_{sucrose} \qquad (4)$$

where y is in μl/50 min and H⁺ in μequiv./50 min.

Analysis was restricted to experiments in which acid secretion had been stimulated with histamine, to maximize y. Table 2 gives the acidities thus calculated for the last period with 0.12M-NaCl before the solution was changed, as a control, and for the third period with 220mM-sucrose. The latter was chosen arbitrarily, to avoid any transitional periods.

TABLE 2

Acidity: effects of solute

Secretory	μequiv. H^+/l
NaCl (120 mM)	228 ± 21
Sucrose (220 mM)	441 ± 57

Data from 7 expts, errors are S.E.M.

The acidity for NaCl secretory in Table 2 is considerably less than the mean from Table 1, but the difference is not significant ($P > 0.05$). On the other hand, the acidity measured with sucrose secretory is significantly higher than its matched NaCl group in Table 2 ($P < 0.005$) or the overall NaCl group in Table 1 ($P < 0.02$). The results with sucrose thus reinforce and extend those obtained with NaCl.

The present study shows that the isolated gastric mucosa yields a response to the nature of the secretory instillate which resembles that obtained in the dog (Moody & Durbin 1965). In the latter, however, the effects were smaller and NaCl and sucrose gave about the same acidity (about 190 mM).

There is reason to expect that bullfrog gastric secretion in the absence of instillate is approximately iso-osmotic with plasma (Makhlouf & Duckworth 1973). It then remains to account for the action of instillates in increasing acidity. One possibility is that both NaCl and sucrose reduce the normal osmotic permeability of the tissue and thereby hamper osmotic equilibration. If such a change occurs, it is readily reversible in the dog (Moody & Durbin 1965).

Perhaps a more attractive viewpoint is that the instillates alter normal osmotic gradients within the mucosa. Instillation of NaCl or sucrose implies the replacement of HCl with a less permeable solute. The diffusion coefficient in free solution of NaCl is about half, and that of sucrose about one-sixth, that of HCl.

This approach follows the analysis of Whitlock & Wheeler (1964), who studied the absorption of NaCl and water by the isolated rabbit gall bladder. Normally this preparation transports a NaCl solution which is iso-osmotic with the luminal contents; however, replacement of NaCl by an osmotic equivalent of sucrose induced a hyperosmotic absorption. In particular, the presence of 85mM-sucrose in the serosal solution increased the concentration of absorbed fluid from 161 to 211 mequiv./l. In this case, the less permeable solute (sucrose) was on the side towards which active transport was directed, as in the present study.

Whitlock & Wheeler used the double-membrane model (Curran 1960; Durbin 1960), as described theoretically by Patlak et al. (1963), to interpret their findings. In reference to Fig. 3, active transport is considered to occur across membrane (1) from the left compartment l to the middle m, while membrane (2) serves to separate the small middle compartment from a large receiving compartment r. Thus the latter could be the serosal interstitial space in gall bladder, or the lumen in stomach.

The choice of reflection coefficients here is not arbitrary, being largely prescribed by experimental results. That of the first membrane for the transported solute, σ_1, must be near unity for effective movement of water to be ensured; the second membrane has to have a reflection coefficient for the transported solute (σ_2) of near zero for a transported fluid isotonic with the normal bathing media to be obtained (Whitlock & Wheeler 1964; Schultz & Curran 1968). Hence this version of the double-membrane model shares some essential elements with the standing-gradient model of Diamond & Bossert (1967).

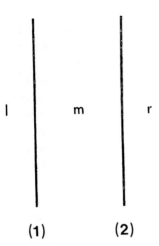

(1)   (2)

FIG. 3. Double-membrane model of transporting epithelium. Left compartment is denoted by *l*, middle by *m* and right by *r*. Active transport is assumed to occur across membrane (1) from *l* to *m*.

According to Whitlock & Wheeler (1964), the double-membrane model can predict the increase in absorbate osmolarity observed with sucrose, provided some other qualifications are met. Important among these is the requirement that the hydrostatic permeability, L_p, of both membranes be large enough for the osmolarity of the transported fluid to approach that of the bathing solutions (in the absence of added solutes such as sucrose).

Are there membranes with such properties? Clearly L_p for membrane (2) could be quite large if this corresponds to intercellular spaces. Hydrostatic pressure proved to be about two orders of magnitude more effective than osmotic pressure in producing net volume flow across dog gastric mucosa (Moody & Durbin 1969); later work suggested that such flows follow an intercellular route (Altamirano *et al.* 1974). Recently Altamirano (personal communication) has measured the difference in hydrostatic pressure between serosal interstitium and lumen of dog stomach, and the resulting fluid move-ment. He estimates an L_p for the intercellular channels more than 10^3 larger than that inferred for the mucosa as a whole from osmotic pressure data.

If membrane (2) represents intercellular spaces, spaces between microvilli, etc., membrane (1) must correspond to the actual site of transport. Here it is more difficult to imagine properties which would yield a large L_p, unless the surface area is greatly elaborated. There is some evidence for the latter, for example in the secreting oxyntic cell of stomach. It may be necessary to isolate the osmotic properties of this membrane before much further progress can be made in fitting models to results.

ACKNOWLEDGEMENTS

The work reported here was supported by the National Institutes of Health (grant HL 06285) and by a Visiting Scientist award (project No. 12V-4579) from the Swedish Medical Research Council. I also thank Fabian Michelangeli and Sharon Paris for their advice and assistance.

References

ALTAMIRANO, M., REQUENA, M. & DURBIN, R. P. (1974) Effects of gastric arterial and venous pressures on gastric secretion in the dog. *Am. J. Physiol.* 227, 152-160

CURRAN, P. F. (1960) Na, Cl, and water transport by rat ileum in vitro. *J. Gen. Physiol.* 43, 1137-1148

DIAMOND, J. M. & BOSSERT, W. H. (1967) Standing-gradient osmotic flow. A mechanism for coupling of water and solute transport in epithelia. *J. Gen. Physiol. 50*, 2061-2083

DURBIN, R. P. (1960) Osmotic flow of water across permeable cellulose membranes. *J. Gen. Physiol. 44*, 315-326

DURBIN, R. P., FRANK, H. & SOLOMON, A. K. (1956) Water flow through frog gastric mucosa. *J. Gen. Physiol. 39*, 535-551

DURBIN, R. P., MICHELANGELI, F. & NICKEL, A. (1974) Active transport and ATP in frog gastric mucosa. *Biochim. Biophys. Acta 367*, 177-189

HOUSE, C. R. (1974) *Water Transport in Cells and Tissues*, Edward Arnold, London

LINDE, S., TEORELL, T. & ÖBRINK, K. J. (1947) Experiments on the primary acidity of the gastric juice. *Acta Physiol. Scand. 14*, 220-232

MAKHLOUF, G. M. & DUCKWORTH, G. R. (1973) Secretion and electrical activity of a unilateral in vitro gastric mucosa. *Gastroenterology 65*, 907-911

MAKHLOUF, G. M., McMANUS, J. P. A. & CARD, W. I. (1966) A quantitative statement of the two-component hypothesis of gastric secretion. *Gastroenterology 51*, 149-171

MOODY, F. G. & DURBIN, R. P. (1965) Effects of glycine and other instillates on concentration of gastric acid. *Am. J. Physiol. 209*, 122-126

MOODY, F. G. & DURBIN, R. P. (1969) Water flow induced by osmotic and hydrostatic pressure in the stomach. *Am. J. Physiol. 217*, 255-261

PATLAK, C. S., GOLDSTEIN, D. A. & HOFFMAN, J. F. (1963) The flow of solute and solvent across a two-membrane system. *J. Theor. Biol. 5*, 426-442

SCHULTZ, S. G. & CURRAN, P. F. (1968) in *Handb. Physiol.* Section 6: *Alimentary Canal*, vol. 3 (Code, C. F., ed.), pp. 1245-1275, American Physiological Society, Washington, D.C.

TEORELL, T. (1940) On the primary acidity of the gastric juice. *J. Physiol. (Lond.) 97*, 308-315

VILLEGAS, L. & SANANES, L. (1968) Independence between ionic transport and net water flux in frog gastric mucosa. *Am. J. Physiol. 214*, 997-1000

WHITLOCK, R. T. & WHEELER, H. O. (1964) Coupled transport of solute and water across rabbit gallbladder epithelium. *J. Clin. Invest. 43*, 2249-2265

Discussion

Michel: Dr Durbin, you assumed that the site of acid secretion had to be at the surface and couldn't be intracellular. Doesn't this depend on the hydraulic conductivity (L_p) of the cell membrane? A hypotonic solution outside a cell with a high enough L_p will affect the intracellular constituents, won't it?

Durbin: It is conceivable that acid could be formed in vesicles inside the oxyntic cell. In that case the acidity may be expected to be iso-osmotic with the cytoplasm and independent of the kind of solute instilled in the lumen. The present results (and previous findings) show that the latter is not the case, hence they argue against formation of acid in vesicles.

Formation of acid directly in the cytoplasm also seems unlikely. The average pH of the oxyntic cell is slightly more alkaline than the pH of blood (F. Michelangeli, unpublished results, 1975). The oxyntic cell cytoplasm is probably not materially different from other kinds of cytoplasm.

Michel: My point was that if acid were formed in vesicles, then if there is a high L_p for the cell membrane and a hypotonic solution is put outside the cell, the intracellular osmotic pressure could quickly equilibrate by water movement across the cell membrane. In this way the hypotonic extracellular solution would exert its effects on the intracellular vesicle.

Durbin: It should be kept in mind that the overall osmotic permeability of gastric mucosa is quite low.

Michel: One must assume the cell membrane has a very low L_p if a vesicular type of mechanism is to be eliminated by this sort of experiment. The possibility that an extracellular hypotonic solution is rapidly diluting the intracellular constituents has to be eliminated if one wants to be sure that vesicles inside the cell are not also subjected to a hypotonic environment.

Maetz: The L_p values are calculated for the whole membrane. The question is whether the barrier to water permeability is the apical or the basal membrane. MacRobbie & Ussing (1961) showed that the basal membrane of the cells of frog skin is probably the one that is permeable to water. Those cells swell rapidly when a hypotonic medium is placed on the serosal side. The skin epithelium is however very impermeable to water on the apical side. Similar studies should be done on the gastric mucosa, to discover which membrane is more permeable. I would guess that it is the basal cell membrane which is the more permeable, while from the apical side the epithelial cells are probably impermeable.

Durbin: Perhaps it is easier to discuss the role of apical and basal membranes in the gall bladder. The exact site of active NaCl transport is not known, but for the purpose of this discussion we can assume it is the lateral surface of the epithelial cell. The cytoplasm of this cell is probably immediately responsive to changes in osmolarity in the luminal solution. That is, the lumen and cytoplasm are iso-osmotic with respect to each other. This is suggested by the fact that the tonicity of the absorbate follows closely the tonicity of the solution in the lumen.

On the other hand, the absorbate formed by active transport at the apical end of the lateral spaces is probably hypertonic to cell and luminal solution.

In a sense, the lateral membranes isolate the 'standing gradient' from the cell interior. It is this gradient which seems to be reduced when a solute like sucrose is substituted for NaCl in the serosal solution. The less permeable solute gives rise to an increase in absorbate osmolarity (Whitlock & Wheeler 1964).

Keynes: I agree with your arguments but I am considerably bothered by the conclusion from them. Diamond (1964a, b) has shown that in gall bladder the tonicity of the bathing medium can be changed by a factor of 8 and that the tonicity of the secretion stays equal to that over the whole of that range. One of the objections against the simple two-compartment model of Curran (1960) is that however hard one tries, one cannot plot a 45° relationship between the osmotic pressure of the secreted fluid and that of the bathing fluid. Yet the experimental observation, with which no one disagrees, is that there is a 45° relationship in the gall bladder.

Durbin: Precisely. But Schultz & Curran (1968) showed that the same result could be obtained from the double-membrane model, provided certain assumptions were made. The latter include the condition that the reflection coefficient for the transported solute at the first membrane (the one responsible for active transport) be unity, and zero at the second membrane.

Keynes: There is a piece of experimental evidence missing still which I hope we shall be able to provide soon. As you said, on the Diamond model the tonicity of the cytoplasm has to follow the tonicity of the bath solution exactly. Yet I don't know of any experimental evidence that it actually does. But there are now microelectrodes which will measure internal sodium, chloride and potassium activity. I have just got a whole lot of mud-puppies (*Necturus*) so that we can work on their gall bladders; these have enormous cells that can be penetrated nicely with microelectrodes, so we won't have the problem of not knowing precisely where the tip of the electrode is. It will be extremely interesting to see whether the prediction of the Diamond model is right. Does the intracellular activity change over an eightfold range the moment the bathing fluid is changed? I am willing to bet that it does not.

Maetz: To estimate net water transfer across the gall bladder, two different techniques have been used which may lead to different results with respect to osmolarity of the fluid secreted by the preparation. Diamond (1964a) used the 'unilateral' preparation with the bladder used as a bag with fluid dripping from it. Whitlock & Wheeler (1964) measured fluid transport by a preparation with fluid bathing both sides. There has been some criticism of the 'unilateral' preparation: Marro & Germagnoli (1966) contended that the absorbate's osmolarity will be recorded invariably as isotonic with that of mucosal solution because of the fairly rapid osmotic equilibration which occurs in the small volume of the serosal solution. Whitlock & Wheeler (1964) observed a hypertonic absorbate. Some epithelia such as fish intestine and fish bladder produce absorbates which are two to six times more concentrated than blood plasma (Skadhauge 1969; Lahlou & Fossat 1971).

Durbin: I agree; the experimental conditions are important. It is also possible that osmotic equilibration could occur by way of the tight junctions and intercellular pathways. These are quite permeable in some epithelia.

Keynes: Hill (1975) argues that equilibration through the tight junctions won't work.

Durbin: To return to the point raised by Dr Maetz, it should be noted that mammalian gastric secretion is only about 5% hypertonic to blood, despite the fact that this fluid can be formed at quite a rapid rate *in vivo*.

Robin: Though you are of course talking of complex epithelial structures, could you conceive of a circumstance where, within the boundaries of a single cell membrane, osmotic gradients could exist at equilibrium?

Durbin: I suppose osmotic gradients at equilibrium are impossible unless a hydrostatic gradient is also present, as in the capillary bed. Of course transient osmotic gradients of permeable solutes can occur as part of a mixing process within the cell. We have to keep in mind the possibility that small differences in hydrostatic pressure may be present in epithelia. These seem to be needed to drive fluid movement as described by the double-membrane model.

Strang: Do you mean could there be a steady state, not an equilibrium, Dr Robin?

Robin: I'll start off with equilibrium.

Maetz: Skadhauge (1969) in my laboratory has adapted eels to media as hypertonic as double-strength sea water (2100 as against 350 mosm). Yet, in their intestinal tracts, these fish absorb water along with salt. For net absorption to take place the ingested water is diluted first down to about 650 mosm by passive entry of water from the body fluids into the intestinal lumen. When this dilution is obtained a steady state is reached that is characterized by a net flow of water equal to zero. The 300 mosm osmotic gradient is called the 'standing gradient'. A net flow of water of 0 corresponds, however, to compensation between water moving passively out into the lumen along the osmotic gradient and water driven by solutes absorbed by the gut according to mechanisms described by Curran's and Diamond's models (Curran & McIntosh 1962; Diamond & Bossert 1967).

Durbin: Is this because the osmotic permeability of these membranes is very low?

Maetz: Yes, the osmotic permeability (P_{os}) of eel's intestine is much higher than in mammals (Skadhauge 1969). In mammals the standing gradient is only about 75, as against 300 in eels adapted to double-strength sea water. In fact efficiency of water absorption against a water concentration gradient depends on the P_{os} of the membrane but also on the efficiency of the sodium and chloride pumps which act as driving forces.

Dickinson: I don't think you have reassured Dr Robin at all, but increased his disquiet!

Maetz: I don't know what the osmolarity of the epithelial cell fluid is, in the case of extreme hyperosmolarity of the absorbate. Skadhauge (1969) suggests that it is iso-osmotic with the body fluids.

Robin: My question was really what happens to a single intestinal cell in those circumstances. Is there a different osmotic pressure in the cytoplasm, compared to the mitochondria?

Olver: I can see with these models how we can end up with hypertonic and isotonic secretions. In order to get a hypotonic secretion, do we have to postulate that solute is reabsorbed at some distal site in the system?

Durbin: I think so, unless you invoke a model other than the one mentioned.

Keynes: One of the points that Diamond originally made was that a backward-facing system on his model will produce a hypotonic secretion. The snag is that one of the fanciest secretory epithelia, the nasal salt gland of sea birds, has a backward-facing epithelium which produces large volumes of an extremely hypertonic solution. This observation is not explained by Diamond's hypothesis at all.

Strang: Would your criticism of Diamond's model be done away with if one assumed a much larger hydraulic conductivity than you did for the walls of the long narrow channel?

Keynes: Yes, that is really what Dr Hill (1975) says in his paper. There is no dispute about the mathematics of Diamond or Segel (1970) but, to make the process work isotonically, one either has to make the hydraulic permeability much bigger than was previously assumed, or alter the dimensions. On the dimensions in the published electron micrographs the L_p still has to go several orders of magnitude beyond what seems possible, or than anyone ever seems to find it.

Strang: Once one has admitted that there are differences in hydraulic conductivity or water permeability in different parts of epithelia, then—considering the difficulty of getting into these long narrow channels experimentally—one ends up in the position that any explanation is possible in the present state of knowledge.

Durbin: There is no question but that the intercellular spaces could have an enormous hydrostatic permeability under favourable conditions, but the transporting membrane itself, either in the double-membrane model or the standing gradient model, must also have a high permeability. At present this is a big problem.

Keynes: Yes. As you said, the cytoplasm has to be equilibrated in osmolarity with the bathing medium as well as the far side. Diamond did some nice measurements of the hydraulic permeability coefficient of the whole gall bladder, which would be the two membranes in series.

Durbin: The difficulty in measuring the osmotic permeability of the gall bladder has been discussed by Wright *et al.* (1972). This parameter was undoubtedly underestimated by previous workers.

Strang: There must presumably be a substantial difficulty in putting the osmotic load into the space actually in contact with the epithelium and knowing what that solute concentration is. We have produced osmotic flows in the lung, using sucrose, to evaluate solvent drag (Olver & Strang 1974), but of course we hadn't the slightest idea, in such a complex branching organ, what the concentration of the solute was at the epithelial surface.

Michel: When we are talking about osmotic permeability we are talking about what Kedem & Katchalsky (1958) designated the L_{pd}. We assume that when we measure L_p by an osmotic method we are dealing with a substance which has a reflection coefficient of 1, i.e. the condition when L_{pd} equals minus L_p. Of course we don't know that a membrane always has a reflection coefficient of 1 throughout. Your evidence that there was a vast difference between hydraulically measured conductivity and osmotically measured hydraulic conductivity, Dr Durbin, could in fact be accounted for by a very small number of very large holes, or areas of the membranes where the osmotic reflection coefficient is much less than 1. Such areas would reduce the value of osmotic permeability well below that of the hydraulically measured permeability.

Durbin: This was the explanation originally advanced by Vargas (1968) and I think it is probably correct.

Olver: Dr Keynes, you said that the dimensions of the system and the area of the channels in which the standing gradients exist must be crucial. How easy is it to get a good estimate of the area term? Could one be several orders of magnitude out in estimating the area?

Keynes: I imagine one could be one or two orders of magnitude out, but the point of the calculations I was quoting was that one would need to be a great deal more out than that. The figures Dr Hill gives, based on the calculations of Segel (1970), are that the length of the channel squared, divided by the diameter, has to be more than 50 cm to give sufficient time for equilibration, with a reasonable figure for L_p. The figure from Diamond's pictures is 0.05 cm. I don't think one could possibly be as far wrong as that.

Olver: That is three orders of magnitude.

Durbin: H. Blom and H. F. Helander (personal communication) in Umeå happen to have been studying this problem. They use the techniques of Weibel (1973) for morphometric analysis of electron micrographs of rabbit gall bladder, and find a value for L^2/r of between 6 and 70 cm: here L is the channel length and r the channel radius. The earlier figures of Tormey & Diamond (1967) were derived from light micrographs, which are inadequate for this purpose. These results of Blom and Helander give some support to the standing gradient model, at least in gall bladder.

Keynes: Hill gives a figure of 1 in insect Malpighian tubules, from the literature.

Durbin: Our estimates of the geometrical parameters may be changing, in short.

Keynes: It seems to me there is too large a gap to bridge.

Maetz: If the liquid in the intercellular region is not iso-osmotic how would it change the calculation? I still believe that the fluid that is secreted in the gall bladder is hyperosmotic. In addition the intercellular surface cannot be properly estimated and is certainly an underestimate. How would these considerations change the whole trend of the calculations?

Staub: In the gastric mucosa or in the gall bladder do the cells swell or shrink depending on which side the osmotic fluid is added?

Durbin: Tormey & Diamond (1967) studied the effects of hypertonic solutions in the lumen of gall bladder; they did not see any change in cell volume.

Keynes: Yes, that is something that has always puzzled me.

Staub: If you add hyperosmotic or hypo-osmotic fluid to the luminal and serosal sides of the cells do their volumes change differently? Would this give you any idea about the water permeabilities of the apical and basal membranes?

Maetz: That question has been well answered in frog skin and bladder. If hypotonic fluid is put in the lumen of the frog bladder and no neurohypophysial hormones are present, the cell stays in a normal state. It is certainly not swollen. But as soon as neurohypophysial hormones are added, the water flow goes up to about three times the cell volume per minute. When that happens even the cell nuclei are tremendously swollen (Carasso *et al.* 1966). If a hyperosmotic fluid is placed on the luminal side, characteristic blisters appear in the region of the tight junction under the influence of neurohypophysial hormones. There is a dramatic decrease in the cell volume, which has obviously completely shrunk. Also the nuclei have completely shrunk (Ripoche & Pisam 1973).

Staub: Why shouldn't the gall bladder and the stomach show the same effect? If the cell membrane is completely impermeable to solute but permeable to water on the luminal side, a hyperosmotic bathing solution should cause the cell to shrink rapidly.

Robin: That depends on how well the cell obeys the Boyle/Van't Hoff Law. Cells have widely divergent osmotic compliances, and volume–pressure curves are not the same for all cells. It also turns out that even cells which come fairly close to obeying the Boyle/Van't Hoff Law don't necessarily obey it in the same way for swelling with hypotonic solutions as they do during shrinkage with hypertonic solutions. So if there is less shrinkage that would be a pretty good indication, but if there isn't much change in volume, that would not prove that the cell was not being manipulated osmotically.

References

CARASSO, N., FAVARD, P., BOURGUET, J. & JARD, S. (1966) Rôle du flux net d'eau dans les modifications ultrastructurales de la vessie de grenouille stimulée par l'ocytocine. *J. Microsc. (Paris)* 5, 519-522

CURRAN, P. F. (1960) Na, Cl and water transport by rat ileum in vitro. *J. Gen. Physiol.* 43, 1137-1148

CURRAN, P. F. & McINTOSH, J. R. (1962) A model system for biological water transport. *Nature (Lond.)* 193, 347-348

DIAMOND, J. M. (1964a) Transport of salt and water in rabbit and guinea-pig gall-bladder. *J. Gen. Physiol.* 48, 1-14

DIAMOND, J. M. (1964b) *J. Gen. Physiol.* 48, 15-42

DIAMOND, J. M. & BOSSERT, W. H. (1967) Standing gradient osmotic flow: A mechanism for coupling of water and solute transport in epithelia. *J. Gen. Physiol.* 50, 2061-2083

HILL, A. E. (1975) Solute-solvent coupling in epithelia: a critical examination of the standing-gradient osmotic flow theory. *Proc. R. Soc. B Biol. Sci.* 190, 99-114

KEDEM, O. & KATCHALSKY, A. (1958) Thermodynamic analysis of the permeability of biological membranes to non-electrolytes. *Biochim. Biophys. Acta* 27, 229-246

LAHLOU, B. & FOSSAT, B. (1971) Mécanisme du transport de l'eau et du sel à travers la vessie urinaire d'un poisson téléostéen en eau douce, la truite arc-en-ciel. *C.R. Hebd. Séances Acad. Sci. Sér. D Sci. Nat.* 273, 2108-2111

MacROBBIE, E. A. C. & USSING, H. H. (1961) Osmotic behaviour of the epithelial cells of frog skin. *Acta Physiol. Scand.* 53, 348-365

MARRO, F. & GERMAGNOLI, E. (1966) Letter to the editor. *J. Gen. Physiol.* 49, 1351-1353

RIPOCHE, P. & PISAM, M. (1973) Ultrastructural modifications of the frog urinary bladder epithelium under the influence of hypertonic media. *Z. Zellforsch. Mikrosk. Anat.* 137, 13-19

OLVER, R. E. & STRANG, L. B. (1974) Ion fluxes across the pulmonary epithelium and the secretion of lung liquid in the fetal lamb. *J. Physiol. (Lond.)* 241, 327-357

SCHULTZ, S. G. & CURRAN, P. F. (1968) in *Handb. Physiol.* Section 6: *Alimentary Canal*, vol. 3 (Code, C. F., ed.), pp. 1245-1275, American Physiological Society, Washington, D.C.

SEGEL, L. A. (1970) Standing-gradient flows driven by active solute transport. *J. Theor. Biol.* 29, 233-250

SKADHAUGE, E. (1969) The mechanism of salt and water absorption in the intestine of the eel (*Anguilla anguilla*) adapted to water of various salinities. *J. Physiol. (Lond.)* 204, 135-158

TORMEY, J. McD. & DIAMOND, J. M. (1967) The ultrastructural route of fluid transport in rabbit gallbladder. *J. Gen. Physiol.* 50, 2031-2060

VARGAS, F. F. (1968) Water flux and electrokinetic phenomena in the squid axon. *J. Gen. Physiol. 51*, 123s-130s

WEIBEL, E. R. (1974) Stereological techniques for electron microscopic morphometry, in *Principles and Techniques of Electron Microscopy*, vol. 3 (Hayat, M. A., ed.), Van Nostrand Reinhold, New York

WHITLOCK, R. T. & WHEELER, H. O. (1964) Coupled transport of solute and water across rabbit gallbladder epithelium. *J. Clin. Invest. 43*, 2249-2265

WRIGHT, E. M., SMULDERS, A. P. & TORMEY, J. McD. (1972) The role of the lateral intercellular spaces and solute polarization effects in the passive flow of water across the rabbit gallbladder. *J. Membr. Biol. 7*, 198-219

Ion transport across amphibian lung

JOHN T. GATZY

Department of Pharmacology, School of Medicine, University of North Carolina, Chapel Hill, North Carolina

Abstract The simple architecture of the amphibian lung makes it possible to study the movement of substances across a barrier with permeability and bioelectric properties that are dominated by the alveolar epithelium. When mounted as a planar sheet between identical Ringer solutions the excised lung of the bullfrog exhibited a transmural electrical potential difference of nearly 20 mV (pleural surface positive) and a resistance of about 700 Ω cm². Unidirectional fluxes of ^{36}Cl, Br^-, I^-, and SCN^- across the short-circuited lung were asymmetrical. The net $^{36}Cl^-$ flow from pleura to lumen matched the short-circuit current after 1.5 h of voltage clamping, followed the kinetics of a saturable process, and was reduced by inhibitors of oxidative metabolism. These results suggest that halide and certain pseudohalide anions are secreted by the frog alveolar epithelium. Fluxes of Na^+, K^+, Ca^+, HCO_3^-, TcO_4^-, SO_4^{2-}, *p*-aminohippurate, gluconate, dinitrophenolate and water were compatible with passive diffusion of the probe molecules across the barrier. Measurements of lung oxygen consumption, ion fluxes and bioelectric properties have helped to pinpoint possible sites and modes of action of airborne agents, such as heavy metals, sulphates and nitrates, that may damage the mammalian pulmonary barrier.

For about 15 years investigators in several laboratories have measured the rates at which solutes and water penetrate the barrier between blood and the fluid-filled air space of the lungs of mammals and reptiles (e.g. Cross *et al.* 1960; Taylor *et al.* 1965; Deitchman & Paganelli 1967; Wangensteen *et al.* 1969). The results of the studies were strikingly similar to those obtained for tracer movement across the epithelia of the gastrointestinal tract and renal tubule, suggesting that the cells which line the alveoli are the major barrier to solution translocation. This viewpoint was reinforced by the observation that small solutes added to the vascular space exerted a much greater osmotic effect in the fluid-filled than in the air-filled lung (Taylor & Gaar 1970). On the other hand, results from dye-dilution studies were consistent with a pulmonary capillary endothelium that was relatively impermeable to small ions such as

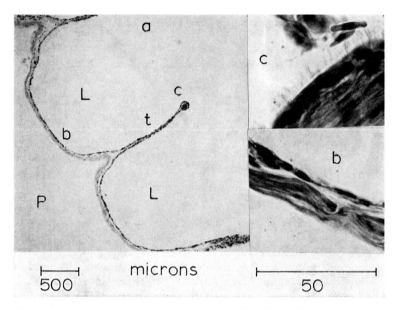

Fig. 1. (a) A cross-section of a portion of the bullfrog lung. The tissue was fixed in formalin and stained with haematoxylin and eosin. L = lumen, P = pleural, t = trabecula; (b) and (c) = regions b and c in (a), shown at higher magnification.

Na^+, and with the notion that the endothelium may make an appreciable contribution to the barrier between blood and air (Chinard 1966).

Even though indirect experiments have been devised to separate the series components of the barrier, parallel flow across the bronchiolar mucosa has not been resolved. The studies in our laboratory attempt to assess directly the permeability of the alveolar epithelium by exploiting the relatively simple architecture of the amphibian lung. Each lung lobe of a frog or toad is a single alveolar sac. The luminal aspect of the organ is covered by a continuous epithelium of one cell thickness. A network of fibrous trabeculae underlie the epithelium, giving the luminal surface the appearance of an open honeycomb. A cross-section of two 'cells' or cups of this comb is presented in Fig. 1a. Both squamous and cuboidal cells make up the epithelium and the cells at the tips of the trabeculae are ciliated (Fig. 1b, c). A connective tissue space with fibres, blood vessels and nerve endings separates the alveolar lining from the thin pleural covering. Since small ions penetrate the mesothelial lining of the peritoneum of the amphibian and mammal very rapidly, it seemed likely that the pleural covering would be similarly 'leaky' and that the only other continuous cell layer, the epithelium, constitutes the major permeability barrier. Findings will be presented later in support of this contention.

TABLE 1

Bioelectric properties of excised epithelia from amphibians and reptiles

Tissue	Transmural p.d. (mV, serosa +)	D.c. resistance (Ω cm^2)
Lung		
bullfrog	19	700
marine toad	6	790
South American bullfrog	7	380
fresh water turtle	9	450
Intestine[a]		
bullfrog	1–3	150
Skin[b]		
leopard frog	56	4000
Urinary bladder		
marine toad	72	1900

[a] Quay & Armstrong 1969
[b] Helman & Miller 1973

BIOELECTRIC PROPERTIES

When the amphibian lung is pinned open and mounted in an Ussing-type apparatus as a planar sheet between identical Ringer solutions, a transmural bioelectric potential difference (p.d.) can be measured (Gatzy 1967). Table 1 lists the p.d. and d.c. resistance for the lungs of several anurans and a freshwater turtle, along with representative figures for several other amphibian epithelia. The values for toad urinary bladder were obtained in this laboratory from tissues mounted in the lung chambers and are compatible with minimal edge damage (Finn & Hutton 1974). From these results we infer that the lung is probably not damaged by the apparatus.

The orientation of the lung p.d. (pleura or serosa positive with respect to lumen) is similar to that measured for the urinary bladder, the skin and all regions of the amphibian gastrointestinal tract. The magnitudes of the p.d. values and resistances suggest that the lung is not as 'tight' an epithelium as the skin or bladder but is considerably less 'leaky' than the intestine. Values for South American bullfrog and the turtle were obtained from only a few animals in questionable condition and may, therefore, be low.

Since bullfrog lung exhibited the highest p.d., it has received the most comprehensive study. Agents that affect the bioelectric properties of this lung are listed in Table 2. In general, those substances which affect the resistance of the lung induce an even greater change in p.d. Since the tissue follows Ohm's

TABLE 2

Agents that affect bioelectric properties of the excised bullfrog lung

Change in transmural p.d. and short-circuit current		
Increase	No effect[a]	Decrease
HgCl$_2$(10^{-7}M)	PbCl$_2$	HgCl$_2$ (10^{-5}M)
amphotericin B (10^{-6}M)	CdCl$_2$	amphotericin B (10^{-4}M)
	aldosterone	dinitrophenol
	vasopressin	NaCN
	amiloride	iodoacetate
	adrenaline (epinephrine)	hypoxia
	histamine	ouabain
	5-hydroxytryptamine	p-chloromercuribenzoate
	acetylcholine	n-ethylmaleimide
	acetazolamide	etacrynic acid
	furosemide	EDTA sodium salt
	p-chloromercuri-	aqueous cigarette smoke
	benzenesulphonate	extract
		proteinase
		collagenase

[a] Both surfaces of the lung were exposed to concentrations of up to 10^{-3}M

law the current needed to reduce the biopotential to zero (short-circuit current) and the p.d. always change in the same direction. Evidence will be presented which indicates that the short-circuit current is an index of Cl$^-$ secretion.

Few compounds raise the open-circuit voltage and short-circuit current of the lung. Low concentrations of HgCl$_2$ or amphotericin B in the mucosal bathing solution routinely induce increases of 25 to 50% by, as we shall see, two separate mechanisms. In contrast, several classes of agents reduce voltage and current. Inhibitors of oxidative, glycolytic and ATP metabolism, penetrant sulphydryl reagents, a divalent cation chelator, proteolytic enzymes and cigarette smoke, along with higher concentrations of HgCl$_2$ and amphotericin B, bring about decreases of at least 50% which are, with the exception of hypoxia, irreversible. For the most part, these results are not surprising since the spontaneous bioelectric p.d. of epithelia is universally dependent on the integrity of energy metabolism and on the continuity of the epithelial cell layer. EDTA and proteolytic enzymes are known to disaggregate cells and, therefore, probably affect the latter property. Other heavy metals, such as lead and cadmium, a poorly permeant sulphydryl reagent (PCMBS) and a number of diuretics, hormones, neurotransmitters, autocoids and carbonate dehydratase (EC 4.2.1.1, carbonic anhydrase) inhibitors that affect Na$^+$ or Cl$^-$ transport and the bioelectric properties of a wide spectrum of epithelia all fail to influence the bullfrog lung.

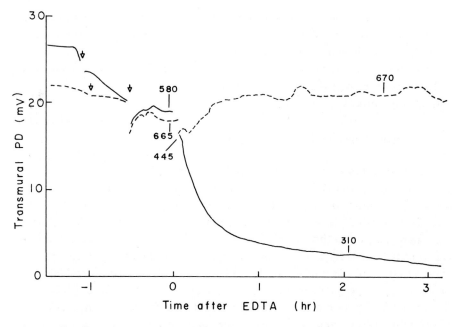

FIG. 2. The effect of 3×10^{-4} M-Na EDTA on bioelectric properties of the excised bullfrog lung. EDTA was added to the mucosal (solid line) or serosal (dashed line) bathing solution at zero time. Downward arrows represent replacement of the bathing solutions with fresh Ringer. Numbers indicate d.c. transmural resistances (ohm cm²).

TABLE 3

The effect of bathing solution composition on bioelectric properties of the excised bullfrog lung

Change in transmural p.d. and short-circuit current after ion replacement in both bathing solutions

Increase	No effect	Decrease
SO_4^- for Cl^-	choline for Na^+	NO_3^- for Cl^-
$CH_3SO_4^-$ for Cl	Na^+ for K^+	SCN^- for Cl^-
gluconate for Cl^-	Na^+ for Ca^{++}	I^- for Cl^-
isethionate for Cl^-	Cl^- for HCO_3^-	
	Br^- for Cl^-	

A similar approach can be used to summarize the effects of changes in bathing solution composition (Table 3). It is apparent that the bioelectric properties of the lung are not affected by cation replacement. Replacement of Cl^- by a group of poorly permeant anions in the luminal (mucosal) or both bathing solutions is always accompanied by an increase. Br⁻ substitutes for Cl⁻ but concentrations of SCN⁻ or I⁻ above 5 mм induce an irreversible fall. Complete replacement of Cl⁻ by NO_3^- also lowers p.d. and short-circuit current but these changes are reversible. Thus, the pattern of response in Table 3 indicates that the bioelectric properties of the bullfrog lung are most consistently linked with the Cl⁻.

SITE OF THE BIOPOTENTIAL AND RESISTANCE

Even though it seemed reasonable to dismiss the contribution of the pleural covering to the permeability of the preparation, a number of experiments were designed to evaluate this supposition. Concentrations of $HgCl_2$ or EDTA were found which induced a nearly immediate fall in tissue p.d. and resistance after they were added to the mucosal solution (Gatzy 1967). A representative experiment for EDTA is illustrated in Fig. 2. Addition of the same concentration to the serosal solution caused gradual changes after a considerable delay or, as in the experiment in Fig. 2, no change at all. It seemed likely that luminal administration afforded direct access to the epithelium but ligands in the pleural covering and connective tissue retarded the deeper penetration of metal or EDTA that was added to the serosal solution. More recently, surgical removal of one-tenth to one-fifth of the pleural covering failed to affect the bioelectric p.d. (Gatzy 1972). Therefore, both direct and indirect evidence favour the idea that the epithelium is the site of the transmural biopotential and resistance.

ION AND WATER TRANSPORT ACROSS THE BULLFROG LUNG

To assess the permeability of the lung to ions and water, unidirectional fluxes of radioactive molecules were measured under short-circuit conditions (Gatzy 1975). Equal rates of penetration in each direction are compatible with passive movement of the probe molecule. Asymmetrical fluxes in the absence of a transmural gradient of chemical and electrical potential are compelling evidence for a mode of translocation that requires energy, such as active transport. Table 4 outlines the flux coefficients that were calculated from the movement of a number of labelled ions and tritiated water. Coefficients for water and each of the cations of the bathing solution are symmetrical and close to values for passive movement across other amphibian epithelia such as toad bladder (Leaf & Hays 1962; Gatzy 1971b) and, where comparisons are possible, for passage between the blood and the fluid-filled air space of the mammalian and turtle lung (Taylor et al. 1965; Deitchman & Paganelli 1967).

TABLE 4

Unidirectional flux coefficients for ion and water movement across short-circuited, excised bullfrog lung

Symmetrical $(k_s \rightarrow_m = k_m \rightarrow_s)$		Asymmetrical $(k_s \rightarrow_m > k_m \rightarrow_s)$
1 to 10 $\times$ 10⁻⁷ cm/s	70 to 700 $\times$ 10⁻⁷ cm/s	
Na^+	HTO	Cl^-
K^+	dinitrophenolate	Br^-
Ca^{2+}	HCO_3^-	I^-
SO_4^{2-}		SCN^-
gluconate		
p-aminohippurate		

The value for K^+ may be low because the lung had not attained specific activity equilibrium after 3 h of exposure to the tracer. However, estimates based on the fraction of total tissue K^+ labelled by ⁴²K indicate that the flux coefficients should not exceed 35 $\times$ 10⁻⁷ cm/s.

The pattern of anion movement across the lung reveals a large number of species with symmetrical coefficients. Among this group are ions that are actively secreted by the renal proximal tubule (p-aminohippurate: PAH) and accumulated by the thyroid (TcO_4). The values for SO_4^{2-} and dinitrophenolate are in reasonable agreement with the results for dog lung (Taylor *et al.* 1965). The rate of HCO_3^- penetration suggests that part of the tracer was moving as CO_2. These suspicions were confirmed when radioactivity in the gas phase above both the sink and source solutions was trapped by 2-aminoethanol. Furthermore, carbonate dehydratase inhibitors reduced both the transmural fluxes by about 50%.

In contrast to the anions with symmetrical unidirectional fluxes, Cl^-, Br^-, I^- and SCN^- move more rapidly from serosa to mucosa. For example, the mean flux coefficients for ³⁶Cl movement from serosa to mucosa and mucosa to serosa were 27.5 ($\pm$ 2.8 s.e.) and 16.9 ($\pm$ 1.5 s.e.) $\times$ 10⁻⁷ cm/s, respectively. Since there was no concentration gradient for any bathing solution constituent and all constituents except chloride appear to move passively, the net flow of Cl^- cannot be coupled to the movement of any other species. These results suggest that the halides and SCN^- are actively secreted into the bullfrog lung lumen.

NET Cl⁻ FLUX AND SHORT-CIRCUIT CURRENT

The net charge flow generated by the transport of an ion or ions across amphibian epithelia such as skin, urinary bladder, gastric mucosa, large intestine and cornea has been shown to be equal to the short-circuit current. Cl⁻ transport across the lung accounted for about half of the current during the first hour of voltage clamping. However, the current gradually fell during this period, so that by 90 min net Cl⁻ flux and short-circuit current were indistinguishable. It appears likely that the asymmetrical flow of an ion from the tissue might account for the early discrepancy.

THE EFFECT OF CL⁻ CONCENTRATION, METABOLIC INHIBITORS AND BR⁻ ON NET CL⁻ FLUX

Although asymmetrical flow in the absence of a gradient of electrochemical p.d. is probably the most rigorous test of active transport, other criteria such as the kinetics of a saturable process, inhibition by blockers of energy metabolism and competition between similar molecules have been described frequently. Fig. 3 depicts the unidirectional and net flux of Cl⁻ across the short-circuited lung plotted as a function of the concentration of Cl⁻ in the bathing solution. It is obvious that both unidirectional fluxes increase with increasing Cl⁻ concentration but the net flow approaches a maximum at 20 μequiv./ml. The net transport of Cl⁻ yields a straight line when plotted according to a linear transformation of the Michaelis–Menten equation. These observations are compatible with the saturation of a fixed number of tissue sites with Cl⁻. The apparent dissociation constant for this reaction (K_m) is 19 mM and the maximum velocity equals 0.3 μequiv. cm⁻² h⁻¹.

As summarized in Table 2, both dinitrophenol (DNP) and low oxygen tension depressed the short-circuit current of the lung. These agents also reduced the net transport of Cl⁻. The results with DNP were clear-cut; only the serosa → mucosa flux was affected. Hypoxia reduced the magnitude of both fluxes to the same value.

Since Br⁻ can replace Cl⁻ without affecting short-circuit current, one might expect Br⁻ to have roughly the same affinity for a halide carrier and to compete effectively with Cl⁻ for transport. Attempts to demonstrate competition were inconclusive. A constant concentration of 30 mequiv. bromide/l shifted the net flux-concentration relationship for Cl⁻ in the appropriate direction but the shift was smaller than anticipated and the calculated K_m for Br⁻ was more than three times the value for Cl⁻. Hence, there is ample evidence for the secretion of Cl⁻ into the lung lumen but it is not clear that other halides are translocated by the same mechanism.

THE SIGNIFICANCE OF CL TRANSPORT BY THE LUNG

The physiological importance of Cl⁻ secretion by the bullfrog lung remains

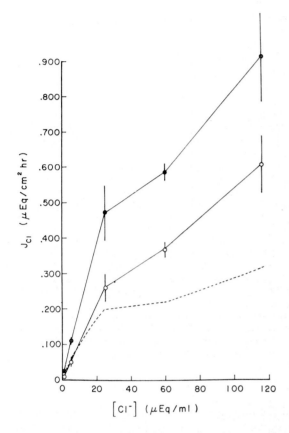

FIG. 3. Influence of the concentration of bathing solution Cl⁻ on unidirectional fluxes of ³⁶Cl across the short-circuited lung. —○— = M → S flux, —●— = S → M flux, and the net flow is represented by the dashed line. Cl⁻ was replaced by gluconate. Each point represents the mean of at least five experiments. Vertical lines represent standard errors. (Reprinted from Gatzy 1975 with the permission of the *American Journal of Physiology*).

obscure. Because the lung evaginates from a region of the gastrointestinal tract near the stomach, halide transport may represent a vestigial gastric function. Although this suggestion cannot be dismissed, other properties of the stomach, such as H^+ secretion and Cl⁻ exchange diffusion, are not shared by the lung (Gatzy 1975).

Alternatively, the secretion of Cl⁻ and, hence, salt may be required for the maintenance of surfactant activity. The observation that the toad lung produces surfactant but does not, according to our measurements, transport Cl⁻ speaks against this proposal.

Finally, Cl⁻ secretion by the fetal mammalian lung has been described

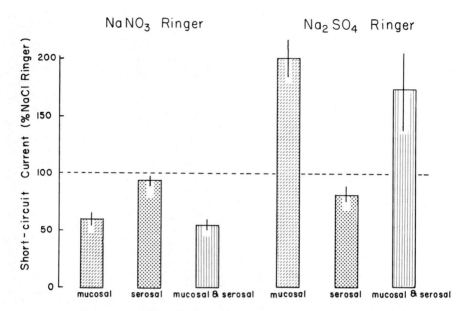

FIG. 4. The effect of NO_3^- or SO_4^{2-} on short-circuit current of the excised bullfrog lung. All of the Cl^- in the bathing solution noted on the ordinate was replaced by the test anion. Short-circuit current is plotted as a percentage of the steady-state value in NaCl Ringer just before the anion replacement. Each bar is the mean of at least three experiments. Vertical lines are the S.E.

(Olver *et al.* 1973), so the bullfrog lung may represent a functional analogue of a step in the development of the mature mammalian lung (Staub 1974). This suggestion is not entirely consistent with our findings that the lungs of the toad and the South American bullfrog do not secrete Cl^-.

THE EFFECT OF AIR POLLUTANTS ON THE LUNG

Measurements of tissue ion composition have demonstrated that the average cell of the bullfrog lung, like most cells, has a high K^+ and low Na^+ and Cl^- content. To effect the transport of Cl^- from serosa to mucosa the pump must be located at the apical border of the epithelial cell layer. We reasoned that alterations in bioelectric properties and Cl^- movement might provide a sensitive assay for airborne agents which act at this site. Studies with nitrate, sulphate and mercury salts will illustrate this point.

The effects of airborne nitrates and, particularly, sulphates on the lung have received increasing attention because of the action of the catalytic converter on car exhaust emissions. Although it is clear that sulphuric acid is irritating

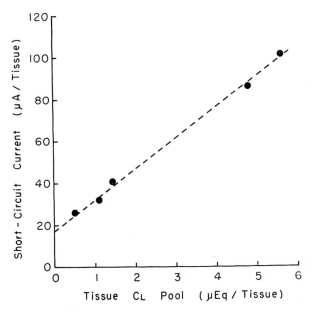

FIG. 5. The relationship of short-circuit current to the tissue Cl⁻ pool of five excised bullfrog lungs. The lungs were incubated for two hours in Na_2SO_4 Ringer in an Ussing-type chamber before the Cl⁻ concentration was measured.

to the respiratory tract, preliminary experiments with the bullfrog model indicate that this lung reacts only to a decrease in pH and not to the chemical nature of the acid. In contrast, nitrate and sulphate salts induce quite different effects on bioelectric properties, as noted in Table 2. These effects are examined in more detail in Fig. 4. Replacement of all the Cl⁻ in the mucosal bathing solution by NO_3^- decreased the short-circuit current by nearly 50% whereas substitution in only the serosal solution was without effect. Since the resistance of the tissue did not change during the fall it seems likely that the inhibition reflects an action on Cl⁻ transport. This possibility is currently under examination.

Replacement of mucosal Cl⁻ by SO_4^{2-} doubled the short-circuit current. This increase was always accompanied by a raised resistance. The increase in resistance is compatible with the fact that the flux coefficient for SO_4^{2-} is about one-fifth of the value for the passive flow of Cl⁻. Even though the rise in short-circuit current might be attributed to a stimulation of active Cl⁻ transport, it is also possible that SO_4^{2-} acts as an 'indifferent', poorly permeant anion. The increase in current would then reflect the passive flow of alveolar cell Cl⁻ across the apical membrane into the lumen. Since removal of

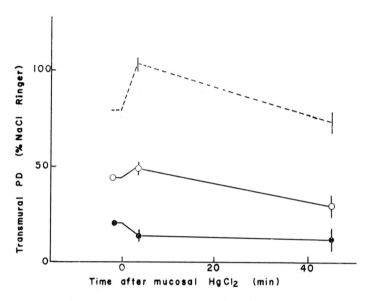

Fig. 6. The effect of metabolic inhibitors on the time-course of the p.d. change induced by mucosal $HgCl_2$ ($10^{-5}M$) followed one minute later by the addition of cysteine ($10^{-4}M$). P.d.'s are plotted as a percentage of the steady-state values in NaCl Ringer before the introduction of inhibitor. —○— = 100% N_2; —●— = dinitrophenol and NaCN ($10^{-4}M$) and the control response is represented by the dashed line. Each point is the mean of at least four experiments.

Cl^- from both bathing solutions does not alter the response, the apical membrane must be more Cl^--selective than the serosal border. The study summarized in Fig. 5 bears on this hypothesis. Lungs from five animals were mounted in the Ussing chambers and incubated in a Na_2SO_4 Ringer solution for two hours. At the end of this period the tissues were removed from the apparatus and analysed for Cl^-. The short-circuit current just before tissue removal is plotted as a function of tissue Cl^- content. The correlation between the parameters is excellent and is consistent with the idea that SO_4^{2-} replacement merely provides a favourable gradient for passive Cl^- movement from the cell into the lumen.

The effects of $HgCl_2$ on the bioelectric properties of the bullfrog lung were mentioned earlier in the discussion of Table 2. The entire spectrum of mercury's effects can be obtained with an intermediate dose ($10^{-5}M$). With this concentration in the mucosal solution, the p.d. and short-circuit current rise transiently and then fall. Resistance continues to drop during the entire course of metal action. If one is interested in examining only the increase in p.d. and short-circuit current, an excess of a mercury complexer, such as

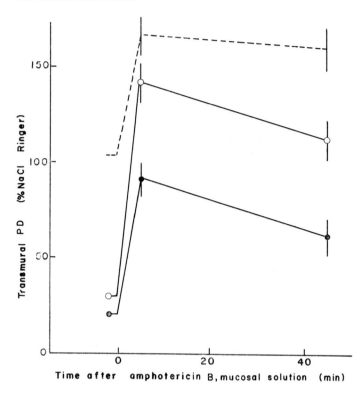

FIG. 7. The effect of metabolic inhibitors on the time-course of the p.d. change induced by the addition of amphotericin B (3×10^{-6}M) to the mucosal solution. Other conditions are the same as in Fig. 6.

cysteine, dimercaprol or albumin, can be added one minute after the introduction of $HgCl_2$ into the bathing solution (Gatzy 1971a). An example of this experiment is shown as the control response in Fig. 6. When the experiment was repeated in the presence of inhibitors of metabolism the mercury-induced increase in p.d. disappeared. To show that the disappearance resulted from inhibition of metabolism rather than deterioration of the epithelium, the experiment was repeated with a low dose of amphotericin B (Fig. 7). This antifungal agent increases the ion permeability of natural and synthetic membranes that contain cholesterol. It is clear that the increased p.d. after amphotericin B was not reduced by pretreatment with inhibitors. On the other hand, replacement of Na^+ in the mucosal solution by Mg^{2+} or choline abolished the response to amphotericin B without altering the $HgCl_2$ effect. Furthermore, the oxygen consumption of the lung was increased about 25% by a low concentration of $HgCl_2$ but was minimally affected by amphotericin B (Gatzy &

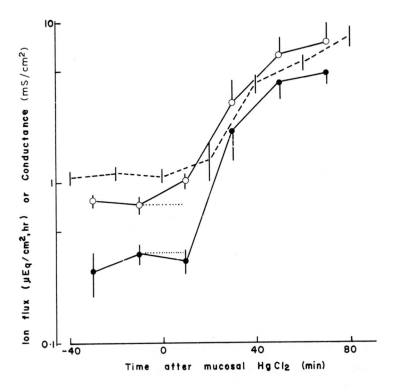

FIG. 8. The effect of mucosal $HgCl_2$ (10^{-5}M) on simultaneous serosal to mucosal fluxes of
^{36}Cl(—○—) and ^{22}Na (—●—) and on d.c. transmural conductance (dashed lines). Con-
ductances were measured at end of each collection from the sink solution. Fluxes are plotted
at the midpoint between collection periods. Each point is the mean of four experiments.
Vertical lines represent the S.E. The ^{36}Cl flux during the first period after the administration
of $HgCl_2$ was significantly increased when calculated as a percentage of the flux before the
addition of $HgCl_2$. The units of conductance are millisiemens/cm² (= $m\Omega^{-1}$ cm^{-2}).

Stutts 1975). The evidence above demonstrates that the increase in p.d. and
short-circuit current induced by $HgCl_2$ is the consequence of an energy-
requiring process, whereas the charge flow after amphotericin B requires
mucosal Na^+ but probably not cellular energy.

It seemed likely that the chloride transport mechanism was the initial target
of $HgCl_2$. This hypothesis was tested by measuring simultaneous fluxes of
^{22}Na and ^{36}Cl across the short-circuited lung. The results for movement in
the serosa to mucosa direction before and after $HgCl_2$ are presented in Fig. 8.
Addition of the metal induced the progressive increase in conductance (fall in
resistance) which was described earlier. Like the open-circuit response, the
short-circuit current under voltage clamping increased by about 30% during

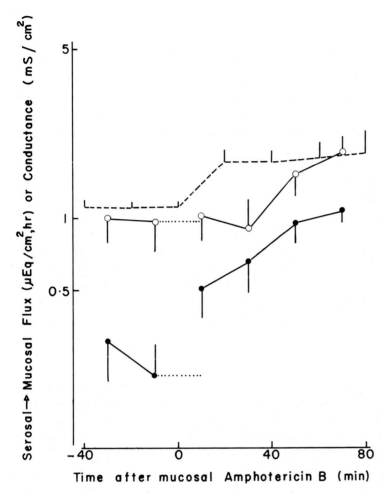

FIG. 9. The effect of mucosal amphotericin B (5×10^{-6}M) on simultaneous serosal to mucosal fluxes of ^{36}Cl (—○—) and ^{22}Na (—●—) and on d.c. transmural conductance (dashed lines). All conductance and ^{22}Na flux points after amphotericin B are significantly greater when calculated as a percentage of the control points before addition of the drug. Only the Cl⁻ point at 70 min was significantly increased. Other conditions are the same as in Fig. 8.

the first 20 min after addition of $HgCl_2$ and then declined throughout the remainder of the experiment. The initial increase in current was paralleled by a selective increase in the flux of Cl⁻. The Na⁺ flux did not increase until the conductance had doubled and the lung was rapidly becoming very leaky to both ions. When the direction of isotope penetration was reversed, changes in Na⁺ and Cl⁻ flux could not be detected during the period of the short-circuit current increase.

Addition of dimercaprol to the mucosal solution one minute after the initial exposure to $HgCl_2$ resulted in an even greater increase in short-circuit current that persisted for an hour. During this time the serosal to mucosal Cl^- flux doubled. Both Na^+ fluxes and the flow of Cl^- in the opposite direction were affected minimally. These results indicate that the initial or low dose effects of $HgCl_2$ result from a stimulation of active Cl^- transport. Higher metal concentrations appear to induce a non-selective increase in ion permeability.

Similar flux studies with amphotericin B revealed immediate selective changes in Na^+ permeability during the increase in short-circuit current. An example is illustrated in Fig. 9. Conductance and serosal to mucosal Na^+ flow increased during the first period of measurement after the addition of amphotericin B and remained raised. Cl^- flux was unaffected for at least 30 min. Identical results were obtained when tracer flowed in the opposite direction. Again, the most plausible locus of drug action is the apical membrane but, in this case, amphotericin B appears to increase the permeability of the barrier to Na^+, thereby increasing the rate of passive entry into the alveolar cell, the bioelectric p.d. and the short-circuit current.

CONCLUSIONS

The excised bullfrog lung is a relatively simple alveolar epithelium that shares many permeability characteristics with the mammalian barrier between blood and air. In addition, an active Cl^- transport mechanism is probably located at the apical membranes of the epithelial cell layer. Studies with airborne agents such as mercury, sulphate and nitrate salts suggest that this border is a primary site of toxic action.

ACKNOWLEDGEMENT

These studies were supported, in part, by Public Health Service Grants HL – 12246, HL – 16674 and GM – 11598.

References

CHINARD, F. P. (1966) in *Advances In Respiratory Physiology* (Caro, C. G., ed.), pp. 106-147, Williams & Wilkins, Baltimore

CROSS, C. E., RIEBEN, P. A. & SALISBURY, P. F. (1960) Urea permeability of the alveolar membrane; hemodynamic effects of liquid in the alveolar spaces. *Am. J. Physiol.* 198, 1029-31

DEITCHMAN, D. & PAGANELLI, C. V. (1967) Solute movement across the alveolar-capillary membrane of the turtle. *Physiologist 10*, 154

FINN, A. L. & HUTTON, S. A. (1974) Absence of edge damage in toad urinary bladder. *Am. J. Physiol.* 227, 950-953

GATZY, J. T. (1967) Bioelectric properties of the isolated amphibian lung. *Am. J. Physiol.* 213, 425-431

GATZY, J. T. (1971a) The effect of mercury and amphotericin B on bioelectric properties of the excised bullfrog lung. *Fed. Proc.* 39, 673

GATZY, J. T. (1971b) The effect of K⁺-sparing diuretics on ion transport across the excised toad bladder. *J. Pharmacol. Exp. Ther.* 176, 580-594

GATZY, J. T. (1972) Volume flow across excised amphibian lung and urinary bladder exposed to heavy metals, in *V Int. Congr. Pharmacol.*, Abstr., p. 78

GATZY, J. T. (1975) Ion transport across the excised bullfrog lung. *Am. J. Physiol.* 228, 1162-1171

GATZY, J. T. & STUTTS, M. J. (1975) Ion transport and O_2 consumption of excised bullfrog lung after treatment with $HgCl_2$ or amphotericin B. *Fed. Proc.* 34, 753

HELMAN, S. I. & MILLER, D. A. (1973) Edge damage effects on electrical measurements of frog skin. *Am. J. Physiol.* 225, 972-977

LEAF, A. & HAYS, R. M. (1962) Permeability of the isolated toad bladder to solutes and its modification by vasopressin. *J. Gen. Physiol.* 48, 527-540

OLVER, R. E., REYNOLDS, O. R. & STRANG, L. B. (1973) in *Foetal and Neonatal Physiology* (Comline, K. S., *et al.*, eds.), pp. 186-207, Cambridge University Press, London

QUAY, J. F. & ARMSTRONG, W. McD. (1969) Sodium and chloride transport by isolated bullfrog small intestine. *Am. J. Physiol.* 217, 694-702

STAUB, N. C. (1974) Pulmonary edema. *Physiol. Rev.* 5, 678-811

TAYLOR, A. E. & GAAR, K. A., JR. (1970) Estimation of equivalent pore radii of pulmonary capillary and alveolar membranes. *Am. J. Physiol.* 218, 1133-1140

TAYLOR, A. E., GUYTON, A. C. & BISHOP, V. S. (1965) Permeability of the alveolar membrane to solutes. *Circ. Res.* 16, 353-362

WANGENSTEEN, O. D., WITTMERS, L. E., JR. & JOHNSON, J. A. (1969) Permeability of the mammalian blood-gas barrier and its components. *Am. J. Physiol.* 216, 719-727

Discussion

Dickinson: What accounts for the potential in the toad, which you showed has no active chloride transport?

Gatzy: The flux of chloride in the passive (mucosal to serosal) direction is quite high relative to the active flow. Since there is no other useful chloride isotope we have to do these studies in paired lobes, so the errors tend to be quite large. There could be a small chloride transport that is not detected.

Olver: Would successive experiments on the same lobes be more sensitive than those on paired lobes, or would the tissue deteriorate too much with time?

Gatzy: I think it is much better to do these experiments with paired lobes. The absolute fluxes across the tissue are so small that washing out the source is a real problem. Isotope penetrates into every aqueous crevice, for example into the electrodes.

Durbin: When you said that substitution of isethionate and other ions did not affect chloride movement, were you talking about the rate coefficient or the net flux of chloride?

Gatzy: I was talking about the bioelectric properties (Table 4, p. 185). Isethionate and gluconate always increased short-circuit current and potential difference. We think that this is because the chloride that remains in the cell diffuses across a selectively permeable apical membrane, giving rise to a diffusion potential. When the tissue is exposed to sulphate Ringer solution for two hours, the concentration of chloride that remains in the tissue is directly related to the short-circuit current (Fig. 5, p. 189). I conclude that the pool of tissue chloride determines the short-circuit current. Although all of the chloride flow could be mediated by the transport mechanism it seems unnecessary to postulate this if passive outflow can account for the observations.

Staub: Did you say that the cells contained a very low concentration of chloride?

Gatzy: Not very low but lower than that of the bathing solution.

Staub: We have measured the chloride content of the lung and find that intracellular chloride is relatively high, being about half the concentration it is in interstitial fluid (Selinger *et al.* 1975).

Gatzy: I don't think it is high. When compared with measurements for amphibian epithelia that is not an unreasonable value.

Staub: Even though the ciliated cells on the ridges occupy only a small part of the lung, this part could be contributing almost all of the chloride transport. Since the alveoli in frog lung are large, is there a way of filling them up individually and measuring short-circuit currents or potentials without touching the ciliated ridges?

Gatzy: An individual alveolar 'cup' is too small to mount in a chamber. One reason why the ridges are not likely to contribute appreciably to chloride transport is that the tissue approaches specific activity equilibrium with chloride and sodium quite rapidly, about as fast as epithelia without trabeculae, such as toad bladder. Since the trabeculae represent an extremely long pathway (up to several millimetres), it seems unlikely that they could make a major contribution to the early tracer pool or to chloride transport that is measured contemporaneously.

Staub: We find that even after two hours the specific activity of chloride in the sheep lung is not equal to that in interstitial fluid or plasma.

Olver: You seem to be put off by the fact that the active transport mechanism may have different affinities for the different halides. You said that transport is unlikely to be by the same mechanism. Why couldn't the same carrier have different affinities for the different halides?

Gatzy: My statement is based on several assumptions. If chloride accounts for a large share of the short-circuit current and biopotential one would expect the bioelectric properties to change when chloride is replaced by an identical concentration of bromide—a halide that, on the basis of competition studies, appears to have a much lower affinity for the chloride transport mechanism. But short-circuit current doesn't change. If halide transport continues to account for most of the short-circuit current, the movement of bromide on the chloride pump would not be large enough to explain the net ion flow.

Keynes: Another chloride isotope, ^{38}Cl, is available but it has a half-life of only about 40 minutes.

Gatzy: As far as I am concerned, that is useless.

Keynes: Precisely for this reason Dr Ellory has been working at Harwell recently on double tracer fluxes. But one needs to be somewhere which has a pile or a cyclotron.

Hughes: Could you use your technique in mammalian bronchiolar or in alveolar tissue?

Gatzy: I don't see how we could use the technique with alveolar tissue. It might be possible with the larger bronchi.

Hughes: Have you got to have a completely undamaged single-cell sheet?

Gatzy: Yes.

Staub: In some animals (pigs and cows) the secondary lung lobules are completely surrounded by connective tissue septae. In these, you could fill one lobule with fluid and measure the p.d. between the inside and outside.

Gatzy: We have begun an attempt to block the bronchus of a terminal alveolar sac with oil, put fluid into the alveolus and then measure with a microelectrode the p.d. between the lumen and the pleural surface.

Dickinson: You said that the toad lung produces surfactant although it may not need it. That is the same lung in which you failed to demonstrate active chloride transport.

Strang: Dr Gatzy also said that although he hadn't demonstrated it, that didn't mean it wasn't there.

Reference

SELINGER, S. L., BLAND, R. D., DEMLING, R. H. & STAUB, N. C. (1975) Distribution volumes of ^{131}I albumin, ^{14}C sucrose and ^{36}Cl in sheep lung. *J. Appl. Physiol. 39*, 773-779

Ion transport and water flow in the mammalian lung

R. E. OLVER

Department of Paediatrics, University College Hospital Medical School, London

Abstract   The coupling of bulk water flow to active ion transport has been described in various epithelia; evidence presented here suggests that this is also a feature of the mammalian lung. Measurements of the ionic composition of lung liquid and its rate of formation in the fetal lamb *in vivo* have made it possible to estimate the net flux of each ion and, with tracer measurements of ion one-way fluxes, to calculate flux ratios. When these are compared with the ratios predicted by the Ussing flux ratio equation it is clear that the secretion of lung liquid is linked to active transport of Cl^- from plasma; sodium moves passively. In addition there is an apparent uphill transfer of HCO_3^- out of lung liquid. In an *in vitro* preparation of adult canine trachea Cl^- is actively transported towards the lumen and is associated with a small net flux of Na^+ in the opposite direction. Addition of acetylcholine increases the net Cl^- flux towards the lumen but reverses the orientation of the net Na^+ flux. Changes such as these may be important determinants of bulk liquid flow *in vivo* as well as *in vitro*.

Liquid covers the entire internal surface of the lung and although it forms a continuum it is quite possible that the composition of this aqueous layer in different areas varies, as does its function. In the trachea and bronchi water flow across the respiratory epithelium may be an important determinant of mucus viscosity, and may serve to lubricate the airways and facilitate coupling between cilia and the mucus layer. In the alveoli an aqueous subphase is theoretically essential for the normal function of the surfactant system and there is evidence to suggest that the ionic composition of the subphase may influence the surface tension properties of the surfactant layer (Frosolono *et al.* 1970). Measurements of ionic composition of liquid draining from the trachea have been made in animals (Boyd 1972) and man (Potter *et al.* 1963) but nothing is known about the site of origin of the liquid, the mechanism of its formation or its control. Although the alveolar lining layer has been sampled by micropuncture (Reifenrath & Zimmermann 1973), analysis of its

199

electrolyte composition has not, as yet, been made. Furthermore, there are technical problems which make it difficult to obtain a sample of the alveolar fluid uncontaminated by plasma in the air-filled lung. No such problems exist in the fetal lung, the potential air spaces of which are expanded by copious amounts of liquid.

This paper is concerned with two types of experiment which are in several ways complementary. The first are those performed *in vivo* in exteriorized fetal lambs in which it has been possible to measure both liquid volume flow and ion fluxes, and to show that the secretion of lung liquid in the fetus is associated with active ion transport. In the second group of experiments the tracheal epithelium of adult dogs has been studied *in vitro* and ion flux measurements have been made under short-circuit conditions. In this preparation it was possible to demonstrate active ion transport and to investigate the effect of agents which may be involved in the control of ion transport, and thus possibly water flow, across the respiratory epithelium.

EXPERIMENTS IN FETAL LAMBS

These studies were performed in lambs of 123–144 days gestation (term: 147 days) with intact placental circulations, exteriorized by Caesarean section. In each animal cannulas were inserted into the trachea and carotid artery to allow for sampling of lung liquid and blood.

The introduction into lung liquid of a known amount of tracer to which alveolar walls are impermeable (inulin, ^{125}I-labelled albumin) makes it possible to measure the volume of lung liquid and its rate of formation. The decline in ^{125}I-labelled albumin concentration in Fig. 1 represents dilution by newly-formed lung liquid and from the intercept of the line at zero time, lung liquid volume can be calculated. Mean values obtained by Normand *et al.* (1971) were (per kg body weight): lung liquid volume 30 ml, secretion rate 2.2 ml/h.

Chemical analysis of lung liquid (Table 1) shows it to differ strikingly from plasma: [Cl^-] is high while [HCO_3^-] and [protein] are low. Lung liquid is clearly quite unlike an ultrafiltrate of plasma.

With a knowledge of the lung liquid secretion rate and its electrolyte composition we can calculate the net flux of each ion from plasma to lung lumen. However, in order to determine whether an ion is actively transported we need to be able to measure the ratio of the one-way fluxes of each ion across the epithelium and to compare it with that predicted by the Ussing flux ratio equation:

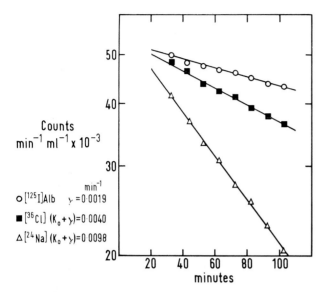

FIG. 1. ^{24}NaCl, Na^{36}Cl and a volume marker (^{125}I-labelled albumin) injected into lung liquid. Log concentration of tracers is plotted against time.

$$\ln \left[\frac{J_{p \to L}}{J_{L \to p}} \right] = \ln \left[\frac{a_p}{a_L} \right] + \frac{ZF}{RT} (\psi_p - \psi_L) + \frac{J_v}{D_s} \int_0^x \frac{1}{A} \, dx \qquad (1)$$

where $J_{p \to L}$ = the one-way flux of the ion from plasma to lung liquid and $J_{L \to p}$ = the one-way flux in the reverse direction; a_p and a_L = ion activity in plasma and lung liquid; $(\psi_p - \psi_L)$ = potential difference between plasma and lung liquid; Z, F, R and T have their usual meaning; J_v = volume flow from plasma (lung liquid secretion rate); D_s = ionic free diffusion coefficient; A = total area available for ion transfer, and x = path length (mean thickness of epithelium). This equation describes passive transfer and relates the measured flux ratio of an ion to the sum of the measured forces acting on it—the right-hand terms. The different terms in the flux ratio equation were evaluated in the following manner: flux ratios were measured in experiments in which isotopes of one or more ions were introduced into lung liquid together with a volume marker. Samples of lung liquid were then taken at intervals over a total period of at least 90 min and the change in concentration of tracers was followed as illustrated in Fig. 1. Since the concentration of tracers in plasma remains at a very low level and their diffusion out of lung liquid follows first-order kinetics, tracer concentration in lung liquid is given by:

$$\ln C_L = \ln C_L^o - t (K_o + \gamma) \qquad (2)$$

TABLE 1

Composition of lung liquid and plasma (mean values in mequiv./kg H_2O except where stated)

	Na^+	K^+	Ca^{2+}	Cl^-	HCO_3^-	pH	Protein (g/100 ml)
Lung liquid	150	6.3	0.86	157	2.8	6.27	0.027
Plasma	150	4.8	2.49	107	24	7.34	4.09

Ca^{2+} activity measured with an Orion Ca^{2+} selective electrode (from Olver & Strang 1974). All other values obtained by chemical measurement (from Adamson et al. 1969).

where C_L^o is the concentration of tracer (C_L) at zero time, $K_o(min^{-1})$ is the transfer constant for outward diffusion across alveolar walls and the rate constant γ (min^{-1}) is the ratio of the secretion rate of lung liquid to its volume. Thus in a plot of log concentration against time as in Fig. 1, the slopes of the tracers equal $K_o + \gamma$. For ^{125}I-labelled albumin, $K_o = 0$ (i.e. its slope is γ) and thus K_o values for the permeant tracers are readily derived.

The one-way flux of an ion out of lung liquid is given by $J_{L \rightarrow p} = K_o C_L V_L$ where C_L is the total concentration of the ion in lung liquid, labelled and unlabelled, and V_L is the volume of lung liquid. The net flux from plasma to lung liquid is given by $J_{net} = J_v C_L$ and the one-way flux from plasma to lung liquid must be $J_{p \rightarrow L} = J_{net} + J_{L \rightarrow p}$, thus $\dfrac{J_{p \rightarrow L}}{J_{L \rightarrow p}} = \dfrac{J_v C_L + K_o C_L V_L}{K_o C_L V_L}$ since $J_v/V_L = \gamma$; this simplifies to:

$$\frac{J_{p \rightarrow L}}{J_{L \rightarrow p}} = \frac{\gamma + K_o}{K_o} \tag{3}$$

In this way it is possible to measure the flux ratio of any ion, whether normally present in lung liquid or not. Table 2 gives the values of flux ratio for Na^+, K^+, Rb^+, Ca^{2+}, Cl^-, I^-, Br^-; in all cases they are greater than 1.0, reflecting net transport from plasma. Where possible, activity ratios were obtained from measurements of chemical concentration in plasma and lung liquid. Values for other ions were obtained by isotope equilibration after injection into the circulation. Table 2 shows that values of activity ratio (a_p/a_L) for all ions other than Na^+ and Ca^{2+} are less than 1.0, that is net transport takes place against a concentration gradient. For the anions, net transport takes place against an electrical gradient as well as a concentration gradient. In all experiments in which potential difference measurements were made, by one KCl-agar bridge being inserted into a small bronchus via the trachea and the other into the circulation, lung liquid was negative with respect to plasma (range 1–10 mV,

TABLE 2

Mean values for flux ratio ($J_{p\to L}/J_{L\to p}$) and activity ratio (a_p/a_L).

	Na^+	K^+	Rb^+	Ca^{2+}	Cl^-	Br^-	I^-
$\dfrac{J_{p\to L}}{J_{L\to p}}$	1.15	1.12	1.15	3.70	1.62	1.18	1.27
$\dfrac{a_p}{a_L}$	1.03	0.75	0.40	2.89	0.68	0·62	0.40

Figures taken from Olver & Strang 1974

mean 4.3 mV $\pm$ 0.45 s.e.). The last term in the flux ratio equation is solvent drag which, as its name implies, refers to the drag effect on solute molecules of bulk water flow. From theoretical considerations (J_v is small in relation to the denominator) and the results of experiments in which osmotic flows were generated across the alveolar epithelium, it was concluded that this force is small—in electrical units less than 1 mV for all ions (Olver & Strang 1974).

In Fig. 2, the measured flux ratios are compared with those predicted for passive diffusion by the sum of the righthand terms in the flux ratio equation. For Na^+ and Ca^{2+} there is good agreement between the two, suggesting that these ions are passively transferred. For K^+, Rb^+ and the halides, the measured forces predict net flux from lung liquid whereas the reverse occurs, showing that the ions are actively transported from plasma to lung liquid. Of these, Cl^- is by far the most important quantitatively and thus most likely to be coupled to bulk water flow. The affinity of the transport mechanism for halides other than Cl^- is similar to that described in the frog stomach (Hogben 1955; Durbin 1964).

The low bicarbonate concentration in lung liquid (Table 1) could be a result of one of three mechanisms:

(*a*) severe restriction to passive diffusion in the face of a volume flow from plasma to the lung interior,

(*b*) active transport of HCO_3^- out of lung liquid,

(*c*) active secretion of H^+ into lung liquid.

We could not measure one-way fluxes with $H^{14}CO_3^-$ because it was not possible to distinguish between movement of the labelled ion and movement as $^{14}CO_2$. We did, however, measure net fluxes of HCO_3^- after addition of isotonic $NaHCO_3$ to lung liquid as illustrated in Fig. 3A. In all cases there was an apparent uphill transport of HCO_3^- out of lung liquid. However, this process is indistinguishable from H^+ secretion into lung liquid. Plots of net flux of HCO_3^- out of lung liquid against lung liquid [HCO_3^-](e.g. Fig. 3B)

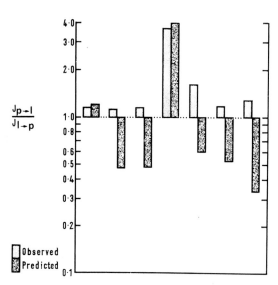

FIG. 2. Comparison of observed flux ratios, $J_{p \to L}/J_{L \to p}$ with ratios predicted from Ussing's equation for passive transfer (1). Each is represented on a log scale as a deviation from 1.0.

showed that if this transport is carrier-mediated it is not saturated at concentrations of up to 60 mequiv./kg H_2O.

Although *transepithelial* HCO_3^- flux has not been demonstrated in the way that is possible with radioactive isotopes, calculation of the total intracellular water volume of the alveolar epithelium demonstrates that the large amounts of HCO_3^- introduced into lung liquid could not have been accommodated inside alveolar cells but must have passed into the interstitium and blood. The same argument could be used when the passage of H^+ in the reverse direction is being considered.

On the basis of these experimental findings we may conclude that the secretion of lung liquid involves the active transport of Cl^- from plasma and is associated with either HCO_3^- absorption from, or H^+ secretion into, lung liquid (nonetheless *net* HCO_3^- movement is from plasma to lung liquid). This would account for the observed electrical potential gradient across the alveolar epithelium down which Na^+ appears to move passively. Water may follow NaCl transport as in other epithelia (Curran & Schwartz 1960; Diamond 1962). Moderate increases in capillary hydrostatic pressure (left atrial pressure 7 cm) do not appear to influence the rate of secretion of lung liquid.

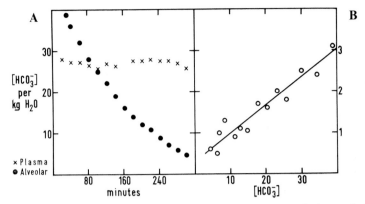

FIG. 3. A: Concentration of HCO_3^- in lung liquid (●) and plasma (×) after injection of isotonic $NaHCO_3$ into lung liquid.
B: Plot of net HCO_3^- flux out of lung liquid (J_{net}) against lung liquid HCO_3^- concentration.

It is possible that the active transport of K^+ is related, at least in part, to the secretion of surfactant. E. J. Mescher *et al.* (1974, unpublished work) have observed that the net flux of K^+ doubles in the last week of gestation in the lamb and parallels the simultaneous increase in surfactant output. They speculate that intracellular K^+ may be lost to lung liquid when lamellar bodies are discharged. Rb^+ could be secreted by the same mechanism since it is known to be able to substitute for K^+ in other systems (Sjodin 1959).

Because these observations were made in the whole lung, it was not possible to determine which part of the pulmonary epithelium is responsible for the secretion of lung liquid. One part of the lung which can readily be studied in isolation from the rest is the trachea.

EXPERIMENTS USING CANINE TRACHEA IN VITRO

Segments of the posterior membranous portion of adult canine trachea were mounted in plastic chambers and bathed on each surface by a modified Krebs-Henseleit solution bubbled with 5% CO_2 and 95% O_2 (pH of solution 7.4) and maintained at 37 °C. Under these conditions the epithelium developed a spontaneous potential difference with the lumen always negative with respect to submucosa (mean 30.7 $\pm$ 2.7 mV S.E.). Initial studies showed that this p.d. was reversibly abolished when 100% N_2 was bubbled through for 20 minutes but did not recover when ouabain (10^{-4}M) was added to the submucosal solution.

Reference to the flux ratio equation suggests that with identical solutions bathing each surface ($a_p/a_L = 1$) and the p.d. held at zero, the ratio of the

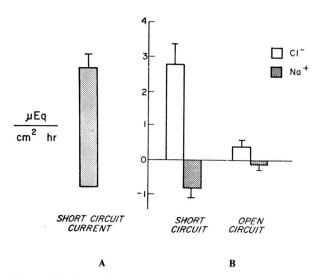

FIG. 4. (A) Short-circuit current, and (B) net fluxes of Cl⁻ and Na⁺ during continuous short-circuiting and under open-circuit conditions. Each column represents the mean value in mequiv. cm^{-2} h^{-1} (+ s.e.). A plot above zero indicates net flux from submucosa to lumen and below zero indicates net flux in the reverse direction.

one-way fluxes should be 1.0 in the absence of significant solvent drag if the ion in question is passively transferred. None of the passive membrane–ion interactions, such as exchange diffusion, can alter this relationship, and any significant deviation therefore indicates active transport (Curran & Schultz 1968). For this reason bidirectional fluxes of Cl⁻, and later Na⁺, were measured during continuous short-circuiting. Under these conditions there was a net flux of Cl⁻ from submucosa to lumen which accounted for 79% of the short-circuit current. The balance was due to a smaller net flux of Na⁺ in the reverse direction (Fig. 4). Addition of acetylcholine (up to 5×10^{-4}M) to the submucosal solution had no significant effect on p.d. or short-circuit current, but even at 5×10^{-5}M it significantly increased the one-way Cl⁻ flux towards the lumen (by 40%), while the one-way Cl⁻ flux in the reverse direction remained unchanged (i.e. net Cl⁻ flux increased). This apparent anomaly was explained by the finding that the one-way Na⁺ flux towards the lumen also increased (103%) and as a result the direction of the net Na⁺ flux reversed and became orientated towards the lumen. These changes in net flux accounted for the lack of change in short-circuit current.

Initial measurements of ion fluxes at spontaneous p.d. suggested that there might be a net flux of Cl⁻ towards the lumen, but neither Cl⁻ nor Na⁺ net fluxes differed significantly from zero ($P > 0.05$). However, addition of as

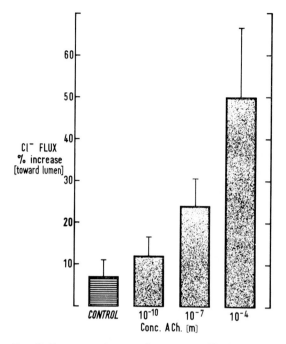

FIG. 5. Percentage increase in one-way Cl⁻ flux from submucosa to lumen (S→L) when acetylcholine was added to the submucosal solution after a control period. The control column represents the increase in one-way S→L flux which occurred during this second period when no acetylcholine was added. Measurements made with open circuit.

little as 10^{-7}M-acetylcholine to the submucosal solution resulted in a significant net flux of Cl⁻ towards the lumen. This effect, and the greater response elicited by 10^{-4} M-acetylcholine (Fig. 5), were blocked by 10^{-3}M-atropine.

DISCUSSION

Neither of these two groups of experiments performed *in vivo* or *in vitro* gives any information as to which cell types are capable of active ion transport. It would be reasonable to suspect that the serous cells of the submucosal glands are the site of active Cl⁻ and Na⁺ transfer but they are unlikely to be the only cells involved. They constitute a minute fraction of the total internal surface of the lung, and in the rabbit, which has no submucosal glands in its tracheobronchial tree, there is good circumstantial evidence of active Cl⁻ transport towards the lumen (Mélon 1968). Furthermore, the observation that lung liquid composition in the fetal lamb remains the same irrespective of how much lung liquid is withdrawn before sampling, suggests that secretory activity is widespread and involves most of the lung. We have found evidence of active ion transport as early as 87 days in the fetal lamb, at a time when the lung epithelium is undifferentiated and contains only cuboidal cells. Thus, potentially at least, all cells of the respiratory epithelium may be capable of active ion transport. Indeed, it may be that active Cl⁻ transport is a feature of all tissues derived from the primitive foregut since it has also been demonstrated in the oesophagus (Powell 1974), stomach (Hogben 1955; Durbin 1964; Kitahara 1967) and bullfrog lung (Gatzy & Gosselin 1966). It is interesting to note that some patients with bronchiolo-alveolar carcinoma, a well differentiated cuboidal tumour of the lung, secrete copious amounts of a liquid which resembles fetal lung liquid (Levinsky & Kern 1952; Storey *et al.* 1953), indicating that some peripherally situated cells in the adult lung may retain (or recall) the ability to transport Cl⁻ actively.

Certain similarities between the fetal lamb lung and adult canine trachea are obvious. Both develop a potential difference (lumen negative) and in both there is active Cl⁻ transport towards the lumen of the lung. In the fetal lamb we have shown this active transport process to be linked to the bulk flow of water, a feature which has not yet been demonstrated in the trachea, although it is suggested by the observation that the fluid collected from the trachea of adult human is similar to fetal lung liquid in that it has a high concentration of Cl⁻ and K⁺ relative to plasma (Potter *et al.* 1963). It is quite possible that in both the fetal and the adult lung, active ion transport, by setting up local osmotic gradients within the epithelium, produces bulk flow of water in the manner suggested by Diamond (1962). In such a system agents which alter net ion fluxes, as does acetylcholine in the trachea, are likely to bring about concomitant changes in the bulk flow of water across the respiratory epithelium. It is also quite possible that in disease states such as cystic fibrosis and status asthmaticus, both characterized by increased mucus viscosity, the control of water flow across the tracheobronchial epithelium is defective. The control of water flow across the alveolar epithelium and the composition of the aqueous subphase of the lining layer may be no less important. Not only is the aqueous subphase necessary for surfactant activity but there is evidence that the low pH of this layer may be an important feature (Frosolono *et al.* 1970). It is interesting to speculate that a liquid similar to that elaborated by the fetal lung, with its low bicarbonate content and low pH, may continue to be produced by alveolar cells after birth. Although techniques exist for sampling the alveolar layer, the relevant analyses which could confirm or deny this hypothesis have yet to be made.

References

ADAMSON, T. M., BOYD, R. D. H., PLATT, H. S. & STRANG, L. B. (1969) Composition of alveolar liquid in the foetal lamb. *J. Physiol. (Lond.)* 204, 159-168

BOYD, E. M. (1972) *Respiratory Tract Fluid*, Thomas, Springfield

CURRAN, P. F. & SCHULTZ, S. G. (1968) Transport across membranes: general principles, in *Handb. Physiol.*, Section 6: *Alimentary Canal*, vol. 3 (Code, C.F., ed.), pp. 1217-1243, American Physiological Society, Washington, D.C.

CURRAN, P. F. & SCHWARTZ, G. F. (1960) Na, Cl, and water transport by rat colon. *J. Gen. Physiol.* 43, 555-571

DIAMOND, J. M. (1962) The mechanism of water transport by the gall bladder. *J. Physiol. (Lond.)* 161, 503-527

DURBIN, R. P. (1964) Anion requirements for gastric acid secretion. *J. Gen. Physiol.* 47, 735-748

FROSOLONO, M. F., CHARMS, B. L., PAWLOWSKI, R. & SLIVKA, F. (1970) Isolation, characterisation and surface chemistry of a surface active fraction from dog lung. *J. Lipid Res.* 11, 439-457

GATZY, J. T. & GOSSELIN, R. E. (1966) Ion transport across the isolated bullfrog lung. *Fed. Proc.* 25, 507

HOGBEN, C. A. M. (1955) Active transport of chloride by isolated frog gastric epithelium. Origin of the gastric mucosal potential. *Am. J. Physiol.* 180, 641-649

KITAHARA, S. (1967) Active transport of Na^+ and Cl^- by *in vitro* non-secreting cat gastric mucosa. *Am. J. Physiol.* 213, 819-823

LEVINSKY, W. J. & KERN, R. A. (1952) Fluid, electrolyte and protein depletion secondary to the bronchorrhoea of pulmonary adenomatosis. *Am. J. Med. Sci.* 223, 512-521

MÉLON, J. (1968) Activité sécrétoire de la muqeuse nasale. *Acta Oto Rhino Laryngol. Belg.* 22, 11-244

NORMAND, I. C. S., OLVER, R. E., REYNOLDS, E. O. R., STRANG, L. B. & WELCH, K. (1971) Permeability of lung capillaries and alveoli to non-electrolytes in the foetal lamb. *J. Physiol. (Lond.)* 219, 303-330

OLVER, R. E. & STRANG, L. B. (1974) Ion fluxes across the pulmonary epithelium and the secretion of lung liquid in the foetal lamb. *J. Physiol. (Lond.)* 241, 327-357

POTTER, J. L., MATTHEWS, L. W., LEMM, J. & SPECTOR, S. (1963) Human pulmonary secretions in health and disease. *Ann. N.Y. Acad. Sci.* 106, 692-697

POWELL, D. W. (1974) Electrolyte transport by rabbit esophagus *in vitro. Fed. Proc.* 33, 215

REIFENRATH, R. & ZIMMERMANN, I. (1973) Blood plasma contamination of the lung alveloar surfactant obtained by various sampling techniques. *Respir. Physiol.* 18, 238-248

SCARPELLI, E. M., GABBAY, K. H. & KOCHEN, J. A. (1965) Lung surfactants, counterions and hysteresis. *Science (Wash. D.C.)* 148, 1607-1609

SJODIN, R. A. (1959) Rubidium and cesium fluxes as related to the membrane potential. *J. Gen. Physiol.* 42, 983-1003

STOREY, C. F., KNUDTSON, K. P. & LAWRENCE, B. J. (1953) Bronchiolar ('alveolar cell') carcinoma of the lung. *J. Thorac. Surg.* 26, 331-406

Discussion

Strang: Ion concentrations in plasma are substantially the same as those in interstitial fluid, aren't they?

Robin: It depends on the protein concentration.

Strang: The expected differences depend on the Gibbs–Donnan equilibrium.

Olver: The differences are certainly minor—the pulmonary capillary endothelium doesn't offer much of a barrier to ionic diffusion.

Dejours: What is the value of P_{CO_2} in lung liquid?

Olver: Between 40 and 50 mmHg (5.33–6.66 kPa).

Dejours: But the bicarbonate concentration in the alveolar liquid is less than 3 mequiv./l.

Olver: The pH of lung liquid is 6.2–6.3. One has, of course, to be careful to take anaerobic samples.

Dickinson: That doesn't seem right to me. The bicarbonate concentration is 1.8 mequiv./l, so the hydrogen ion activity should be more than eight times that in plasma.

Olver: The pH is about 6.2–6.3, i.e. there is a tenfold difference in bicarbonate concentration and a tenfold difference in $[H^+]$ between plasma and lung liquid, as one would expect. There is no anomaly there.

Strang: The pH is that expected from a solution of 2–4 mM-bicarbonate in equilibrium with 5% CO_2. The liquid has been titrated and the titration curve indicates that there is very little buffer.

Maetz: In one experiment you increased the bicarbonate content of the luminal fluid and the bicarbonate flux increased. Does the chloride flux also change then? If there is an exchange between bicarbonate and chloride, chloride would be driven out faster. This works quite well in fish.

Olver: We haven't looked at that. Bicarbonate is certainly of some interest and we must try to return to it.

Keynes: In the short-circuit experiments you got something like a fivefold increase in the net chloride flux in the trachea, Dr Olver. That is a much bigger effect than in any other system I know of. People in this field have hardly looked at what short-circuiting does to the ion flux. In frog skin the sodium flux nearly doubles. In rumen epithelium, on which I have worked, there is active transport of chloride, sodium and potassium and various other things as well, but there is no change in the flux when one short-circuits. What this means, if one applies Ohm's law and starts making electrical models, is that the internal resistance of the chloride pump is much smaller relative to the shunt resistance than it is in the other systems.

Guyton: What about the possibility of back leakage?

Olver: The net flux is the difference between the two one-way fluxes, influx and back flux. The main effect is to increase the submucosa to lumen flux of chloride.

Michel: In the fetal lamb experiments you calculated the flux from plasma to lung liquid as the net flux plus the one-way flux from lung liquid to plasma. Could unstirred layers lead to this being an underestimate?

Olver: Yes, despite our efforts to mix the liquid. Of course unstirred layers are much more important with rapidly moving tracers than with relatively slow-moving tracers, and chloride is moving slowly.

Dejours: The bicarbonate concentration and pH of the lung liquid are among the lowest of any body fluid. How do you explain the low bicarbonate concentration?

Olver: In spite of what seems to be an active transfer of bicarbonate out of lung liquid, or active hydrogen ion secretion into it, there is still a net transfer of bicarbonate from plasma to lung liquid. Lung liquid contains 2 to 3 mequiv. bicarbonate per kilogram of water and there is a continuing secretion of lung liquid into the lung lumen.

Dejours: Is there any lactic acid in the liquid which could displace CO_2?

Adamson: There is no CO_2 gradient across the fetal lung blood barrier. The mean pH of lung liquid is 6.27 (Adamson *et al.* 1969) and the low amount of bicarbonate can be explained by the Henderson-Hesselbach equation, assuming a Pco_2 of 40 mmHg (5.33 kPa).

We couldn't find any lactate in lung liquid. The buffer values of lung liquid show one peak which is at the pK of the carbonic acid system. Although there is only about 2.8 mmol bicarbonate, its effective buffering capacity at the pH of lung liquid is about the same as 20 mequiv. bicarbonate at the pH of normal blood.

Dickinson: The anion gap wasn't greater than expected?

Adamson: It all balances out.

Robin: Is there any way of interfering with delivery of ATP to the exteriorized lung and still maintaining the sheep in a more or less viable state?

Olver: It is difficult to examine metabolic inhibitors in the intact lamb *in vivo*. We have looked at the effect of cyanide, which one might think is pretty potent stuff, on lung liquid secretion. There is dilution of albumin as lung liquid secretion progresses but if we add 2 mM-KCN to lung liquid, reversal of the direction of bulk flow takes place in every case. However, we can't exclude an effect on epithelial structure and the possibility of passive leakage being increased, but the effect is so rapid that perhaps there is no structural damage.

Staub: Did the tracer albumin concentration in circulating blood rise rapidly?

Olver: We didn't detect any, which of course doesn't necessarily mean there wasn't any leakage, because dilution in the extracellular fluid would have made it difficult to pick up the albumin.

Robin: Was there any shift in pH at this time?

Olver: We didn't look for that.

Robin: Would it be worth trying antimycin A? It is a more specific inhibitor of oxidative phosphorylation than cyanide, being more or less a specific inhibitor of cytochrome *b*. You might get a more precise way of inhibiting ATP provision without necessarily clobbering a large number of biochemical pathways with cyanide.

Olver: That is a good idea. We haven't done that.

Keynes: Does acetazolamide do anything to this system?

Olver: Preliminary studies have shown that it reduces the potential difference across the canine trachea. Dr Adamson has looked at acetazolamide in the intact fetal lung. It has an effect, as he will describe later (this volume).

Maetz: The possibility of back flow of chloride through the tight junctions has been mentioned. Diamond and his colleagues have demonstrated the occurrence of such back flows of ions in the gall bladder (see review by Moreno & Diamond 1975). They suggest that junctional proteins have fixed charges, either negative or positive depending on the pH or the presence of bivalent ions.

Olver: So if the channels have negative charges on them, sodium will go through quite happily and chloride won't?

Maetz: Yes.

Olver: Are you referring to charges within the channels or at the mouths of the channels?

Maetz: In the channels, along the whole tight junction.

Olver: If they extend out onto the surface of the epithelium at the mouths of the pores, for example, one would expect anions to be retarded, and that is exactly what we find. The permeability of the epithelium to chloride is much lower than that to sodium. We have looked at other cations, and at halides other than chloride, and their permeability sequences are compatible with the idea that there are fixed negative charges on the mouths of these aqueous channels.

Maetz: One way to change the electric charges in these channels is to remove calcium or add it, because these ions will fix negative charges quite easily. Or one could also play with the pH.

Olver: We played around with both early on and didn't get any noticeable effects. Changing the pH dramatically is difficult to do *in vivo* without killing the animal. One has to get the pH down to about 2.0 to get a change in the permeability sequences.

Staub: What is the electrical resistance across the tracheal membrane?

Olver: About 300 Ω cm^2, which is a middling resistance. It is lower than Dr Gatzy showed in amphibian lungs but it is not as low as in intestine, where it is under 100 Ω cm^2.

Hugh-Jones: Does iodide have an effect?

Olver: We haven't done replacement experiments, except rather crudely. Tracer iodide and bromide are both actively transferred but whether this is by the same carrier mechanism as chloride, we don't know.

Hugh-Jones: Clinically it was always held that iodide was one of the few drugs that really increased water secretion, when used as an expectorant. I don't know whether that is true.

Olver: With acetylcholine and various other agents the rate of production of fluid from the trachea in intact animals increases. Of course we don't know, over the short term anyway, whether that is due to an increase in ciliary action or to a real increase in water flow.

Hugh-Jones: In Miami Marvin Sackner has been doing work on ciliary action and the rate of ciliary movement of mucus up the trachea, using Teflon discs. Bronchodilator drugs increase that movement, but I don't know what effect they have on serosal fluid composition.

Dickinson: Has anybody tried, for example, dropping fluid into a lobe of human lung, sucking it out again rapidly and analysing it? One could then find out whether the adult alveolar epithelium secretes acid.

Crosbie: We injected radioactive labelled water into the external jugular vein and were able to detect the water in the expired air 10 seconds later; so it was coming out of the blood into the expired air just like a gas.

Olver: Although fetal lung hasn't got as good a blood flow as the air-filled lung, tritiated water put into the lung liquid also goes out fast and is flow-limited unless one takes measures to increase pulmonary blood flow.

Keynes: Would microelectrodes that would directly measure chloride activity be useful? If they can be put on the inner surface of the lung, this might be the technique you are looking for.

Olver: This is one direction we are taking. We would like to by-pass the trachea and bronchi and get into the terminal units from the outside. There are certain technical problems, as you can imagine. *In vivo,* a tremendous amount of movement of the lung is due to the action of the heart, although there is no breathing to contend with in the fetus. In the early stages of embryological development of the lung in mice and chicks, in which we are interested, this problem wouldn't exist. The lungs can be excised and they grow quite nicely in artificial media.

Dejours: Did you look mainly at the fetus near term?

Olver: Yes, but we have looked earlier in gestation as well. The furthest back we have gone is 79 days, just over halfway through gestation.

Strang: The 79-day liquid isn't quite identical to the mature liquid, is it?

Olver: No. We think the bicarbonate concentration is higher and the chloride concentration lower at the earlier gestation times, which might well mean that the transport system is less efficient than in the more mature fetus.

Hughes: Have you looked at the effect of oxygen tension on secretion rates in the fetal lamb? In adult terms these secretion rates approach four litres a day, so something switches that secretion off after birth.

Olver: Clearly something has to change, and the dramatic rise in Pao_2 at birth could be important in this context.

Agostoni: Incidentally, there is some scanty evidence that pleural liquid is alkaline with respect to plasma and its bicarbonate concentration is high (Agostoni 1972).

I wonder what happens when the lung liquid with low bicarbonate is reabsorbed. Could this help in determining the kinetics of the absorption of the lung liquid in the newborn? Have you followed the changes in pH or of bicarbonate in the blood after the first breath?

Olver: No.

Adamson: Neither have I.

Strang: Although it has a low pH, the amount of acid present in this liquid is small. With the buffers that are in blood and extracellular fluid one could not detect the transfer to them of such a small amount of acid.

Dickinson: The large amounts of liquid that can go into the adult lungs suggest that the osmotic permeability could be high. We still have no answer to the question, what turns the secretion of lung liquid off?

Strang: We haven't any measurements of osmotic permeability as such but, under all conditions that we have attempted to look at, the calculated pore radius of the air-breathing lung is larger than in the fetus. In all these experiments a net volume flow of liquid takes place from the air spaces to the blood. If this represents the normal state of affairs in the air-breathing lung it would probably end up by making an ion transport pump ineffective. Although the ions might be transported to the inner surface of the lung, they would leak back rapidly through the fairly open fluid-filled pathways. In other words, if the passive permeability to chloride was increased enough there would be no net volume flow of water.

Robin: Colin (1856) poured 25 litres of warm water down the trachea of an adult (or at least non-fetal) horse and much of that must have reached the alveoli; as the lungs were found to be dry, it was apparent that the water passed from the lungs into the blood.

Staub: He didn't pour it down the trachea; it took 2 hours to give it.

Adamson: Some human infants are born with bronchogenic cysts. In postnatal life, these cysts remain fluid-filled, presumably with fetal lung liquid. I have analysed a sample of liquid from one of these cysts but unfortunately I could not get a corresponding plasma sample. The chloride concentration was around 120 mmol/l, not as high as I would have expected. Encysted lobes will stay filled with liquid for a long time and if the whole lung changes, as Dr Strang suggests, there should be reabsorption of the liquid.

Olver: This would be a part of the lung that has not been exposed to any expansion and the intercellular junctions will not have been stretched.

Dickinson: But the cause might not be a mechanical one. Could it, for instance, be a change in the Po_2, which is a very spectacular change?

Egan: In the adult collapsed lung which is degassed, the alveolar Po_2 is very low. The pulmonary artery Po_2 is not much different in fetal life than in adult life. If the secretion of fetal lung liquid was controlled just by oxygen, one would think that adults would start to secrete such a liquid with atelectasis. When we did the static inflation experiments on mature lamb fetuses, both nitrous oxide and oxygen seemed to turn off the active chloride pump. The liquid started getting absorbed. I think the real question is, is the pump still going? If an increase in passive permeability persists, and an active pump is transporting chloride ions into alveoli, it may do no good because the passive permeability to chloride is so great that back diffusion prevents a net secretion of water. That could be an explanation but it seems inefficient.

Staub: Have you done direct puncture of alveoli?

Olver: No, not yet. There are technical problems.

Staub: Cortisol affects lung maturation and the secretion of surfactant. Is the chloride pump sensitive to endocrine control?

Maetz: When adrenalectomized eels are moved from fresh water to sea water, they cannot adjust unless cortisol is injected. As suggested earlier (p. 120), something like an endocrine control must fairly rapidly change the whole system during birth. Not only does secretion have to be switched off, but the existing lung liquids have to be reabsorbed quickly. Could some hormone intervene which makes the whole system reverse? A rapidly acting hormone is needed, mediated by the cyclic AMP system, for example.

Dickinson: But cortisol is not a rapidly acting hormone.

Maetz: No.

Widdicombe: The luminal side of the basement membrane in the respiratory tract has motor nerves which are probably cholinergic. Secretion in the respiratory tract epithelium, that is goblet cells in birds and probably goblet cells and mucus glands in mammals (cat), is also under cholinergic control—at least there is one motor pathway, cholinergic, going to the epithelium (P. S. Richardson & R. Phipps, unpublished work, 1975). Do you think from your experiments, Dr Olver, that the doses of acetylcholine that you use might act via this control system? Dr Gatzy didn't find any action of acetylcholine in the frog alveolar system; this might suggest that your acetylcholine results apply only to the respiratory tract and not at the alveolar level. Furthermore, the respiratory tract secretion in mammals (cat) is both adrenergic and cholinergic, with β receptors. Have you tried β stimulants in your perfused preparations?

Olver: Yes, terbutaline increases the net chloride flux towards the lumen dramatically in the isolated canine trachea.

Widdicombe: That fits well with the known pharmacology of airway mucus secretion.

Olver: Dibutyryl cyclic AMP also increases net chloride flux. These results are from preliminary experiments that haven't been followed up yet. The best evidence is with acetylcholine.

Maetz: In sea water fish, adrenaline augments water permeability and blocks the chloride pump. Prostaglandins also block the chloride pump, but they do not interfere with water permeability. I suggest that for a short time there may be a change in endocrine control which may, at birth, induce reversed water movement.

Olver: Prostaglandins actually reverse secretion in the intestine, don't they?

Keynes: They do the same as cholera toxin.

Olver: So there are plenty of agents which can bring about a reversal of ion transport processes. In the trachea we have shown net flux of chloride towards the lumen in one set of circumstances, but in other circumstances there might be net flux in the opposite direction with coupled water flow.

Strang: Does any epithelium other than the gill undergo reversal as part of its physiological adaptation?

Maetz: In salt-loaded animals—amphibians and mammals—the intestinal tract works 'in reverse' and excretes water and salt (Ferreira & Smith 1968; Richet & Hornych 1969).

Olver: Secretion into the intestinal lumen can occur as a purely passive mechanism, can't it? If venous pressure on the serosal surface is increased there is a net flux of fluid and electrolytes into the lumen.

Maetz: It is certainly not passive in this case. The concentration is high.

Robin: Does the osmolarity of the plasma change dramatically at about the time the lung expands and begins to lose its water? That would be a simple kind of mechanism for reabsorption.

Olver: I don't think that follows. If the fluid is isotonic with plasma, absorption won't change the tonicity.

Robin: If you set up a temporary osmotic gradient by having a sharp increase in free water clearance, at least you could explain loss of some of the water and I suppose some of the ions could go by bulk flow.

Olver: The problem as we saw it a couple of years ago was that we might be able to account for forces that would move the water but we couldn't account for how the ions got out unless there was some increase in permeability. This goes back to what Ted Egan was talking about (this volume, pp. 101–110).

Robin: Did you measure the osmolalities in the plasma at the time lung liquid was lost? If we could explain the loss of liquid at the beginning, it could be the first step.

Olver: I don't know of any evidence that in the immediate newborn period the osmolality is any different from that in the fetus.

Guyton: I would like to explore the mechanical changes at birth. Dr Strang, you told us that lymph flow in the fetal lung is twice that in the adult lung, but does lymph flow increase in the lung immediately after birth? Fetal lymph flow cannot be compared fairly with adult lymph flow.

Strang: When breathing begins by positive pressure ventilation the lymph flow goes up as much as five times, for four to six hours. We haven't measured it right through but in animals at different ages. It then falls back, after six hours, and certainly by 12 hours, to about half the fetal flow (Humphreys *et al.* 1967).

Durbin: Isn't that good evidence for a change in hydrostatic permeability, if driving forces are unchanged?

Strang: Not really. When the fetus takes large breaths after birth pleural pressure falls with every breath and that constitutes a driving force for liquid movement.

Guyton: What I am trying to get at is that respiratory movement should be a powerful force for activating the lymphatic pump.

Staub: The external forces on lymphatics only seem to work when the tissue is very wet; once all of the excess water is removed in the newborn, the lymphatics only pump out what is filtered. The fluid is actively transported by contraction of the lymphatics, but filling may be passive.

Adamson: It has been assumed that there is no prenatal breathing pattern. We have monitored the fetus for 30 days or more before delivery (Maloney *et al.* 1975) and regular breathing patterns as reported by Dawes (1972) occur with pressure oscillations of up to 60–70 cmH$_2$O (5.9–6.9 kPa) in the fluid-filled compartment. Certainly pressure varies quite widely prenatally.

Dickinson: Both the adult and the fetal lung epithelium might be secreting isotonic protein-free fluid at approximately the same rate. We know that the epithelium is extraordinarily impermeable, at least to large molecules, early on. If permeability increased substantially at birth, for mechanical reasons, and if a highly negative interstitial pressure was there to suck fluid in against the colloid osmotic pressure gradient, would this be a reasonable explanation for the event?

Guyton: You are saying that the rate of secretion may not change at birth, but that an absorption factor may be added that wasn't there before.

Olver: This goes back to increasing the shunt out of the lungs back into plasma. One wouldn't need much of a change in pore radius to nullify the effect of an active chloride system completely. One of the prerequisites of an efficient system is that back flux shouldn't be too excessive.

Guyton: Your cyanide data showed a turnaround in the flow of fluid, Dr Olver.

Maetz: There was no air at that time.

Guyton: Presumably there was also no active transport in either direction.

Hugh-Jones: Are you reasoning, Dr Guyton, that the breathing movements actuate the lymph pump, which is why there is increased flow directly after birth which then decreases for the entirely opposite reason?

Guyton: My reasoning couldn't explain Dr Strang's finding that lymph flow fell by half after about six hours. However, it could explain the initial increase in lymph flow, with the first respiratory movements activating the lymphatic pump, creating a more negative interstitial fluid pressure, creating more absorption, and therefore giving still more lymph flow.

Staub: Drinker (1945) found, in anaesthetized dogs in which the lymphatic system was depressed, that increased breathing caused a temporary increase in lung lymph flow.

In unanaesthetized adult sheep which were breathing 10% oxygen, which increases alveolar ventilation, we found that the change in breathing had no effect on lung lymph flow. The lungs in these animals had normal water content. We believe the lymphatics act as a skimming pump rather than as a suction pump.

Guyton: You are saying that fluid is removed from the lung during the skimming process? If there is any positive correlation between volume and pressure, pressure must decrease as the fluid is removed from the lungs. Consequently, the interstitial fluid pressure would have to decrease.

Staub: Yes, we believe that the interstitial pressure at the site of the lymph capillaries is subatmospheric. Dr R. D. Bland in our institute is looking at the rate of fluid removal from the alveoli into the interstitium of the lungs of newborn rabbits after the onset of breathing. Before birth there were no interstitial free fluid cuffs around the blood vessels. Within 5 minutes of the onset of air breathing, he found large fluid cuffs. Apparently, the fluid is sucked out of the alveoli quite rapidly.

Guyton: Another mechanical effect at birth is a change in the mean volume of the lungs. How does the mean volume increase? Permutt *et al.* (1961) showed that the blood vessels enlarge when the lungs expand; therefore, it is reasonable that the interstitial spaces will also expand.

Dickinson: Permutt has a model of spherical objects which can expand in a cylinder and move a piston up and down. When these objects, which might be alveoli, expand then inevitably the solid tissue pressure between them goes up. Since the total pressure is unchanged the interstitial fluid pressure must go down. Suction will be exerted on the interstitial space by the expansion of the alveoli.

Guyton: Permutt said that as the alveoli become larger, the spaces between the alveoli must also become larger.

Staub: Yes, but the spaces are mostly filled by the highly compliant blood vessels.

Guyton: The same must happen in the interstitial spaces, and the pressure should fall.

Maetz: The fluid has to go across the epithelium. Could it be that during this short time there is slight disruption of the tight junctions by the fluid pushed there and that the junctions quickly get repaired?

Schneeberger: Using peroxidase (EC 1.11.1.7) in newborn mice less than an hour old, we observed epithelial junctions that were as impermeable to the tracer as were those of adults. The Stokes–Einstein radius of peroxidase is about 3.55 nm. We found no tracer in the alveolar lumen.

Dickinson: But perhaps you should have got them half a minute after birth instead of an hour.

Normand: When it is put into fetal lung Evans' blue appears in the lymph as soon as positive pressure ventilation is started. A lot of it would be unbound but I don't know what size it is. The concentration in the lymph is about a third or a fifth of what it is in the alveolar lumen (Humphreys *et al.* 1967).

Michel: The Stokes–Einstein radius of Evans' blue unbound to albumin is about 1.31 nm (Levick & Michel 1973).

Durbin: Didn't you tell us that during birth there was a big increase in pore radius, Dr Egan?

Egan: It goes up to 4 nm. Another point that has to be made, at least in humans, is that there is a big movement of plasma out of the vascular space in the first hours after birth. The haemoglobin concentration goes up without any evidence of a new release of red blood cells. There is a shift of about 10% of the blood volume to the extravascular space in the first hour or two after birth. This is presumably moving to an interstitial space but whether this interstitial space is in the lung or not is completely unknown. Part of the high lymph flow at the start of breathing could conceivably be due to shifts of fluid from the capillaries to the interstitial space in the lung, along with the fluid movement from the alveoli into the interstitial space. It could be a bit more complicated than the assumption that all of the lymph flow and all of the changes in the interstitial space at the onset of ventilation are just due to fluid movement from the alveolar space into the interstitial space.

Staub: But lung fluid content decreases continuously after birth until it reaches the adult level.

Egan: Yes, but it is interesting that the changes in plasma volume follow the changes in the lung weights very closely. I don't know whether they are related. They may be simultaneous and unrelated events. Tremendous changes are going on in the pulmonary vascular system. The flow increases dramatically, the pressure has dropped. It may be much more complicated than just lung liquid absorption. Obviously that has to be going on but there may be other things as well.

References

ADAMSON, T. M., BOYD, R. D. H., PLATT, H. S. & STRANG, L. B. (1969) Composition of alveolar liquid in the foetal lamb. *J. Physiol. (Lond.) 204*, 159-168

AGOSTONI, E. (1973) Mechanics of the pleural space. *Physiol. Rev. 52*, 57-128

COLIN, G. (1856) *Traité de Physiologie Comparée des Animaux Domestiques*, pp. 39-41, Baillière, Paris

DAWES, G. S. (1972) Breathing and rapid-eye-movement sleep before birth, in *Foetal and Neonatal Physiology* (Comline, K. S. *et al.*, eds.), pp. 49-62, Cambridge University Press, London

DRINKER, C. K. (1945) *Pulmonary Edema and Inflammation*, Harvard University Press, Cambridge, Mass.

FERREIRA, H. G. & SMITH, M. W. (1968) Effects of saline environment on sodium transport by the toad colon. *J. Physiol. (Lond.) 198*, 329-343

HUMPHREYS, P. W., NORMAND, I. C. S., REYNOLDS, E. O. R. & STRANG, L. B. (1967) Pulmonary lymph flow and the uptake of liquid from the lungs of the lamb at the start of breathing. *J. Physiol. (Lond.) 193*, 1-29

LEVICK, J. R. & MICHEL, C. C. (1973) The permeability of individually perfused frog mesenteric capillaries to T1824 and T1824-albumin as evidence for a large pore system. *Q. J. Exp. Physiol. 58*, 67-85

MALONEY, J. E., ADAMSON, T. M., BRODECKY, V., CRANAGE, S., LAMBERT, T. F. & RITCHIE, B. C. (1975) Diaphragmatic activity and lung liquid flow in the unanaesthetised fetal sheep. *J. Appl. Physiol. 39*, 423-428

MORENO, J. H. & DIAMOND, J. M. (1975) in *Membranes—A Series of Advances*, vol. 3 (Eisenman, G., ed.), Pergamon, Oxford; Dekker, New York

PERMUTT, S., HOWELL, J. B. L., PROCTOR, D. F. & RILEY, R. L. (1961) *J. Appl. Physiol. 16*, 64

RICHET, G. & HORNYCH, A. (1969) The effect of an expansion of extracellular fluids on the net Na flux in the jejunum of rats. An experimental model for the study of the third factor. *Nephron 6*, 365-379

Carbonate dehydratase (carbonic anhydrase) and the fetal lung

T. M. ADAMSON and B. P. WAXMAN

Department of Paediatrics, Monash University, Melbourne

Abstract Carbonic anhydrase activity (carbonate dehydratase, EC 4.2.1.1) has been detected in the fetal lungs of stillborn human infants and rhesus monkeys, but a role for this enzyme in the fetal lung has not been elucidated. *In utero* the mammalian lung develops as a liquid-filled structure, the liquid being secreted by the lung. In the fetal lamb this liquid, when compared with plasma, has a high chloride and a low bicarbonate concentration, suggesting a possible role for carbonate dehydratase. Studies on 10 fetal lambs confirmed the presence of carbonate dehydratase in the lung. Levels at 60–66 days were negligible and rose to 0.30 Meldrum Roughton units/mg protein at about 140 days (term 147 days), with little change after birth. In another six fetal lambs at 135–136 days, inhibition of this enzyme with 100 mg acetazolamide suppressed the mean rate of secretion of lung liquid by 64.5% ($P < 0.005$), which correlated with a significant drop in chloride concentration ($P < 0.001$). This magnitude of change in secretion after acetazolamide is of the same order as that occurring in the secretion of cerebrospinal fluid when carbonate dehydratase is inhibited. This observation supports the hypothesis that carbonate dehydratase in fetal lung affects the secretion of lung liquid, although its mechanism is as yet unknown.

My task here is to review current knowledge about carbonic anhydrase (carbonate dehydratase, EC 4.2.1.1) and the fetal lung, and attempt to define what role this enzyme may play in fetal lung development. Carbonate dehydratase activity was first detected in the lungs of pre-term human infants by Berfenstam in 1952. In 1961 Fisher showed that the fetal lung of the rhesus monkey contained small amounts of the enzyme and that this changed little throughout gestation, but increased twofold from term to one year. However, a role for the enzyme was not identified by either worker.

Our interest in carbonate dehydratase and the fetal lung arose because fetal lung liquid had a high Cl^- and low HCO_3^- concentration when compared with plasma (Adamson *et al.* 1969). Circumstantial evidence at the time suggested that these two factors should be related. Firstly there is the observation that in most organs in which an acid fluid is secreted, or where there is active transport of HCO_3^- and Cl^-, carbonate dehydratase is found, and in these organs its role in secretion can be demonstrated (Maren 1967; Carter, 1972). Secondly, from an embryological aspect the lining epithelium of the lung arises as a diverticulum of the foregut, other derivatives of which (salivary glands, stomach and pancreas) all have a secretory role, and in each of which carbonate dehydratase is present (Maren 1967; Carter 1972). Lastly, there is evidence obtained from phylogenetic studies. The pharyngeal mucosa has a great propensity for forming highly vascular structures designed for gaseous exchange (Hughes 1967), and carbonate dehydratase is found in each of these structures, these structures being the pharyngeal epithelium of primitive vertebrae (Jennings 1962), the branchial epithelium of the fish gill, where its function in electrolyte exchange has already been demonstrated (Maetz 1971), and the gas gland cells of the teleostean swim bladder (Fänge 1966).

CARBONATE DEHYDRATASE ACTIVITY IN FETAL LUNG

In our lung liquid experiments, as in other recent studies (Adamson et al. 1973; Normand et al. 1971; Olver et al. 1973), we used the fetal lamb. It was first necessary, therefore, to confirm whether carbonate dehydratase was present in such lungs. Ten fetuses were studied in all, in three groups: at 60–66 days, 81–101 days, and 134–141 days (term 147 days). Lungs for analysis were obtained from fetuses delivered by hysterotomy. In each case the lung before excision was perfused via the aorta, to minimize contamination of lung tissue carbonate dehydratase with erythrocyte carbonate dehydratase. Lung tissue samples were taken from left and right upper and lower lobes; carbonate dehydratase activity was then determined by Maren's micro method (Maren 1960) and expressed as Meldrum Roughton units at $0°C$. The mean contamination of the lung tissue homogenate with erythrocyte enzyme was 60%, and the lung tissue activity was calculated by a modified method of Ballantine & Maren (1955), allowing for erythrocyte carbonate dehydratase.

In the fetuses of 60 to 66 days' gestational age enzyme activity was negligible; by 81 to 101 days (Fig. 1) it had risen to a mean of 5 Meldrum Roughton units (MRU)/g wet weight, and this increased four- to fivefold by 134 to 141 days (28.8 MRU/g wet weight). After birth there was an apparent doubling in the activity (52.9 MRU/g wet weight), but when this activity was expressed as MRU/mg protein (Fig. 2), there was no apparent change from 134–141 days (mean activity 0.30 MRU/mg protein) to after birth (mean 0.35 MRU/mg protein). This discrepancy between wet weight and protein determinants can be explained by the dilution effect of lung liquid. For in the fetus the volume

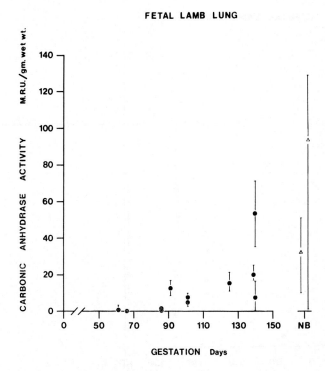

Fig. 1. Carbonate dehydratase (carbonic anhydrase) activity in fetal lung (MRU/g wet weight) and gestational age (days). Each point is the mean and the bars are the ranges of values obtained from four separate homogenates for each animal. NB designates newborn values.

of this liquid is substantial, being around 30 ml/kg body weight near term (Normand *et al.* 1971; Olver & Strang 1974), and it can account for 50–70% of the total weight of the fetal lung. As this liquid contains no carbonate dehydratase (B. Waxman, unpublished work) and only a small amount of protein (30 mg/100 ml) (Boston *et al.* 1968), the fetal lung filled with liquid and the neonatal lung filled with air can be compared only by comparing their protein or DNA content. These levels of enzyme activity are comparable to those in lungs of pre-term human infants (Berfenstam 1952) and fetal rhesus monkeys (Fisher 1961). They are also comparable to the levels in the infant monkey (Fisher 1961) and the adult rat and dog (Travis *et al.* 1966), when allowance is made for the high ratio of lung wet weight to dry weight in the fetus.

Recent work on the secretion of lung liquid (Olver *et al.* 1973; Olver & Strang 1974) shows that the lining epithelium is the site of ionic exchange. If

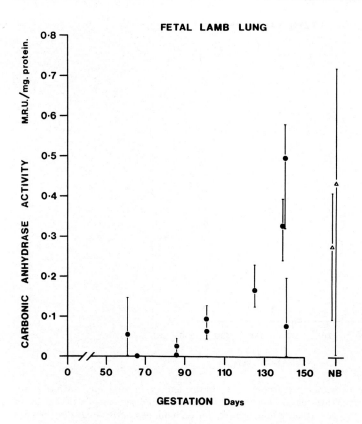

FETAL LAMB LUNG

FIG. 2. Fetal lung carbonate dehydratase (carbonic anhydrase) activity (MRU/mg protein) and gestational age (days). Each point is the mean and the bars are the ranges of values obtained from four separate homogenates for each animal. NB designates newborn values.

carbonate dehydratase is involved in the secretion, the enzyme should be located in this layer. Such a location would explain in part the rise in activity seen with increasing gestational age, for during the later part of gestation the mitotic indices of this layer are two to three times higher than those of stromal cells (Sorokin *et al.* 1959), and the epithelium changes from columnar to squamous. Epithelial cells are therefore increasing in number while reducing in size, which would tend to increase the amount of enzyme present compared with total protein content. Moreover, the lining epithelium near term constitutes only 20% of the total lung tissue mass (Weibel 1973). If carbonate dehydratase is solely distributed in this layer then relative activity of the enzyme per milligram of epithelial cell protein will be fivefold that seen in the whole lung. This level of activity is about half that found in the kidney cortex of the fetal lamb near term (B. P. Waxman, T. M. Adamson & T. F. Lambert, 1972, unpublished work), and is sufficient to have an effect on secretion.

ACETAZOLAMIDE AND THE SECRETION OF LUNG LIQUID

Effect on the rate of secretion

The presence of carbonate dehydratase in the fetal lung of the lamb has been confirmed, but is it involved in the secretion of lung liquid? To answer this question, we developed a partially exteriorized fetal lamb model, similar to that described by Normand et al. (1971). In each experiment a baseline measurement of lung liquid secretion was obtained over a three-hour period, using a marker dilution technique (Normand et al. 1970)—^{125}I-labelled human serum albumin (HSA) was used in this experiment. After the control period, lung carbonate dehydratase was inhibited by the addition of 100 mg acetazol-amide intratracheally; this was thoroughly mixed with lung liquid to ensure its uptake by the lining cells. In all fetuses the validity of the assumption that the enzyme was taken up by the lining cells was confirmed, in that at the end of the experiment enzyme activity was reduced by about 90 % in fetal lung, kidney cortex and erythrocyte. Carbonate dehydratase activity in maternal erythrocytes was not significantly altered. After the addition of acetazolamide, lung liquid secretion was monitored for a further 3 h and the two rates of secretion were compared.

In the eight lambs of 135–136 days' gestation the mean control volume of lung liquid $\pm$ s.E. was 27.9 $\pm$ 2.1 ml/kg body weight, while the mean production rate $\pm$ s.E. was 2.75 $\pm$ 0.25 ml kg^{-1} h^{-1} or 9.9 ml/h. These values are similar to those reported by other workers in acute experiments (Normand et al. 1971; Olver & Strang 1974). The production rates are also close to the daily rates obtained from chronic preparations where the effluent from the fetal lamb trachea was collected for 10–20 days (Platzker et al. 1972; Adamson et al. 1973). The similarity of these production rates, whether direct collections for several days were used, or a radioactive dilution technique lasting only hours, suggests that lung liquid secretion is relatively constant and that substantial volumes of liquid are transferred daily.

Fig. 3 shows the result of a typical experiment in which lung carbonate dehydratase was inhibited. The samples taken in the first 30 min after ^{125}I-labelled HSA or acetazolamide had been added were disregarded when the regression lines were calculated, so that any effects of mixing could be avoided. In this experiment lung liquid production in the control period was 3.79 ml

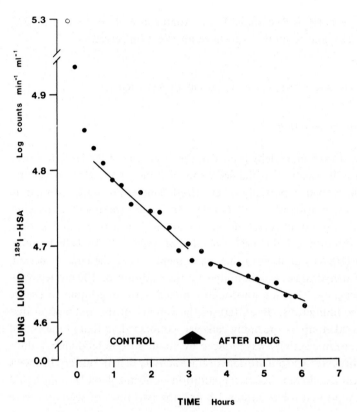

FIG. 3. Effect of intratracheal acetazolamide on the production rate of lung liquid in the fetal lamb (135 days; 2.65 kg). Each point represents 0.5 ml of lung liquid: (○) before mixing (in 30 ml of lung liquid), and (●) after mixing. Samples in first 30 min after addition of ^{125}I-labelled HSA or acetazolamide were disregarded in the regression line analysis, to avoid mixing effects. Values for lung liquid production rate obtained from regression lines were: control, 3.79 ml kg^{-1} h^{-1}; after drug, 1.54 ml kg^{-1} h^{-1}; % reduction, 59.5% ($P <$ 0.001). Acetazolamide, 100 mg, was added at 3.1 h.

kg^{-1} h^{-1}; after acetazolamide was added it dropped to 1.54 ml kg^{-1} h^{-1}, a reduction of 59.5%.

The validity of the use of regression line analysis in the calculation of production rates, as outlined by Normand *et al.* (1971), has recently been reviewed by Olver & Strang (1974). The assumption that albumin does not cross the fetal lining barrier is essential for this technique. Normand *et al.* (1971) showed that alveoli of the fetal lung are impermeable to inulin (Stokes–Einstein radius about 1.4 nm) and to large molecules, including albumin (Stokes–Einstein radius about 3.4 nm). This conclusion is supported by our findings in that activities of ^{125}I-labelled HSA in all serial samples of fetal blood were not

TABLE 1

Effect of intratracheal acetazolamide on the production rate of lung liquid in the fetal lamb

	Mean ± S.E. (n = 6)	Range
Acetazolamide, dose (mg/kg)	30.0 ± 2.3	22.2 – 37.7
Lung liquid production rate (ml kg^{-1} h^{-1})		
(*a*) Control	2.75 ± 0.25	1.66 – 3.79
(*b*) After drug	1.09 ± 0.26	0[a] – 1.79
(*c*) % change	64.5 ± 12.0	18.8 – 100[a]
(*d*) Significance	*P* < 0.001	Only one N.S.

[a] One preparation had a production rate not significantly different from zero and hence a reduction of 100%. Fetal physiological parameters are normal throughout.
N.S.: not significant

significantly different from background, which confirmed that all ^{125}I-labelled HSA remained in the lung compartment.

Table 1 presents the data from six fetuses in which acetazolamide was added to lung liquid. The mean reduction (± S.E.) in secretion was 64.5 ± 12.0%. In all but one preparation, where the reduction was 18.8%, the change in the secretion rates was highly significant ($P < 0.001$). In each period the linearity of the regression lines was confirmed: in control periods $r = 0.84$ (S.E. $= 0.02$), and after drug administration $r = 0.70$ (S.E. $= 0.1$).

This magnitude of change in secretion after acetazolamide is comparable to the 45-60% reduction in cerebrospinal fluid secretion that occurs when choroid plexus carbonate dehydratase is inhibited (Holloway & Cassin 1972; Maren & Broder 1970). Likewise, in other tissues in which carbonate dehydratase has a secretory role, a similar order of reduction occurs after inhibition of the enzyme (Maren 1967; Carter 1972), supporting the hypothesis that this enzyme plays a part in lung liquid secretion.

Effect on lung liquid composition

If the overall secretion rate can be affected by inhibition of acetazolamide, what effect is there on ionic composition? In the experiments just described, three ions were analysed—Na$^+$, K$^+$ and Cl$^-$. The concentrations of each were measured for 3 h after inhibition with acetazolamide and compared with the control period values. Fig. 4 shows results from a typical experiment, while Table 2 summarizes results from six similar preparations. Neither [Na$^+$] nor

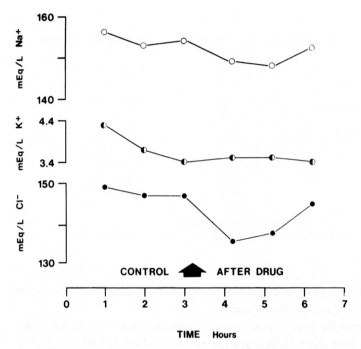

FIG. 4. Effect of intratracheal acetazolamide on concentrations of Na$^+$, K$^+$ and Cl$^-$ in lung liquid of fetal lamb (135 days; 3.25 kg). Acetazolamide added at 3.2 h.

[K$^+$] showed any significant change, but [Cl$^-$] fell significantly at 1 h, ($P < 0.001$) and at 2 h ($P < 0.01$), but not at 3 h ($P < 0.05$). This reduction in the concentration of chloride correlated with the reduction in lung liquid secretion ($r = 0.77$) and was similar to the effects of acetazolamide on cerebrospinal fluid secretion (Maren & Broder 1970).

The mechanism by which acetazolamide affects lung liquid secretion is not known. Other workers have emphasized the lack of specificity of carbonate dehydratase inhibitors and their effect on ion transport. Hogben (1967), working on gastric mucosa, concluded that such inhibitors affect the transport of chloride ions in a way unrelated to their effect on carbonate dehydratase. This hypothesis is supported by the inhibitory action of acetazolamide on anion transport that occurs in the cornea (Kitahara *et al.* 1967) and common bile duct (Chenderovitch 1972), both of which are devoid of carbonate dehydratase. Other workers have suggested that acetazolamide can produce vasoconstriction in the choroidal arteries (Macri *et al.* 1966), but no similar action has been suggested for pulmonary arterioles. In our study acetazolamide crossed the lung blood barrier and significantly inhibited enzyme activity in

TABLE 2

Effect of intratracheal acetazolamide on Na^+, K^+ and Cl^- concentration in lung liquid in the fetal lamb

Control (mmol/l)	Hours after acetazolamide		
	1	2	3
Na^+ (n = 2)	151 ± 2	148	149	148
K^+ (n = 6)	5.7 ± 0.3	5.7 ± 0.5	5.8 ± 0.5	5.6 ± 0.6
Cl^- (n = 6)	144 ± 1	134 ± 2	137 ± 2	141 ± 3
		$P < 0.001$	$P < 0.001$	N.S.

N.S.: not significant

erythrocytes and the kidney cortex. However, no changes were observed in fetal pH, Pco_2 or Po_2 which could have caused pulmonary vasoconstriction.

In 1972 Carter reviewed the role of carbonate dehydratase and ion-transporting epithelia, and showed that in many tissues the enzyme and the acid or alkaline secretion do not have the straightforward association that was once thought to exist between them. In some bicarbonate-secreting tissues such as the ileum carbonate dehydratase seems to be virtually absent. Conversely, in some tissues containing carbonate dehydratase the dominant transporting process appears to involve neither H^+ nor HCO_3^- but rather K^+ or Cl^-.

In any attempt to postulate mechanisms by which carbonate dehydratase may act in the lung, recent work on gastric acid secretion may be helpful. An interplay has been demonstrated between a HCO_3^--stimulated, Mg^{2+}-dependent adenosinetriphosphatase (ATPase, EC 3.6.1.3) and carbonate dehydratase in ionic exchange (Durbin & Kasbekar 1965; Narumi & Kanno 1973), while a Na^+–K^+-dependent ATPase is involved in H^+ secretion (Mozsik et al. 1974). Hence carbonate dehydratase, which is known to be both membrane-bound and intracytoplasmic (Carter & Parsons 1971), may act in two ways: as a membrane-bound anion pump in association with Mg^{2+} ATPase, and secondly as an intracellular buffer, partly to stabilize the intracellular pH during periods of intense metabolic activity (Carter 1972) and partly to neutralize the effects of H^+ secretion. Whether such a system is applicable to secretion of liquid in fetal lung is open to question, for the parietal cell of the gastric mucosa is not seen in the lung and there is no net acid secretion (Adamson et al. 1969).

In this paper it has been assumed that carbonate dehydratase is located in the epithelial layer. However, histochemical confirmation of such a location in the fetal lung is lacking, as is information as to whether it is an isoenzyme of high or low activity. From an ultrastructural aspect, cells involved in secretion tend to possess microvilli, have an indented cell border, and contain glycogen or numerous mitochondria. Cells with these characteristics are found in the lining epithelium of the fetal lamb at around 100 days of gestation, while later in gestation they are seen in the bronchiolar epithelium (D. Alcorn, unpublished work). We can only speculate about whether these cells are the site of secretion of lung liquid, but it is of interest that this cell appears to be absent in the adult lung, a time when lung liquid secretion is thought to have ceased.

CONCLUSION

From the information available it seems likely that carbonate dehydratase is involved in fetal lung liquid secretion. However, much remains unanswered for no information is available on whether other enzyme systems are involved or on how and where carbonate dehydratase acts. It has been postulated that lung liquid secretion ceases in postnatal life, yet the air-breathing lung contains carbonate dehydratase. Clearly, more information is required before we can define what role this enzyme plays in fetal lung development.

ACKNOWLEDGEMENTS

This work was supported by a grant from the National Health and Medical Research Council of Australia. B. P. Waxman was aided by an A. M. S. A. Lilly Research Fellowship.

References

ADAMSON, T. M., BOYD, R. D. H., PLATT, H. S. & STRANG, L. B. (1969) *J. Physiol. (Lond.)* *204*, 159-168
ADAMSON, T. M., BRODECKY, V., LAMBERT, T. F., MALONEY, J. E., RITCHIE, B. C. & WALKER, A. (1973) in *Foetal and Neonatal Physiology* (Comline, K. S. *et al.*, eds.), pp. 208-212, Cambridge University Press, London
BALLANTINE, E. J. & MAREN, T. H. (1955) *Am. J. Ophthalmol. 40*, 148-154
BERFENSTAM, R. (1952) *Acta Paediatr. 41*, 310-315
BOSTON, R. W., HUMPHREYS, P. W., NORMAND, I. C. S., REYNOLDS, E. O. R. & STRANG, L. B. (1968) *Biol. Neonatorum 12*, 306-335
CARTER, M. J. (1972) *Biol. Rev. 47*, 465-513
CARTER, M. J. & PARSONS, D. S. (1971) *J. Physiol. (Lond.) 215*, 71-94
CHENDEROVITCH, J. (1972) *Am. J. Physiol. 223*, 695-706
DURBIN, R. P. & KASBEKAR, D. K. (1965) *Fed. Proc. 24*, 1377-1381
FÄNGE, R. (1966) *Physiol. Rev. 46*, 299-322
FISHER, D. A. (1961) *Proc. Soc. Exp. Biol. Med. 107*, 359-363
HOGBEN, C. A. M. (1967) *Mol. Pharmacol. 3*, 318-326
HOLLOWAY, J. S., JR., & CASSIN, S. (1972) *Am. J. Physiol. 223*, 503-506
HUGHES, G. M. (1967) *Comparative Physiology of Vertebrate Respiration*, Heinemann, London
JENNINGS, J. B. (1962) *Biol. Bull. (Woods Hole) 122*, 63-72
KITAHARA, S., FOX, K. R. & HOGBEN, C. A. M. (1967) *Nature (Lond.) 214*, 836-837

MACRI, F. J., POLITOFF, A., RUBIN, R., DIXON, R. & RAU, D. (1966) *Int. J. Neuropharmacol.* 5, 109-115

MAETZ, J. (1971) *Phil. Trans. Roy. Soc. Lond. B Biol. Sci.* 262, 209-249

MAREN, T. H. (1960) *J. Pharmacol. Exp. Ther.* 130, 126-129

MAREN, T. H. (1967) *Physiol. Rev.* 47, 595-781

MAREN, T. H. & BRODER, L. E. (1970) *J. Pharmacol. Exp. Ther.* 181, 212-218

MOZSIK, G., NAGY, L., TARNOK, F., VIZI, F. & KUTAS, J. (1974) *Experientia (Basel)*, 30, 1024-1025

NARUMI, S. & KANNO, M. (1973) *Biochim. Biophys. Acta* 311, 80-89

NORMAND, I. C. S., REYNOLDS, E. O. R. & STRANG, L. B. (1970) *J. Physiol.* 210, 151-164

NORMAND, I. C. S., OLVER, R. E., REYNOLDS, E. O. R. & STRANG, L. B. (1971) *J. Physiol. (Lond.)* 219, 303-330

OLVER, R. E., REYNOLDS, E. O. R. & STRANG, L. B. (1973) in *Foetal and Neonatal Physiology* (Comline, K. S., *et al.*, eds.), Cambridge University Press, London

OLVER, R. E. & STRANG, L. B. (1974) *J. Physiol. (Lond.)* 241, 327-357

PLATZKER, A. C. G., KITTERMAN, J. A., CLEMENTS, J. A. & TOOLEY, W. H. (1972) *Pediatr. Res.* 6 (*Suppl.*), 406/146 (Abstr.)

SOROKIN, S. P., PADYKULA, H. A. & HERMAN, E. (1959) *Dev. Biol.* 1, 125-151

TRAVIS, D. M., WILEY, C. & MAREN, T. K. (1966) *J. Pharmacol. Exp. Ther.* 151, 464-481

WEIBEL, E. R. (1973) *Physiol. Rev.* 53, 419-495

Discussion

Schneeberger: Large amounts of glycogen are characteristic of fetal lung cells. Except for two mitochondria, I didn't see many specialized organelles in your pictures, Dr Adamson. Peroxisomes are present early in fetal development in these cells (Schneeberger 1972), but there is very little rough endoplasmic reticulum and the Golgi apparatus is small. This would indicate to me that these are undifferentiated cells.

Adamson: The type II cell which was mentioned earlier might be involved in secretion but it is not seen in the fetal lamb at 100 days of gestation, when lung liquid is being secreted.

Maetz: In fish, glycogen is present in the gas gland of the swim bladder. Removal of gas from the swim bladder induces carbon dioxide secretion and simultaneous disappearance of glycogen from the gland. Carbonate dehydratase intervenes in the response to this stimulus because acetazolamide simultaneously blocks gas secretion and glycogen disappearance (Maetz 1956). Concerning the effects of sulphonamides, one has to be careful however, as in some tissues where no carbonate dehydratase is present, such as frog cornea, methazolamide produces a depression of chloride transport (Kitahara *et al.* 1967). Some actively transporting membranes seem to contain carriers which are sensitive to sulphonamides, maybe because their active site resembles the active site of carbonate dehydratase. Such a direct effect of sulphonamides on a cell membrane has recently been described by Motais *et al.* (1975) in the red cell. In their experiments benzolamide, a notoriously slowly penetrating sulphonamide, is used. This substance acts within 2 s on the $Cl^--HCO_3^-$ exchange across the membrane, while its half-time for penetration and contact with the cytoplasmic carbonate dehydratase would be 2 to 3 min. Moreover, benzolamide also blocks the reverse exchange, in some experimental conditions where external HCO_3^- is exchanged against internal Cl^-, a situation where cytoplasmic carbonate dehydratase remains inoperative. Benzolamide also blocks Cl^--CCl^- exchanges. A direct effect of sulphonamides on plasma membranes has also been suggested by Schultz *et al.* (1974) to explain the inhibitory effects of acetazolamide on sodium absorption by the rabbit ileum, a tissue also devoid of carbonate dehydratase.

Dickinson: The swim bladder is in fact maintained by oxygen secretion, isn't it, rather than by carbon dioxide secretion?

Maetz: The first gas to be secreted is carbon dioxide; then oxygen appears. Its origin is oxyhaemoglobin which is dissociated by the Bohr effect and by the Root effect peculiar to fish (see Maetz 1956).

Olver: Dr Adamson, have you measured bicarbonate concentrations in lung liquid after addition of acetazolamide?

Adamson: That would have been a logical thing to do. Unfortunately, we were only able to measure the pH in one experiment, and the change went the way we would have expected. That is, the pH and the bicarbonate concentration rose, and by three hours had returned to the resting level.

Olver: The changes in ion composition seem very definite but what do you do about controls for lung liquid secretion rate? In our experience, secretion tends to fall off with time in acute experiments. The points you showed in Fig. 3 could perhaps have been a continuous curve rather than two separate lines. Obviously you couldn't go back and do a control experiment after you had added acetazolamide, so did you have other controls?

Adamson: Unfortunately we didn't. When we try and fit a regression line for the whole experiment it doesn't fit nearly as tightly as two individual lines. Certainly the physiological parameters of fetal Po_2, Pco_2, blood pressure and heart rate didn't seem to deteriorate over time. However I accept that a control should have been done in which acetazolamide was not added to lung liquid.

Keynes: Did you say there was no evidence as to whether the carbonate dehydratase has high activity or low activity?

Adamson: We didn't look specifically to find what isoenzyme it is, nor am I aware that anyone else has any information on the fetal lung. Fisher (1961) in his study on fetal and neonatal rhesus monkey did not mention isoenzymes.

Keynes: What about the adult lung?

Adamson: I am not aware that anyone has actually defined isoenzymes in the adult lung.

Keynes: It might not even help if one did know the answer. Carter & Parsons (1971) pointed out that the distribution of the high activity and low activity forms of carbonate dehydratase doesn't make any sense at all, in relation to bicarbonate transport or chloride transport.

Maetz: High activity isoenzymes have recently been described by Girard & Istin (1975) in eel gills. These enzymes are different from those found in the red cells. Gills from sea-water- and fresh-water-adapted fish are also characterized by enzymes with significantly isoelectric points.

Keynes: Are the isoenzymes located in the membrane?

Maetz: No, in the cytoplasm. Girard & Istin could extract them completely in the supernatant. In the swim bladder, however, the enzymes seem to cling to the membrane, and they had great difficulty in getting them away from the microsome fraction (M. Istin & J. P. Girard, unpublished).

Keynes: That doesn't seem to fit with the other evidence that acetazolamide is working at the surface.

Adamson: Fain & Rosen (1973) have recently reported that in the amphibian reptile lung, carbonate dehydratase is in the endothelial cells. That would not quite fit my hypothesis. I am not sure about the methods used.

Dejours: How do you measure the rate of flow?

Adamson: By the technique originally described by Normand *et al.* (1970), and the rate of flow is obtained from the slope of the regression line.

Dejours: Do you introduce a catheter?

Adamson: No. Initially a cannula is tied in the lamb trachea, creating a closed compartmental system. We mix the samples thoroughly and take only small amounts for analysis of activity. There is no free flow of fluid from the lung.

Crosbie: Fig. 3 had at least two exponential components. Was the first exponential due to a mass mixing effect, after which you chose the second one?

Adamson: Yes, we used values obtained after 30 min; the first one is due to mixing.

Strang: The best evidence that the impermeant tracer is genuinely diluted by newly formed liquid and is not mixing after the first 30 min is that two impermeant tracers with different diffusion coefficients give the same result, and also that the result obtained tallies very closely indeed with direct measurements of flow.

References

CARTER, M. J. & PARSONS, D. S. (1971) The isoenzymes of carbonic anhydrase: tissue, subcellular distribution and functional significance, with particular reference to the intestinal tract. *J. Physiol. (Lond.) 215*, 71-94

FAIN, W. & ROSEN, S. (1973) Carbonic anhydrase activity in amphibian and reptilian lung, a histochemical and biochemical analysis. *Histochem. J. 5*, 519-528

FISHER, D. A. (1961) Carbonic anhydrase activity in fetal and young Rhesus monkeys. *Proc. Soc. Exp. Biol. Med. 107*, 359-363

GIRARD, J. P. & ISTIN, M. (1975) Isoenzymes de l'anhydrase carbonique d'un poisson euryhalin. Variations en relation avec l'osmorégulation. *Biochim. Biophys. Acta 381*, 221-232

KITAHARA, S., FOX, K. R. & HOGBEN, C. A. M. (1967) Depression of chloride transport by carbonic anhydrase inhibition in the absence of carbonic anhydrase. *Nature (Lond.) 24*, 836-837

MAETZ, J. (1956) Le rôle biologique de l'anhydrase carbonique chez quelques téléostéens. *Bull. Biol. Fr. Belg. Suppl. 40*, 1-129

MOTAIS, R., COUSIN, J. L. & SOLA, F. (1975) Les échanges transmembranaires de Cl^- et de HCO_3^- dans le globule rouge: mise en évidence d'une action directe des inhibiteurs de l'anhydrase carbonique sur le mécanisme de transfert. *C.R. Hebd. Séances Acad. Sci. Sér. D Sci. Nat. 280*, 1119-1122

NORMAND, I. C. S., REYNOLDS, E. O. R. & STRANG, L. B. (1970) Passage of macromolecules between alveolar and interstitial spaces in foetal and newly ventilated lungs of the lambs. *J. Physiol. (Lond.) 210*, 151-164

SCHNEEBERGER, E. E. (1972) Development of peroxisomes in granular pneumocytes during pre- and postnatal growth. *Lab. Invest. 27*, 581

SCHULTZ, S. G., FRIZZELL, R. A. & NELLANS, H. (1974) Ion transport by mammalian small intestine. *Annu. Rev. Physiol. 36*, 51-91

Lung carbonate dehydratase (carbonic anhydrase), CO_2 stores and CO_2 transport

LEON E. FARHI, JOHN L. PLEWES and ALBERT J. OLSZOWKA

Department of Physiology, State University of New York at Buffalo, Buffalo, New York

Abstract   A study of CO_2 storage in excised, exsanguinated lungs revealed that CO_2 stores include a compartment which reaches equilibration very rapidly (< 3 s) and a slower compartment which equilibrates with a half-time of approximately 15 s. Inhibition of carbonate dehydratase (carbonic anhydrase, EC 4.2.1.1) does not change the slope of the total CO_2 dissociation curve of the lung but does increase the slow compartment at the expense of the fast. CO_2 diffusion across the pleura is approximately 20 times faster than that of O_2, a relationship that is not affected by inhibition of carbonate dehydratase. The role of tissue CO_2 stores in limiting respiratory fluctuations of P_{CO_2} or pH in arterial blood is only minor and may be of significance only in rapid, deep inspiration. CO_2 uptake or release by the stores is out of phase with blood CO_2 exchange. As a consequence, the time course of CO_2 exchange at the mouth during expiration cannot be used to predict alveolar or capillary CO_2 exchange.

It is ironic that the very organ entrusted with maintaining appropriate arterial oxygen and carbon dioxide levels was designed by nature in a manner that precludes it from maintaining its own P_{O_2} and P_{CO_2} at fixed values. The reciprocating action of the ventilatory system is doubtless an efficient means of warming and humidifying inspired gas while conserving water, but it imposes cyclic variations in alveolar gas tensions that are transmitted—albeit damped to some extent—to the arterial blood. Because of the characteristics of the haemoglobin dissociation curve, the normal oscillations of arterial P_{O_2} are of no consequence; no such statement can be made for CO_2, for which a tidal variation of only 2 torr (0.3 kPa) corresponds to one-fourth the resting venous–arterial partial pressure difference. This implies that CO_2 elimination must be significantly lower at some parts of the respiratory cycle than at others and that there may be measurable differences in plasma hydrogen ion concentration. As might be expected, this statement has led a number of investigators to question whether there are mechanisms that effectively damp CO_2 oscillations. The possible role of lung tissue as a buffer was recognized by DuBois *et al.* in the first published report on the CO_2 dissociation curve of mammalian lung (DuBois *et al.* 1952). Later discovery of measurable levels of carbonate dehydratase (carbonic anhydrase, EC 4.2.1.1) in lung tissue (Berfenstam 1952; Chinard *et al.* 1962; Maren 1967) made this possibility more attractive, and the hypothesis was tested by a number of authors (Hyde *et al.* 1968; Sackner *et al.* 1964). On the basis of the accumulated evidence, DuBois (1968) stated that tissue CO_2 storage could be expected to reduce respiratory CO_2 oscillations by only 10–20%. Nevertheless, during some prolonged respiratory manoeuvres, such as rebreathing, the effects are much more important, a fact that prompted us to question whether time is not one of the important variables in this equilibrium.

In this communication we shall present new findings on the dynamics of CO_2 and bicarbonate storage in the lung, with specific reference to the role of carbonate dehydratase, and discuss possible effects on CO_2 exchange, arterial blood composition, and changes within the cell. Finally we shall analyse the implications of this storage in terms of some physiological measurements and assumptions.

CO₂ DISSOCIATION CURVE OF LUNG TISSUE

The measurements, reported in detail elsewhere (Plewes 1975), were made on excised exsanguinated dog lungs, suspended in an airtight drum, in which the pressure was cycled between -3 and -10 cmH$_2$O (-0.3 and -1 kPa) below atmospheric pressure. The trachea was tied around a tube that protruded through the drum lid and could be connected to one of several anaesthesia bags. A mass spectrometer was used to monitor gas composition in the drum and at the tracheal opening. After the lung had rebreathed in one of the bags long enough to achieve a steady state, it was switched into another bag. Analysis of gas at the tracheal opening showed that:

(1) A true equilibrium can be achieved only when the CO_2 level in the lung + bag system is the same as in the surrounding gas. In all other cases, bag P_{CO_2} changes continuously and approaches drum P_{CO_2} at an exponential rate, regardless of whether drum P_{CO_2} is higher or lower than that in the lung. We shall return to this finding later but must indicate here that the variations in P_{O_2} and P_{N_2} were much smaller, in spite of a bag–drum difference severalfold larger than for CO_2. This rules out leakage as the possible cause of lung P_{CO_2} changes.

(2) It is possible to distinguish clearly a slow compartment in the readjustment of lung CO_2 stores. This process has a half-time of approximately 15 s. The

half-time of the fast compartment is too short to be measured accurately by this technique.

(3) The slope of the dissociation curve of the slow compartment is independent of Pco$_2$, while that of the fast compartment falls as Pco$_2$ rises.

(4) Carbonate dehydratase inhibition decreases the size of the fast compartment and increases that of the slow compartment in such a fashion that the total CO$_2$ store is not altered significantly.

(5) There are no significant differences when the experiments are conducted at either 22° *or* 37° C.

Fig. 1 summarizes these findings.

The existence of a fast and a slow compartment can be interpreted in a number of ways. One possibility is that all parts of the lung can bind CO$_2$ at the same rate, but that it takes longer for carbon dioxide to reach some of the storage sites (e.g. because some areas are further away from the alveolar wall and capillaries); the opposite view is that CO$_2$ reaches all storage sites instantaneously, and it is taken up at two different rates. Presumably the truth lies somewhere between the two extremes. Fortunately the exact manner in which CO$_2$ is distributed does not influence the way the lung stores affect CO$_2$ transfer from capillary to environment, the question to which we shall now address ourselves.

LUNG TISSUE, CARBONATE DEHYDRATASE AND CO$_2$ EXCHANGE

It is obviously impossible to determine the effects of inhibiting carbonate dehydratase in the lung without changing the activity of that enzyme in blood. As a matter of fact, one would expect that the blood effects would predominate. An alternative approach to the question is to use the data available to predict the behaviour of the system, a path that is reasonably safe in view of the fact that all the necessary basic information is at hand. The mathematical model we have used takes into account pulmonary blood flow, lung volumes (functional residual capacity, dead space, tidal volume), respiratory frequency, and metabolic level (O$_2$ uptake and CO$_2$ output) and predicts the course of a number of variables during the respiratory cycle in a uniformly ventilated and perfused lung.

Fig. 2 is a plot of end-capillary Pco$_2$ versus time in a resting man. The 'normal' curve takes into account CO$_2$ storage in the lungs as it would normally occur, and is very similar to that presented by DuBois and his colleagues a quarter of a century ago without the help of sophisticated computers (DuBois *et al.* 1952). The second curve deals with a lung having the same metabolism, perfusion and ventilation, but in which carbonate dehydratase has been

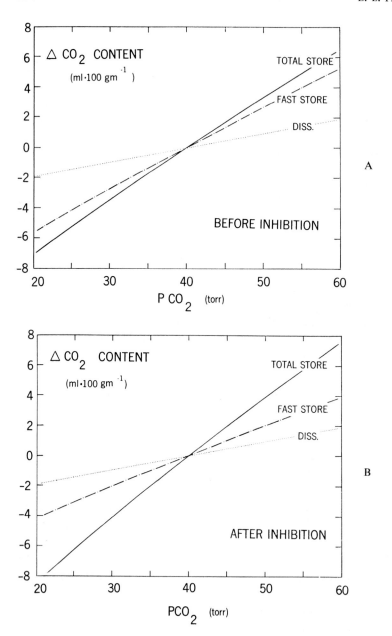

Fɪɢ. 1. Dissociation curve of lung tissue. Changes in CO_2 content are expressed in reference to the CO_2 content at a P_{CO_2} of 40. 'Total store' line and 'fast store' line are experimental. Line for dissolved CO_2 ('Diss.') is calculated. The slow store is the difference between the 'total' and the 'fast store' lines.

A: Normal lung; B: After carbonate dehydratase inhibition.

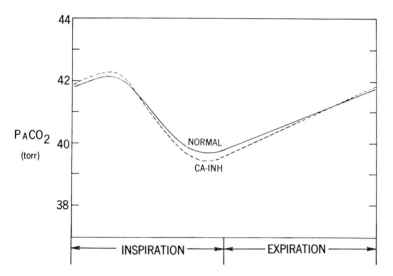

FIG. 2. Oscillations in alveolar Pco₂ during a respiratory cycle. Changes in alveolar Pco₂ (during a single respiratory cycle) are calculated from our experimental results using a mathematical model. The normal lung is represented by the solid line. Oscillations in a lung in which lung carbonate dehydratase activity has been inhibited are shown by the dotted line.

inhibited. Changes in plasma hydrogen ion concentration during a breath are also minimal. The difference between the extreme values (41.3 and 39.8 nanomoles per litre) would increase only from 1.5 to 2 if carbonate dehydratase activity in lung parenchyma were inhibited.

An increase in carbon dioxide elimination by a factor of 10 (coupled with appropriate changes in cardiac output and ventilation) increases only to a limited extent the buffering role of pulmonary tissue in terms of either CO_2 or $[H^+]$ excursions.

Having failed to demonstrate any major role of lung carbonate dehydratase on arterial blood during normal breathing, we must ask whether the role of that enzyme is to protect the lung itself rather than blood. Obviously, the CO_2 tension of lung tissues is essentially that of alveolar gas, and on the basis of the results presented above, it seems fair to conclude that the swings in tissue Pco₂ are only marginally reduced by the presence of carbonate dehydratase. If we accept Hyde's suggestion (Hyde et al. 1968) and assume that lung cells have a pH of approximately 7.00 at a Pco₂ of 40—certainly a reasonable value—we can calculate the hydrogen ion concentration of cells during the respiratory cycle on the basis of the lung dissociation curve and the time constants we have measured. At rest this concentration varies between 79.4 and 83.2 nmol/l, while the corresponding exercise figures oscillate between

75.2 and 87. Paradoxically, one could expect carbonate dehydratase inhibition to decrease the amplitude of these oscillations, since in the absence of the enzyme there could be only minor variations in carbonic acid level. Thus, the role of lung carbonate dehydratase seems to be minimal in moderating P_{CO_2} and $[H^+]$ excursions in lung tissue as well as in blood.

CARBONATE DEHYDRATASE AND TRANSPULMONARY DIFFUSION OF CO_2

Enns has demonstrated that CO_2 diffusion can be facilitated by bicarbonate (Enns 1967), a process which requires hydration of CO_2 on one side and dehydration of H_2CO_3 on the other. Our experiments have allowed us to determine the rate of CO_2 diffusion between alveoli and pleura and compare it to that of O_2, N_2, and Ar, measured simultaneously. Much to our surprise we have found that CO_2 diffuses about 20 times faster than O_2, a figure that would be predicted on the basis of the physical solubility of the gases involved. The same conclusion can be reached by comparing CO_2 to either N_2 or Ar. Furthermore, carbonate dehydratase inhibition has no effect on this rate of CO_2 movement. Obviously the normal CO_2 diffusion pathway—from pulmonary capillary to alveolar gas—differs considerably from the one we have studied. Extrapolation of our findings to the alveolar–capillary tissue layer may therefore be unwarranted but should be considered in view of the fact that carbonate dehydratase seems to play no part in transpulmonary CO_2 movement.

CO_2 EXCHANGE DURING THE RESPIRATORY CYCLE

Alveolar gas exchanges CO_2 with both the pulmonary capillary bed, which acts as a source, and with lung tissues, which serve as a store. The time course of the two processes is quite different and sheds some light on the role played by the tissues.

Basic to this analysis is a description of the cyclic changes in alveolar P_{CO_2}. The dilution of alveolar gas by inspired air, which occurs during most of inspiration, causes a modest decrease in alveolar P_{CO_2}. Because the venous–arterial CO_2 difference is small, even such a limited drop in alveolar P_{CO_2} results in a measurable increase in venous–arterial CO_2 difference and therefore in CO_2 elimination from blood. This can be viewed as some sort of regulatory feedback since the secondary alteration in CO_2 elimination tends to moderate the initial P_{CO_2} changes.

Although the variations in arterial P_{CO_2} are important in terms of the $(\bar{v}-a)$ CO_2 difference, they are of little significance in terms of the carbon dioxide

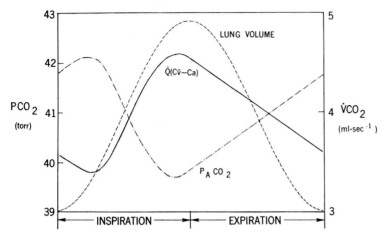

FIG. 3. Oscillations of flux of CO_2 as seen by the body during a respiratory cycle. Changes in flux of CO_2 [$\dot{Q}(C\bar{v}\text{-}Ca)$] as seen by the body are shown in relation to the oscillations in lung volume and in alveolar P_{CO_2} (tidal volume = 580 ml; functional residual capacity = 3000 ml). Note that this CO_2 flux is in phase with changes in lung volume.

concentration in alveolar gas. It follows that during inspiration the flux of incoming fresh air must be loaded with about 5% CO_2. It is during this phase of the cycle that the combined blood and tissue stores are taxed to the utmost, and in fact, during parts of inspiration, supply more CO_2 to the alveolar gas than does the blood itself. Since the rate at which the stores unload depends on the rate of change of alveolar P_{CO_2}, which it is useful to minimize, one can easily perceive the need for large, responsive stores. We can therefore distinguish between two mechanisms that tend to maintain alveolar–arterial P_{CO_2} constancy during the breath. One is the readjustment in CO_2 exchange with blood, essentially in phase with lung volume, which comes into play only at the expense of changes in $\dot{V}_{CO_2}$ (Fig. 3). The second mechanism is the influx of CO_2 from the stores, in phase with gas flow (Fig. 4). Because the amplitude of the oscillations of the second component is so much larger than that of the first, the cyclic pattern of CO_2 elimination in the alveolar gas will show a definite peak, lagging only slightly behind inspiratory flow.

CO₂ STORES AND MEASUREMENT OF ALVEOLAR–ARTERIAL GAS EXCHANGE

One of the tenets of respiratory physiology is that composition of gas at the mouth late in expiration reflects alveolar gas and hence arterial blood tensions; we have no quarrel with this proposition in the narrow terms we have stated it. It seems, however, useful to examine critically here what may appear at

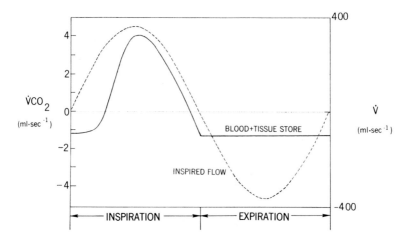

FIG. 4. Variations in flux of CO_2 to and from blood and tissue stores during a respiratory cycle. Changes in flux of CO_2 into and from tissue and blood stores are shown during a single respiratory cycle, in relation to the oscillations in flux of gas into or out of the lung. When $\dot{V}CO_2$ is > 0, flux of CO_2 is from blood and tissue stores into the alveolar gas. When $\dot{V}CO_2$ < 0, flux of CO_2 is into blood and tissue stores from the incoming blood (i.e., recharging the stores).

In this case, CO_2 flux is in phase with flow and out of phase with volume.

first to be a logical extension of the idea, namely that *gas exchange* at the mouth reflects *gas exchange* in the alveoli and in the pulmonary circulation. This is perhaps best shown in Fig. 5 in which CO_2 exchange is plotted as a function of time during a respiratory cycle. Line A represents blood flow multiplied by venous–arterial CO_2 difference. It is therefore the CO_2 elimination as it is seen by the body economy, concerned only with the composition of the blood entering and leaving the lung. The upper boundary of the unshaded area between lines A and B represents a slightly different flux, namely that across the capillary wall; the difference between this flux and the flux represented by line A is due to the unloading of CO_2 stores from the capillary blood volume. This occurs because as alveolar P_{CO_2} decreases during inspiration, mean capillary P_{CO_2} drops and some CO_2 leaves the blood; the converse occurs during expiration. The lined area depicts the contribution of tissue stores during inspiration. During expiration, the uptake of CO_2 by tissue stores is as shown by the stippled area. Both changes are in phase with changes in blood stores. Line B shows the combined influx into alveolar gas from all sources, and finally curve C shows CO_2 elimination into the atmosphere. It is clear that at any point in expiration, P_{CO_2} may well be essentially the same throughout the system, but CO_2 elimination at the mouth bears no resemblance to either CO_2

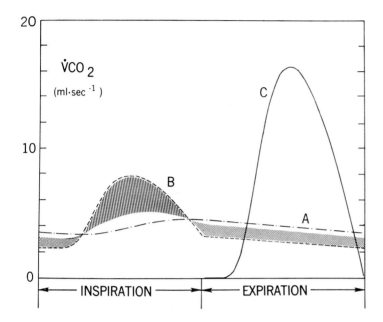

FIG. 5. CO_2 fluxes during a respiratory cycle. Line A represents CO_2 flux as seen by the body
$[\dot{Q}(C\bar{v}\text{-}Ca)]$. Line B represents the CO_2 flux into alveolar gas. The lined area during inspira-
tion represents the volume of CO_2 transferred from the tissue store into the alveolar gas.
The unshaded area between lines A and B represents the volume of CO_2 transferred from
the blood store into alveolar gas.
  The stippled area during expiration represents the CO_2 stored in tissue, the unshaded area
represents CO_2 in blood.
  Curve C represents CO_2 flux as measured at the mouth during expiration.

influx into the alveoli or CO_2 loss from blood at that time or during the preceding inspiration. In fact it is obvious that line C, the only one we really
measure, is 90° out of phase with blood and 180° out of phase with the alveolar
gas curve. The above analysis has serious practical implications. As an example, Kim *et al.* (1966) followed respiratory gas exchange at the mouth and
used this to calculate pulmonary blood flow by a non-invasive technique. The
basic reasoning was that as long as O_2 uptake remained constant, R, the
respiratory gas exchange ratio, was directly proportional to CO_2 output and
therefore to the product of pulmonary blood flow multiplied by venous–arterial
P_{CO_2} content difference. The last term would drop to zero if alveolar–arterial
P_{CO_2} were brought transiently to venous level. On this basis, it is necessary
only to plot P_{CO_2} versus R during a prolonged expiration and extrapolate to an
R of 0 to obtain the calculated value for the oxygenated venous P_{CO_2}. In
Fig. 6 we have plotted P_{CO_2} versus R, calculating the latter on the basis of

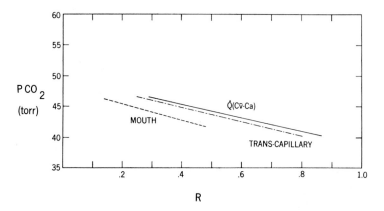

FIG. 6. P_{CO_2} versus R during expiration. R is calculated using the appropriate CO_2 flux—either that seen by the body $[\dot{Q}(C\bar{v}\text{-}Ca)]$, the true transcapillary CO_2 flux $[\dot{Q}(C\bar{v}\text{-}Ca) - \Delta$ blood stores$]$, or the CO_2 flux at the mouth. At a P_{CO_2} of 45, measured R (mouth) is 0.22, while R calculated from $[\dot{Q}(C\bar{v}\text{-}Ca)]$ is 0.45.

venous–arterial CO_2 difference, of expired gas, and of transcapillary gas flux. The differences, which are due entirely to CO_2 storage, are truly staggering.

CONCLUSIONS

Although there is now ample evidence that lung tissue can store CO_2, the role of this phenomenon appears rather limited during normal breathing, at rest or during exercise. The only significant benefit appears to be a moderate protection of alveolar–arterial P_{CO_2} during deep, rapid inspiration. Even a hard-boiled respiratory physiologist must question whether this rare occurrence justifies the need for lung carbonate dehydratase. Whether this enzyme subserves another function or is a phylogenetic or ontogenetic vestigial remnant is a question worth asking.

ACKNOWLEDGEMENTS

Research supported in part by NIH Grant HL 14414-03. Dr Plewes was a Fellow of the Medical Research Council of Canada.

References

BERFENSTAM, R. (1952) Carbonic anhydrase in fetal organs. *Acta Paediatr.* *41*, 310-315
CHINARD, F. P., ENNS, T. & NOLAN, M. F. (1962) The permeability characteristics of the alveolar capillary barrier. *Trans. Assoc. Am. Physicians Phila.* *75*, 253-261

DuBois, A. B. (1958) Significance of carbonic anhydrase in lung tissue, in *CO₂: Chemical, Biochemical & Physiological Aspects*, NASA SP-188, pp. 257-259

DuBois, A. B., Fenn, W. O. & Britt, A. G. (1952) CO₂ dissociation curve of lung tissue. *J. Appl. Physiol. 5*, 13-16

Enns, T. (1967) Facilitation by carbonic anhydrase of CO₂ transport. *Science (Wash. D.C.) 155*, 44-47

Hyde, R. W., Puy, R. J. H., Raub, W. F. & Forster, R. E. (1968) Rate of disappearance of labelled carbon dioxide from the lungs of humans during breathing holding: a method for studying the dynamics of pulmonary CO₂ exchange. *J. Clin. Invest. 47*, 1535-1552

Kim, T. S., Rahn, H. & Farhi, L. E. (1966) Estimation of true venous and arterial Pco₂ by gas analysis of a single breath. *J. Appl. Physiol. 21*, 1338-1344

Maren, T. H. (1967) Carbonic anhydrase: Chemistry, physiology and inhibition. *Physiol. Rev. 47*, 595-781

Plewes, J. L. (1975) Carbonic anhydrase in lung tissue. Ph.D. thesis, State University of New York at Buffalo

Sackner, M. A., Feisal, K. A. & DuBois, A. B. (1964) Determination of tissue volume and carbon dioxide dissociation slope of the lungs in man. *J. Appl. Physiol. 19*, 374-380

Discussion

Keynes: Early in World War II, when it was realized that the sulphonamides were inhibitors of carbonate dehydratase, Roughton and others used groups of volunteers dosed with sulphonamides to see whether they would show respiratory distress. As far as I remember, they found no effects in resting man but there was some effect after severe exercise. Other experiments must have been done since then.

Farhi: The problem is that the experiments deal mainly with carbonate dehydratase in the red cells. There is no doubt that it can be inhibited but there is a very narrow range in which inhibition is physiologically effective and yet safe.

Keynes: Is the conclusion still that no respiratory distress occurs except during severe exercise?

Farhi: High levels of exercise can be reached before the blood fails to exchange completely in the pulmonary capillary.

Robin: Isn't it true that the uncatalysed reaction for the hydration or dehydration of carbon dioxide is a fairly rapid one and that carbonate dehydratase only speeds it up 400 times? I thought that this was a reserve reaction for times when blood remains for only a short time in the pulmonary capillary. Haven't enzyme kineticists come to the same conclusion from a consideration of the reaction rates of the catalysed and uncatalysed reactions?

Farhi: Actually, the half-time of the uncatalysed hydration reaction is 25 s. The enzyme speeds it up by a factor of 13 000. The uncatalysed dehydration reaction is 400 times faster than hydration.

Robin: It may be very important in specific tissues.

Farhi: Yes, it may be important in the metabolism of the tissue itself, or perhaps it is left over from *in utero* days.

Dejours: Twenty-three years ago, DuBois *et al.* (1952) introduced the concept of 'equivalent lung volume', a volume which is bigger than the actual lung volume and which includes the capacity of the capillary blood and tissue for CO_2. Do you think that this concept remains valid?

Farhi: Absolutely. The extra lung volume represented by CO_2 in blood and tissue is 800 ml, about a quarter of the functional residual capacity. In other words it is as though the lung were 25% bigger for carbon dioxide than for oxygen.

Dejours: To say that what happens at the mouth has nothing to do with what happens in the lung seems too strong a statement. Don't you agree that the pressure of CO_2 in the end-expiratory gas at the mouth has something to do with the CO_2 pressure at an earlier stage in the lung?

Farhi: The carbon dioxide at the mouth is a good representation of the carbon dioxide in the alveoli and in the pulmonary capillaries *in terms of partial pressure.* I have no quarrel with that. But it is not true for gas exchange. Only part of the carbon dioxide going out of the blood during expiration reaches the mouth. What I am saying is that the partial pressures are the same in the alveolar gas and in the capillary but the rate of exchange is not.

Dejours: You mentioned the diffusion of carbon dioxide out of the lung through the pleura, but doesn't the pleura itself contain carbonate dehydratase?

Farhi: Yes, you are right.

Staub: For facilitated diffusion to occur, the enzyme should be distributed evenly along the pathway. If it is confined only to the boundaries, it has no significant effect.

Hughes: In life, lung tissue is actually metabolizing. If its metabolic rate is different from that imposed by ventilation and perfusion, wouldn't that have some effect?

Farhi: The lungs we dealt with experimentally were exsanguinated and suspended in a box. They didn't have any blood flow. If artifacts are introduced by lung metabolism, we hope that we have cancelled out the error by looking at the same number of experiments where CO_2 partial pressure increases as where it decreases.

Maetz: Aren't there artificial membranes where carbonate dehydratase can be fixed? I think these membranes will activate CO_2 transfer.

Farhi: Facilitation of CO_2 across liquid layers that contain bicarbonate and carbonate dehydratase certainly occurs. My question is, how important is this mechanism in terms of the gas transfer that was studied? Perhaps it isn't important at all.

Lee: How is the short time constant for CO_2 obtained?

Farhi: The time constant of the fast compartment was too fast to be measured.

Lee: I ask because a number of years ago we found something that we couldn't really analyse properly but which we explained intuitively. In resting individuals the blood flow, being pulsatile, perfuses the lung only episodically in certain areas, so in parts of the lung, during parts of each cardiac cycle, blood will either not be flowing or not be there. When we measured lung capillary blood flow with nitrous oxide in the body plethysmograph we got the blood flow rate *in toto*. Then if we played about with the inspired gases we could look at oxygen going in and carbon dioxide coming out, individually. Oxygen was linearly related to blood flow—it was flow-limited—and carbon dioxide came out initially at the same rate as the blood flow and then flattened out. The curve had a time constant of about 1 or 2 s. We thought that this was because, in the areas which had been perfused episodically, the lung tissue acted as a storage condenser and took up CO_2, discharging it later into the alveoli even though no blood flow could be taking place at this time. But we were not clever enough to know whether this was assisted by carbonate dehydratase or not (Bosman *et al.* 1965).

Farhi: I accept your statement that a capacitance effect is the most logical explanation. Whether it is all due to the presence of carbonate dehydratase I cannot say.

Lee: All I am saying is that the tissue volume of the lung is large enough to store a considerable volume of CO_2 in solution, which could later diffuse out into the alveoli, just like a condenser discharging.

Farhi: And of course the cardiac cycle has just the right frequency for this.

Dickinson: Would the effect of carbonate dehydratase or lack of it be much augmented by much more rapid and deep breaths during exercise?

Farhi: Yes. With exercise something else favours storage. That is, the store of carbon dioxide in the capillary blood is not negligible. You are correct in saying that if there is any buffering effect of lung due to stores, it is during a quick and deep inspiration where a large flux of gas has to be brought up almost instantaneously. I have no figures yet on the pulsatile cardiac cycle. The model we used assumed continuous lung perfusion. Exercise has minimal effects, 10 or 15% from peak to peak, on changes in the P_{CO_2} or in pH of blood. At an oxygen uptake of 2.4 l/min we would expect the oscillation in alveolar P_{CO_2}, normally 7.5 torr (1 kPa), to rise to 8.3 torr (1.1 kPa) after enzyme inhibition. The corresponding figures for swings in blood $[H^+]$ are 4.7 and 5.3 nmol/l.

Dickinson: One can see, teleologically, some advantages in having wide swings of arterial P_{CO_2} during breathing. There would be fluctuation of P_{CO_2} acting on arterial chemoreceptors. It has been suggested that oscillating P_{CO_2} could be a stimulus for exercise hyperventilation, in which case it would be useful to allow a big swing. In addition, if there were extensive buffering capacity, I suppose the lung would be less effective at removing CO_2 overall, and the body would have to run with a higher mixed venous P_{CO_2}. Would you agree with this?

Farhi: To a moderate extent, yes. You are saying that when the P_{CO_2} is high at the end of expiration, then not much CO_2 is eliminated and part of the blood flow is wasted. And because of the shape of the CO_2 dissociation curve, end inspiration and expiration are not averaged exactly, and there is a loss of efficiency. It is not much though.

Staub: I would have thought, considering the volume of blood on the left side of the circulation as well as the mixing in the left ventricle, that the fluctuations of oxygen and carbon dioxide in alveolar gas would be markedly damped by the time the blood reached the carotid bodies.

Farhi: Bondi & Van Liew (1972) found a swing of 2 to 3 mmHg (0.3–0.4 kPa).

Staub: That is as much as you found in the alveolar gas.

Farhi: This is correct. In actual experiments they found CO_2 oscillation of that magnitude in artificially ventilated dogs.

Staub: I still would not expect the fluctuations in systemic arterial blood to be as large as those in the alveolar gas.

Dickinson: Is there not some evidence from recordings from single nerve fibres that chemoreceptors have their discharge rates influenced by the rate of rise of P_{CO_2}?

Michel: Changes in pH in carotid artery blood have been clearly demonstrated by Semple (Band *et al.* 1969), and the rate of change in carbon dioxide stimulates the chemoreceptors most effectively.

Dejours: That is absolutely right. Also the respiratory reflexes caused by the change in the afferent discharge in the chemoreceptor fibres apparently depend on the phase at which this change occurs during the respiratory cycle. If the hypercapnic increase in the afferent discharges occurs during inspiration, the respiratory effect will not be the same as if it occurred during expiration.

The exact function of carbonate dehydratase in the fish gill and in the mammalian lung is not clear to me. What sorts of concentration are present in fish gill, in the adult mammalian lung, and in the fetal lung?

Farhi: In the adult rat lung it is about 30 units, which is about 1% of the concentration in blood, and about one third of 1% of that in the stomach. In other species, it may reach as high as 10%.

Adamson: In the fetal lamb, there is about 100-fold difference between the level in the lung and in the red blood cells, when the former is expressed as Meldrum-Roughton units/g wet weight, and the latter as units/g red blood cells.

Maetz: The fish gill has about the same activity as pure red blood cells and thus exhibits extremely high concentrations of carbonate dehydratase. The pseudobranchs contain the highest concentration ever recorded of this enzyme (Maetz 1956).

Dickinson: Does this fit with a particular hypothesis, Dr Dejours?

Dejours: Yes; from what Dr Farhi said the enzyme has nothing much to do with alveolar–capillary CO_2 exchange. There is very little in the lung tissue, except in the blood.

Maetz: Turtle bladder contains extremely little carbonate dehydratase, yet it has a definite function in acid–base balance, by way of bicarbonate exchange in that tissue.

Farhi: The turtle carries huge amounts of bicarbonate just stored for emergency in the coelomic sac, doesn't it?

Robin: It has 120 mequiv./l bicarbonate. The pH is about 8.2, so the first part of your statement is correct. Whether it is kept for an emergency or not, no one knows.

References

BAND, D. M., CAMERON, I. R. & SEMPLE, S. J. Q. (1969) Oscillations in arterial pH with breathing in the cat. *J. Appl. Physiol. 26*, 261-267

BONDI, K. R. & VAN LIEW, H. D. (1973) Fluxes of CO_2 in the lung gas studied by arterial pH. *Fed. Proc. 31*, 348

BOSMAN, A. R., LEE, G. de J. & MARSHALL, R. (1965) The effects of pulsatile capillary blood flow upon gas exchange within the lungs of man. *Clin. Sci. 28*, 295-309

DuBois, A. B., BRITT, A. G. & FENN, W. O. (1952) Alveolar CO_2 during the respiratory cycle. *J. Appl. Physiol. 4*, 535-548

MAETZ, J. (1956) Le rôle biologique de l'anhydrase carbonique chez quelques téléostéens. *Bull. Biol. Fr. Belg. Suppl. 40*, 1-129

General discussion II

Dejours: Earlier Dr Olver and Dr Strang said that lung liquid has nothing to do with amniotic fluid, but amniotic fluid has something to do with lung liquid. Dr Adamson has found 3 mequiv. bicarbonate per litre in the lung liquid, but there is 20 mequiv./l in amniotic fluid. Could somebody say something about the dynamics of changes in the constituents of amniotic fluid in relation to those in lung liquid?

Adamson: No one knows where the amniotic liquor comes from. You are quite right that there is about 20 mmol/l bicarbonate in amniotic liquid. The osmolarity is 262 compared with 294 for the lung liquid. Lung liquid must contribute to amniotic liquor, otherwise the investigation of the lecithin/sphingomyelin ratio for assessing lung maturity would not be valid. There must also be a contribution from fetal urine, but we don't know what contribution each makes to amniotic liquor. When a fetal lamb is followed *in utero* and lung liquid is run off into a bag, which prevents it from getting into the amniotic liquor, one still sometimes sees liquor at the time of Caesarean section. However it seems to be much more gelatinous than normal amniotic liquor, and of a different constituency.

Egan: In a human fetus with renal agenesis, typically oligohydramnios appears—there is very little amniotic liquor. Yet these children die of pulmonary hypoplasia. On the other hand, if such a fetus happens to be one of twins, amniotic liquor is presumably contributed by the normal twin because the lungs are normally formed and the infant dies of renal failure. A very few cases have been reported by Dr David Smith (Thomas & Smith 1974). There must be some relationship between amniotic liquor and lung development, although the amniotic liquor does not contribute to the lung liquid as far as we

251

can tell. The presence of amniotic liquor may well be important in the normal development of the fetal lung, but the relationship between them is unknown.

Adamson: The lamb fetus can produce up to 0.25 l of lung liquid a day when it weighs not much more than 1 kg. This is a quite fantastic volume when one considers the sort of water loss this means to the animal. It is not a net loss, because a lot of this will be swallowed and then reabsorbed back into the fetus.

Strang: There is evidence that the urine contributes in a major way to amniotic fluid (Alexander *et al.* 1958).

Robin: Wouldn't that complicate the problem that Dr Dejours raises, unless fetal urine has a very high bicarbonate ion concentration? If it resembles adult urine, it should have a very low bicarbonate ion concentration and a low pH. Dr Dejours tells us that it has a bicarbonate ion concentration of about 20 mequiv./l.

Strang: I think that is about the concentration in fetal urine.

Egan: Fetal urine has an almost neutral pH.

QUANTITY OF LUNG LIQUID

Staub: Why does the fetal lung form 0.25 l of liquid per day instead of a few millilitres? It is an enormous production rate for such a small organ.

Adamson: The fetal lung starts off as a cord of cells which at some stage becomes a tube. Does this mean that the cells would have to be a secreting organ at that stage?

Staub: I don't doubt that the lung liquid keeps the bronchi open. But I still don't see why there is so much liquid produced.

Strang: As far as I know there is a lumen in the fetal lung at all times.

Adamson: At some initial stage it is just a cord.

Strang: It depends how big a space you accept as a lumen; there is, as far as I know, some space between the epithelial cells at all stages of development. In embryonic explants of lung, holes can be seen even at the earliest stages (De Jong & De Haan 1943).

Adamson: We have been interested in the role of lung liquid in lung growth between 100 and 130 days of gestation, when alveolar formation is marked in the fetal lamb (D. Alcorn *et al.*, 1975, unpublished work). We compared normal (control) lungs at 130 days with lungs that had been ligated and with lungs that had been drained of lung liquid from 110 to 130 days. The ligated lungs were much larger than the control lungs, while the drained lungs were smaller than the control lungs. Alveolar volume appears to be increased in the ligated lungs, as are alveolar numbers and the total air space compared with the controls. In the drained lungs the alveolar number, alveolar surface area and total air space are all decreased compared with controls. Intriguingly, the numbers of type II cells were markedly higher in the drained lung than in the controls. Whether this was a cortisone effect we couldn't say.

Olver: Is the lung epithelium thicker in the drained lung? I have always liked to think that hydrostatic pressure set up by lung liquid secretion is responsible for the thinning of the alveolar epithelium which occurs as term approaches.

Adamson: Electron microscope and scanning electron microscope pictures certainly show that the epithelium is thicker, while bronchial cells appear increased in number. The work we have published on lung liquid composition throughout gestation was also done on lungs chronically drained into a bag (Adamson *et al.* 1975). The only ion to show an increase in concentration with time in fetal lung liquid was potassium.

Olver: At what period of gestation was this?

Adamson: There seemed to be a fairly slow rise over the period from 100 to 130 days. The interesting thing is that type II cells increased markedly in this model, which may have some relevance to your observations.

Olver: E. J. Mescher *et al.* (unpublished work, 1974) didn't find any change in net secretion of potassium until about the last week of gestation, when it doubled in association with a sharp increase in surfactant output. It wasn't gradual at all.

Staub: Were all these lungs fixed by inflating at low volume?

Adamson: The lung liquid removed at Caesarean section was replaced with fixative.

Staub: Did you keep the lungs that had been drained at low volume?

Adamson: Yes, they were kept at low volume, in a collapsed state.

Dickinson: What is the transpulmonary pressure in the fetal lung? Do you know the pleural pressure?

Strang: There is a negative pressure of about 0.5 to 1 cmH_2O (0.05–0.1 kPa), i.e. if a cannula is put in the trachea and attached to a transducer, and the chest is then opened, the pressure rises to about 1 cmH_2O.

Agostoni: The positive pressure you found in the trachea when you opened the chest wall is just due to the weight of the liquid-filled lung. If the lung were surrounded by water at the opening of the chest wall the positive pressure found in the trachea should be simply that of the hydrostatic factor and no more: i.e. the lung of the fetus at the resting volume of the respiratory system does not recoil inwards (Agostoni 1959; Avery & Cooke 1961).

Strang: I accept that criticism.

Dickinson: The fact that lung liquid comes out in little bursts makes it seem as if the fetus kept its larynx shut. Indeed the ambient pressure might average 1 or 2 cmH_2O (0.1 or 0.2 kPa) in normal circumstances. Dr Adamson is suggesting that developmentally this is a very clotted tissue. All the cells are sticking together in the wrong places and the maintenance of a very small gradient, even perhaps 1 or 2 cmH$_2$O, might be useful.

Strang: Experiments reported by Adams suggest that the fetal larynx does open and close. He did cineradiographic measurements after injecting radio-opaque dye into the trachea and followed the movements of the glottis (Adams *et al.* 1967).

Dickinson: Something along these lines would explain why the fetus needs to produce a fairly substantial volume of fluid.

Strang: The liquid can be envisaged as a sort of template around which the architecture of the lung is built; perhaps a positive liquid pressure is needed to keep the surfaces apart.

Staub: In organ culture will the fetal lung develop to the stage of alveolar formation? Does it lose its cuboidal epithelium?

Dickinson: There is no pressure at all in organ culture.

References

ADAMS, F., DESILETS, D. T. & TOWERS, B. (1967) Control of flow of fetal lung liquid at the laryngeal outlet. *Respir. Physiol. 2*, 302-309

ADAMSON, T. M., BRODECKY, V., LAMBERT, T. F., MALONEY, J. E., RITCHIE, B. C. & WALKER, A. M. (1957) Lung liquid production and composition in the 'in utero' foetal lambs. *Aust. J. Exp. Biol. Med. Sci. 53*, 65-75

AGOSTONI, E. (1959) Volume-pressure relationships of the thorax and lung in the newborn. *J. Appl. Physiol. 14*, 909-913

ALEXANDER, D. P., NIXON, D. A., WIDDAS, W. & WOHLZOGAN, F. X. (1958) General variations in the composition of the foetal fluids and foetal urine in sheep. *J. Physiol. (Lond.) 140*, 1-13

AVERY, M. E. & COOK, C. D. (1961) Volume-pressure relationships of lungs and thorax in fetal, newborn and adult goats. *J. Appl. Physiol. 16*, 1034-1038

DE JONG, B. J. & DE HAAN, J. (1943) Organ and tissue differentiation in perfused cultures of explants from the oesophago-stomach-trachea complex of young chicken embryos. *Acta Neerl. Morphol. 5*, 26

THOMAS, I. T. & SMITH, D. W. (1974) Oligohydramnios, cause of the non-renal features of Potter's syndrome, including pulmonary hypoplasia. *J. Pediatr. 84*, 811-814

Mechanism of alveolar flooding in acute pulmonary oedema

NORMAN C. STAUB, MARLYS GEE and CAROL VREIM

Cardiovascular Research Institute and Department of Physiology, University of California, San Francisco, California

Abstract In severe pulmonary oedema, the alveoli fill rapidly with fluid of essentially the same protein composition as free interstitial fluid. The usual explanation is that the normally 'tight' alveolar epithelial intercellular junctions suddenly become freely permeable to proteins. But the pathophysiological basis for such a change is unknown. In seven anaesthetized dogs one lower lobe was filled with iso-osmotic fluid containing ^{125}I-labelled albumin. The calculated alveolus–blood albumin permeability over three hours averaged 0.06×10^{-7} cm/s. It *decreased* nearly 50% when the alveolar tracer concentration was tripled for three more hours. At autopsy, large interstitial free fluid cuffs around blood vessels and airways were found. Isolated lung lobes were filled with isosmotic fluid containing tracer albumin at 10 and 20 cmH$_2$O (0.98–1.96 kPa) airway pressure. Free interstitial fluid cuffs developed within 30 and 10 minutes, respectively. The tracer protein concentration in the cuff fluid averaged 0.9 that of the alveolar fluid. It is postulated that the terminal airway epithelium is normally permeable to protein and water. In acute pulmonary oedema alveolar flooding may occur along the same pathway after the loose interstitial tissue space is fluid-filled and its pressure exceeds that in the airway. The anatomical site of the bulk fluid and protein leak has not been identified.

Much fluid can accumulate in the lung's interstitium without flooding the alveoli (Staub *et al.* 1967). It is generally believed that the alveolar epithelial membrane, in spite of its attenuated appearance by electron microscopy, forms a substantial barrier preventing alveolar flooding. But, when alveolar flooding does occur, the fluid contains plasma proteins in concentrations ranging from 0.3–1.2 times that of plasma (Staub 1974). Alveolar oedema fluid is not similar in protein content to the active secretion by the distal air space that lines the epithelium of the fetus (Adamson *et al.* 1969). It is probably a gross leak of interstitial fluid (Hayward 1955). We can ask two questions: where does the fluid leak into the alveoli occur, and what initiates it?

The most likely pathway is directly through the alveolar epithelium. Either

255

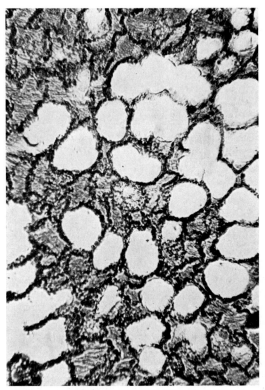

Fig. 1. Intermediate stage of alveolar flooding in acute pulmonary oedema. Some alveoli are completely fluid-filled; others are normal. There does not appear to be any gas trapping (frozen dog lung, 20μm thick section).

the forces that hold the cell junctions tightly together (zonulae occludentes) are altered (Clemens & Willnow 1958; Schneeberger-Keeley & Karnovsky 1968; Nicolaysen 1971), or there is physical rupture of the epithelium due to a hydrostatic pressure difference, although this latter possibility seems unlikely. Fig. 1 shows a histological section from a dog lung rapidly frozen during alveolar flooding. At that time, we believed that our finding that the alveoli filled up individually without any trapping of gas meant flooding had to occur at the level of the individual alveolus (Staub *et al.* 1967).

But if that is so, what initiates the process? It occurs both in high vascular pressure oedema and in increased microvascular permeability oedema.

Other features of alveolar flooding that need to be explained are the apparent acceleration of weight gain seen in isolated perfused lungs during alveolar flooding (Nicolaysen 1971) and the slow clearance of alveolar fluid in contrast to the rapid clearance of interstitial fluid (Courtice & Simmonds 1954).

An alternative mechanism is that fluid leaks backward from some site upstream from the alveoli (Whayne & Severinghaus 1968). We dismissed this possibility too readily in our earlier thinking. In support of the airway leakage concept are the reports of extensive perivascular and peribronchial oedema after fluid-filling of the lungs via the trachea (Gruenwald 1961; Moolten 1967; Muggenburg et al. 1972), suggesting a pathway of relatively low hydraulic resistance between the lumen of the airways and the lung's interstitium. Further, Macklin (1954) postulated that the active liquid secretion of the alveolar pneumonocytes was reabsorbed into the lung interstitium at the level of the respiratory bronchiole.

If fluid can flow from the airways into the interstitium, perhaps it can flow in the opposite direction when the hydrostatic pressure gradient is reversed, as may occur when interstitial oedema develops.

With this nebulous idea in mind, we have done some experiments to determine whether there is any support for the transairway leakage theory.

IDENTITY OF FREE INTERSTITIAL AND ALVEOLAR FLUID

Although alveolar fluid in oedema contains substantial amounts of protein, no one had obtained interstitial fluid of the lung with which to compare alveolar fluid. We therefore made these measurements in our laboratory. Anaesthetized dogs were given alloxan, 100 mg/kg intravenously, to produce acute, severe pulmonary oedema. When airway foam appeared, the thorax was opened and the alveoli were directly punctured with sharpened micropipettes so that fluid samples could be obtained. The lungs were excised and frozen. In a cryostat, the frozen fluid was chipped from the perivascular and peribronchial cuffs. These microsamples were analysed for total proteins by the Lowry method (Lowry et al. 1951) and for the albumin fraction by cellulose acetate electrophoresis.

Table 1 summarizes the results. The total protein and albumin concentrations of interstitial fluid and alveolar fluid were essentially identical. Our conclusion is that the alveoli flood rapidly through pathways that do not sieve proteins. We have not yet obtained comparable data for the oedema caused by increased microvascular hydrostatic pressure.

PROTEIN PERMEABILITY OF THE NORMAL ALVEOLAR MEMBRANE

Investigators have found that the alveolar membrane is much less permeable to solutes than is the pulmonary microvascular membrane (see Table 14 in Staub 1974). Judging from the tight junctions seen by electron microscopy

TABLE 1

Protein composition of alveolar fluid and interstitial free fluid in alloxan-induced acute pulmonary oedema in anaesthetized dogs

Condition	No. of animals	Interstitial fluid		Alveolar fluid	
		TP^a	A	TP	A
		(g/100 ml)		(g/100 ml)	
Severe terminal oedema^b	14	4.7	0.50	5.2	0.49
		±0.7	±0.06	±0.8	±0.07

^{a} Total protein (TP) measured by Lowry method (Lowry *et al.* 1951) on 1-μl samples.
  Albumin fraction (A) measured by cellulose acetate electrophoresis.
^{b} Values are group averages ± one standard deviation.

(Pietra *et al.* 1969) and the marked restriction to the diffusion of small molecules such as sucrose (Taylor & Gaar 1970), the normal alveolar membrane ought to be completely impermeable to protein molecules, such as serum albumin. This is also the conclusion to be reached from the findings of Normand *et al.* (1971) in the lungs of fetal sheep. On the other hand, Schultz *et al.* (1964) and Goetzman & Visscher (1969) showed a small but measurable albumin permeability in the isolated, perfused dog lung.

In our laboratory, the apparent albumin permeability of the alveolar membrane of a fluid-filled lobe was measured in intact, anaesthetized dogs. The lobe was degassed by occluding it after 100% O_2 ventilation, then filling it to its approximate FRC volume (250 ml) with Krebs–Henseleit buffer containing a tracer quantity of radioiodinated serum albumin. The uptake rate of the albumin into circulating blood was measured for 3 h while the lobe was tidally ventilated with fluid (40 ml/10 min). Additional radioactive albumin was then added to the ventilation fluid and the plasma uptake rate was measured for another 3 h. Fig. 2 shows an example of one experiment. Although the concentration of radioactive albumin in alveolar fluid was increased nearly threefold after the third hour, nevertheless the rate of tracer uptake into the blood was not markedly altered. The discrepancy is not due to poor mixing, because in a separate study good mixing was found after four ventilation cycles (40 min). In control experiments the tracer uptake rate was constant for up to 8 h.

Table 2 summarizes results from seven experiments. In every animal, the calculated alveolar to plasma permeability coefficient decreased during the second three-hour period. The average decrease was about 50%. The experiments with fluid-filled lung lobes are crude and the possibility of direct injury to the alveolar membrane during the experiment cannot be ruled out.

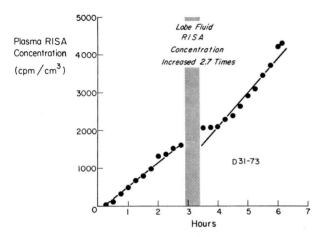

FIG. 2. Time course of a tracer quantity of radioiodinated serum albumin (RISA) in circulating blood plasma after one lower lobe (dog lung) had been filled with Krebs–Henseleit buffer containing tracer. At three hours, additional RISA was added to increase the alveolar concentration to 2.7 times that during the first three hours.

TABLE 2

Calculated alveolar membrane permeability coefficient to radioactive albumin as a function of its alveolar fluid concentration in anaesthetized dogs

Condition	No. of animals	Concentration[a]	Permeability coefficient $(10^{-7}\ cm/s)$
Fluid-filled, left lower lobe			
(a) 0–3 h	7	1	0.061 ± 0.051
(b) 3–6 h	7	2.6 ± 0.4	0.034 ± 0.034

[a] Relative concentration of tracer albumin in alveolar fluid.

Nevertheless, the observations do not readily fit into the standard two-compartment model used to calculate membrane permeability and, therefore, our interest was stimulated so much that we decided to study the phenomenon of perivascular cuff formation during tracheal fluid filling in more detail.

INTERSTITIAL FLUID CUFF FORMATION

Fig. 3 demonstrates interstitial fluid cuffs adjacent to blood vessels and airways in the lung. The picture is from a lung with interstitial oedema rather than from one with tracheal filling. The reason is that the latter does not show adequate contrast for publication. Nevertheless, the cuffs are identical in location and size.

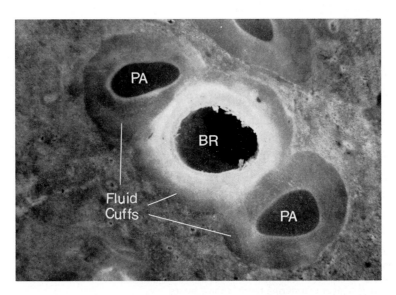

FIG. 3. Freshly frozen section of dog lung, showing perivascular and peribronchial interstitial free fluid cuffs in acute pulmonary oedema. Bronchus (BR); pulmonary arteries (PA).

We first determined the rate of formation and volume of the cuffs. Six isolated dog lung lobes were filled with Krebs–Henseleit buffer to airway pressures of 10 or 20 cmH_2O (0.98–1.96 kPa); then, after 10–90 min, the lungs were frozen. Random sections were cut in the cryostat and the blood vessels and their cuffs were photographed. By a point-counting method, followed by analysis of the homogenized lobes for haemoglobin, water content and dry weight, the absolute volumes of the perivascular cuffs were determined at different time intervals. Fig. 4 shows the interesting result of this experiment. The rate of cuff formation was faster when the lungs were at a higher inflation pressure, which seems in keeping with the view that the perivascular interstitial pressure of extra-alveolar blood vessels is decreased with lung inflation, especially when the blood vessels are unable to fill (Howell *et al.* 1961). Even at 10 cmH_2O airway pressure, however, measurable interstitial cuffs were formed within 30 min, and at the end of 90 min the volumes of fluid cuffs at both pressures were substantially the same, averaging 2.8 ml fluid/g dry blood-free lung weight. We conclude that the interstitial cuffs are of substantial volume and formed at a reasonably rapid rate in the dog lung.

In the mouse, interstitial fluid cuffs form rapidly (< 5 min) even at 10 cmH_2O airway pressure. It is of interest that in the fetal lamb and rabbit there are no perivascular cuffs. But these develop rapidly after the onset of breathing, that

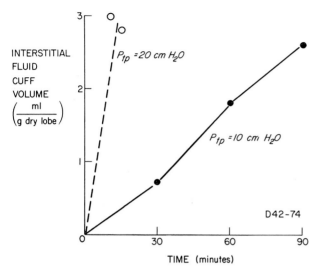

FIG. 4. Time course of increase in interstitial free-fluid cuff volume in isolated, fluid-filled, dog lung lobes at two different transpulmonary pressures (P_{tp}).

is, as soon as the lungs are well-inflated with air and can develop a subatmospheric peri-airway pressure.

Finally, 10 isolated degassed lung lobes were filled with Krebs-Henseleit buffer containing tracer radioiodinated albumin at airway pressures of 10, 20 and 30 cmH$_2$O. Again, the lungs were frozen, but this time microsamples were obtained of the frozen free interstitial fluid and of frozen fluid in small airways. The radioactive albumin concentrations were compared. The results are summarized in Table 3 for each level of airway pressure. On average, the concentration of tracer albumin in the fluid cuffs was 90% of that in the terminal airway fluid. We conclude from this that the interstitial cuff fluid flows through pathways which show little sieving of protein molecules.

DISCUSSION

The findings we have presented are obviously preliminary and inconclusive, but they are sufficiently intriguing and, we hope, controversial enough to stimulate further work on the permeability of the various membranes separating the lung interstitium from the gas phase.

The critical experiment would be to demonstrate the actual pathway for fluid and protein. We believe this could best be done by autoradiography. Unfortunately, there are numerous technical difficulties, not the least of which

TABLE 3

Radioactive albumin concentration (concn.) in airway fluid and interstitial free-fluid cuffs in isolated, dog lung lobes

Airway fluid pressure (cmH₂O)	Duration (min)	Concn. in interstitium/conc. in airway fluid
10	30–120	0.91
20	10–30	0.86
30	30	0.90

Average 0.90
± s.d.   ±0.04

is the method of fixation of the lung. We know from our recent experience of the autoradiography of radioactive albumin in lung lymphatics (Nicolaysen *et al.* 1975) that the best fixation method is undoubtedly rapid freezing, followed by drying. Unfortunately, we cannot freeze the fluid-filled lung very quickly. Slow freezing allows the formation of large ice crystals which makes the resolution of intercellular junctions, for example, difficult.

Finally, to return to the problem of alveolar flooding in pulmonary oedema, we propose the following as an alternative to direct flooding through breaks in the alveolar membrane. As interstitial oedema develops and fills the tissue space around the airways and blood vessels, the interstitial fluid pressure rises from some subatmospheric value, perhaps similar to pleural pressure, until it reaches or slightly exceeds that in the airways. Fluid begins to leak through the low resistance pathways (probably the intercellular junctions of the epithelium in the terminal airways) and then flows retrograde into alveoli.

This fanciful scheme is somewhat analogous to a bathtub overflowing. It does not imply (although it does not exclude) direct damage to the alveolar epithelium. What is more, it provides a reasonable explanation of the abrupt onset of alveolar flooding and the slow clearance of alveolar oedema fluid.

ACKNOWLEDGEMENTS

This work was supported in part by US Public Health Service Grants HL6285 and HL14201 (Pulmonary SCOR).

References

ADAMSON, T. M., BOYD, R. D. H. PLATT, H. S. & STRANG, L. B. (1969) Composition of alveolar liquid in the foetal lamb. *J. Physiol. (Lond.) 204*, 159
CLEMENS, H. J. & WILLNOW, R. (1958) Vorkommen, Lokalization und Bedeutung von sauren Mucopolysacchariden in der Lunge. *Ergeb. Ges. Tuberk. Lungenforsch. 14*, 651

COURTICE, F. C. & SIMMONDS, J. (1954) Physiological significance of lymph drainage of the serous cavities and lungs. *Physiol. Rev. 34*, 419

GOETZMAN, B. W. & VISSCHER, M. B. (1969) The effects of alloxan and histamine on the permeability of the pulmonary alveolocapillary barrier to albumin. *J. Physiol. (Lond.) 204*, 51

GRUENWALD, P. (1961) Normal and abnormal expansion of the lungs of newborn infants obtained at autopsy. I. Expansion of lungs by liquid media. *Anat. Rec. 139*, 471

HAYWARD, G. W. (1955) Pulmonary oedema. *Br. Med. J. 1*, 1361

HOWELL, J. B. L., PERMUTT, S., PROCTOR, D. F. & RILEY, R. L. (1961) Effects of inflation of the lung on different parts of the pulmonary vascular bed. *J. Appl. Physiol. 16*, 71

LOWRY, O. H., ROSEBROUGH, N. J., FARR, A. L. & RANDALL, R. J. (1951) Protein measurement with the Folin phenol reagent. *J. Biol. Chem. 193*, 265-275

MACKLIN, C. C. (1954) The pulmonary alveolar mucoid film and the pneumonocytes. *Lancet 1*, 1099

MOOLTEN, S. E. (1967) Pulmonary lymphatics in relation to pulmonary clearance, interstitial fluid and the pathogenesis of emphysema, in *Current Research in Chronic Obstructive Lung Disease*, pp. 191-221, publication No. 1787, United States Department of Health, Education & Welfare, Washington, D.C.

MUGGENBURG, B. A., MANDERLY, J. L., PICKRELL, J. A., CHIFFELLE, T. L., JONES, R. K., LUFT, U. C., MCCLELLAN, R. D. & PFLEGER, R. C. (1972) Pathophysiologic sequelae of bronchopulmonary lavage in the dog. *Am. Rev. Respir. Dis. 106*, 219

NICOLAYSEN, G. (1971) Increase in capillary filtration rate resulting from reduction in the intravascular calcium ion concentration *Acta Physiol. Scand. 81*, 517

NICOLAYSEN, G., NICOLAYSEN, A. & STAUB, N. C. (1975) A quantitative radioautographic comparison of albumin concentration in different sized lymph vessels in normal mouse lungs. *Microvasc. Res. 10*, 138

NORMAND, I. C. S., OLVER, R. E., REYNOLDS, E. O. R., STRANG, L. B. & WELCH, K. (1971). Permeability of lung capillaries and alveoli to non-electrolytes in the foetal lamb. *J. Physiol. (Lond.) 219*, 303

PIETRA, G. G., SZIDON, J. P., LEVENTHAL, M. M. & FISHMAN, A. P. (1969) Hemoglobin as a tracer in hemodynamic pulmonary edema. *(Science Wash. D.C.) 166*, 1643

SCHNEEBERGER-KEELEY, E. E. & KARNOVSKY, M. J. (1968) The ultrastructural basis of alveolar capillary membrane permeability to perioxidase used as a tracer. *J. Cell Biol. 37*, 781

SCHULTZ, A. L., GRISMER, J. T., WADA, S. & GRANDE, F. (1964) Absorption of albumin from alveoli of perfused dog lung. *Am. J. Physiol. 207*, 1300

STAUB, N. C. (1974) Pulmonary edema. *Physiol. Rev. 54*, 687

STAUB, N. C., NAGANO, H. & PEARCE, M. L. (1967) Pulmonary edema in dogs, especially the sequence of fluid accumulation in the lungs. *J. Appl. Physiol. 22*, 227

TAYLOR, A. E. & GAAR, K. A., JR. (1970) Estimation of equivalent pore radii of pulmonary capillary and alveolar membranes. *Am. J. Physiol. 218*, 1133

WHAYNE, T. F., JR. & SEVERINGHAUS, J. W. (1968) Experimental hypoxic pulmonary edema in the rat. *J. Appl. Physiol. 25*, 729

Discussion

Dickinson: Apart from the lack of sieving one might imagine that the liquid enters the alveoli osmotically. In the experiments on isolated dog lungs you used isotonic saline, didn't you?

Staub: We used Krebs–Henseleit buffer, which is iso-osmotic with plasma.

Strang: What stops the liquid going in there in the normal lung?

Staub: The pressure gradients are in the wrong direction. The alveolar air pressure is higher than the interstitial fluid pressure.

Strang: I am a little worried about that. It is difficult to stop liquid flow completely with gas pressure.

Fishman: The observations on filling a lung with liquid are interesting but I fail to see what they have to do with pulmonary oedema. The genesis of most forms of pulmonary oedema—particularly haemodynamic pulmonary oedema—is an orderly process in which interstitial oedema invariably precedes alveolar oedema. This is not the sequence that pertains to the dog lungs that you described, Dr Staub. Nor does this model raise the same questions about the routes taken by water and macromolecules in passing from capillary lumens to interstitial and alveolar spaces. Indeed, the model seems only applicable to drowning in a sea of albumin.

Staub: I am putting this forward as a viable alternative to the more likely explanation that individual alveolar epithelial cell junctions open.

Lee: You are postulating that the oedema fluid comes in from the terminal bronchioles. If you put Evans' blue into the circulation of your animals, then from serial frozen sections by the techniques you have used you ought to be able to see where the protein is coming from. Have you done that?

Staub: Yes and no. We have looked at the time course of fluorescent protein accumulation in the normal lung. Unfortunately, the resolution of frozen sections in the fluorescence microscope is not adequate to allow us to find individual points of fluid leakage (Nicolaysen & Staub 1975). We have not done experiments in oedema with alveolar flooding. However, in the normal lung we can see the fluorescent albumin in the intercellular junctions of the airway epithelium. It does not penetrate through the tight junctions. We would like to examine this phenomenon in pulmonary oedema.

Lee: You said that there was no sieving of protein in oedema. There certainly is a difference between the handling of protein put into the airways in certain circumstances. For instance, if albumin labelled with radioactive iodine is put into the peripheral airways in the normal state, its absorption time into the blood stream is about 12–13 hours. When we did this in an animal which had distemper the protein was into the circulation in about 20 minutes (Gillespie & Lee 1967).

Staub: I don't doubt that in some conditions, for example respiratory tract burns or toxic gas inhalation, the alveolar epithelial membrane literally disintegrates.

Robin: In your paper on the sequence of pulmonary oedema (Staub *et al.* 1967), you showed diffuse alveolar swelling with both kinds of pulmonary oedema. I think you measured the width of swelling of alveolar epithelial cells and concluded that the change in diffusion pathway was not sufficient to impair oxygenation. So how do you explain alveolar epithelial cell oedema if you are filling a bathtub of alveolar epithelial cells which merely act as containers?

Staub: I wish we had actually done what you say we did. We measured the full thickness of the alveolar wall. In the early phase of interstitial pulmonary oedema, the alveolar walls were not detectably thickened. All the fluid seemed to be accumulating in the large perivascular cuffs. When the cuffs became grossly enlarged, the alveolar wall became thicker. We assumed that meant fluid was accumulating in the alveolar wall interstitium as the fluid pressure rose in the perivascular cuffs. I don't see any conflict between fluid accumulating in the alveolar wall and fluid leaking out of the airways. The same rise in perivascular fluid pressure would cause both events.

Robin: Wouldn't you think that in pure interstitial oedema the alveolar epithelial cells might well be compressed and get thinner?

Staub: No, not unless the alveoli got larger. They get smaller when there is flooding. I presume that the alveolar epithelial cells would get thicker as the surface area decreased, if the volume remained constant.

Hughes: You are suggesting that in fluid-filled lobes the albumin passes through the smaller airways. Perhaps you could dissect out the small airways and study their permeability characteristics.

Staub: I asked several pathologists whether they had found any difference in the intercellular junctions between epithelial cells of the airways. Dr Lynne Reid has reviewed some of her material and told me this week that the epithelial cell junctions looked about the same all along the airways.

Schneeberger: The broncho-alveolar junctional area appears to be involved in a two-way traffic of alveolar macrophages. However, I can't add any information on the ultrastructure of these junctions.

Olver: Are there any epithelial junctions that are normally as permeable as you are postulating these intercellular junctions must be?

Staub: I don't know. That is why I asked earlier why the electrical resistance across the trachea was so low.

Olver: It is not very low.

Staub: It wouldn't take many holes to produce this effect.

Olver: But they would be rather unusual junctions for an **intact** epithelium.

Durbin: In the experiments where you put albumin into the alveolar space, were you measuring disappearance of albumin from the lung or its appearance in the blood?

Staub: During the experiment we measured the uptake in blood, and terminally we measured the residual amount in the lung. We accounted for all the tracer albumin.

Durbin: Does the increase in albumin concentration give enough osmotic flow to create solvent drag against the normal diffusion stream and thus lower the apparent permeability?

Staub: The concentration of the tracer albumin was very low. It had no osmotic effect. There was no other albumin in the alveolar fluid.

Michel: Another possibility accounting for this sort of phenomenon is that, at very low concentrations, albumin appears to interact with capillary walls and change their permeability properties (Mason *et al.* 1973).

Staub: The plasma albumin concentration was normal.

Michel: But we are talking about an alveolar epithelium which might be behaving in the same sort of way.

Staub: Normally, there is no albumin on the air-space side of the alveolar epithelium.

Michel: In adding the tracer amounts of albumin you may be lowering the permeability of that membrane.

Olver: Presumably tracer albumin may get stuck to the alveolar walls.

Staub: A large fraction of the radioactive albumin supplied commercially is not labelled.

Olver: Are your control and experimental situations exactly the same? Was there any washing period in the middle of the control period, for example?

Staub: The lung was tidally ventilated with fluid throughout the experiment. We have omitted all uptake results from the 40-minute wash-in period when we were changing the concentration of alveolar tracer protein.

Maetz: In our laboratory, P. Payan and J. P. Girard (unpublished work) have recently perfused isolated heads of trout in their studies of gill perfusion. If labelled albumin alone was used to measure perfusion space, a considerable amount of label was seen to stick to the endothelial lining of the blood vessels. Cold albumin has to be added to decrease the specific activity of the label. As adsorption is occurring at a finite number of sites, the number of sites with radioactive albumin is low. In your experiments, Dr Staub, you observed that the disappearance rate of labelled albumin from the lung decreased when the concentration of (radioactive) albumin was increased experimentally. I suggest that this may simply be the result of adsorption processes at a limited number of sites in the lung wall. With an increased concentration of albumin, you obtained a decrease in the relative quantity of label attached to the lung wall.

Michel: The concentrations which act on capillary walls and appear to be adsorbed are in the range between 0.01 and 0.1% albumin.

Staub: I don't see how this adsorption phenomenon would have any significance in terms of the bulk flow of albumin we found going into the interstitial free fluid cuffs.

Egan: In some of the adult sheep I described the results are similar to those you have just presented, Dr Staub. The concentration of albumin in the alveolar fluid decreases when the pressure is high. We felt that we had disrupted the epithelium of the lung. A pressure of 10 cmH_2O (0.98 kPa) in the airway of a fluid-filled lung without an air–gas interface is at the top of lung volume. It is almost 100% of lung capacity, and 20 cmH_2O (1.96 kPa) is hyperinflated.

Staub: In our experience with pressure volume curves of fluid-filled lungs, 10 cmH_2O is not total lung capacity, although 20 cmH_2O is.

Egan: We reached total lung capacity in some isolated lungs with as low as 8 cmH_2O (0.78 kPa), the same values as published by Radford (1964). We did not see albumin moving across at low lung volumes. There was a predictable variation in relative rates of diffusion of several tracers, at low lung volumes, which would indicate that the epithelia up and down the airways were very tight and were not allowing albumin, the largest tracer, to move across at any site. It was only at very high lung inflations that albumin moved across the epithelium, and I think this is an abnormal situation. I wondered whether the inflations in your animals reflected an over-distended, fluid-filled lung.

Staub: Didn't you refer earlier to transpulmonary pressures of 41–45 cmH_2O (4.02–4.41 kPa) as opposed to 24–35 cmH_2O (2.45-3.43 kPa)?

Egan: That was for gas inflation of the lung and it is needed to overcome the surface tension forces of a gas–liquid interface. Obviously pressure–volume relationships are very different in the liquid-filled lung.

Waaler: You showed us pictures of lungs where oedema was developing, with some alveoli being filled and some neighbouring ones still being empty. You also suggested that the oedema fluid entered the alveoli via the small bronchi. Shouldn't the pattern then be one of all the alveoli belonging to one small bronchus filling at once? Have you any evidence that this is what happens?

Staub: That was our original reasoning. We didn't think that the alveolar fluid would appear in individual alveoli if it were flowing retrograde down the airways. However, if fluid is trickled down the airways in very small quantities, one can get filling of individual alveoli or small groups of alveoli associated with a single terminal airway. Apparently because of surface tension effects, the fluid fills some alveoli completely but leaves adjacent alveoli air-filled.

Keynes: Could there be a mechanism by which the individual alveoli are marginally stable because of surface tension effects? The first stage in pulmonary oedema would be that the interstitial spaces fill up, as you showed, and then a certain number of individual alveoli would suddenly become unstable and shut or collapse. Might not quite different forces then operate across the walls of those particular alveoli, explaining why an alveolus would then proceed to flood?

Staub: We thought that the alveolar air–liquid interface collapsed and sucked liquid through the alveolar membrane. But, in lungs with high alveolar surface tension, the alveoli collapse, yet they are not fluid-filled because the alveolar epithelium has a low permeability to everything except water.

In pulmonary oedema, of course, the membrane must be freely permeable because the concentration of protein in alveolar liquid is the same as in the free interstitial fluid. Dr Olver said that it must be unique to have epithelium with holes of this size. I agree, but they must exist. The problem is, where are the holes? Do they somehow develop suddenly in the tight alveolar epithelial junctions or were they present normally in the terminal airways?

Olver: I would be surprised if there were holes that size under normal conditions. I agree that holes of that size may occur in pulmonary oedema or when the epithelium is damaged.

Hugh-Jones: You are suggesting that cuffing occurs around the airways and then the liquid overflows into the alveoli, Dr Staub. Have you observed this at different levels down the lung? The hydrostatic pressure should increase. The elephant's lung, for example, has an enormous hydrostatic pressure and the alveolar lining epithelium at the bottom probably differs from that at the top. That would be against your theory and in favour of a theory that the liquid goes straight through the alveoli.

Staub: I am not sure why that would be against my theory. In the normal lung there is no difference in water content up and down the lung. The inter-stitial fluid resistance is so high, compared to the lymphatic resistance, that fluid is drawn off to the lymphatics. There is also a reverse osmotic gradient between the top and the bottom of the lung—at least there should be but I don't know whether anybody has actually measured it.

Hugh-Jones: The alveoli are a bit bigger and the capillaries tend to be closed at the top, don't they? Further down there is a higher hydrostatic pressure and one would expect that there would be a greater tendency for cuffing to occur at the bottom.

Staub: In oedema the cuffing is much greater at the bottom of the lung.

Hugh-Jones: What I am getting at is that if you measured hydrostatic pressure down the lung you might be able to see exactly at what point the overflow is occurring.

Staub: It occurs first at the bottom and works its way up the lung.

Hugh-Jones: In what anatomical location is this actually happening?

Staub: Unfortunately, we have not done experiments to locate the exact site of leakage. From Macklin's observations (1954) we infer that the site of leakage is in the terminal or respiratory bronchioles.

Hugh-Jones: You ought to be able to see the site of leakage as you go down the lung.

Staub: I agree, but we haven't done that experiment.

Guyton: If we assume for a moment that the openings occur in the alveolar septal membranes, wouldn't the liquid still appear primarily in the perivascular spaces? In other words, can the experiments delineate whether the openings are around the perivascular spaces or whether they are in the septal membrane epithelium?

Staub: Unfortunately, we have not been able to design an experiment that would clearly separate these possible sites of leakage.

Lee: The kind of oedema you are talking about is end-state oedema but oedema of the lung occurs before water appears in the alveoli. At what stage is the gel saturated? When is there free fluid in the interstitium? Or is there always free fluid there?

Dickinson: The gel can't be fully saturated.

Lee: So at what point is the water free water and not hidden away in the gel?

Staub: I don't think anybody has obtained free fluid from normal lung interstitium. In oedema, the earliest accumulation of free fluid is in the perivascular loose connective tissue. This appears when the lung water content has increased by about 10%.

Guyton: One can remove Wharton's jelly from the umbilical cord and hydrate it to increase its volume. When the volume has increased more than 30 to 50% one begins to see small pockets of what looks like free water. Thus, the fibrillar network of the gel seems to disrupt at that degree of swelling. In electron micrographs of oedematous lungs almost empty vacuoles are also seen in the perivascular cuffs.

Staub: If the perivascular spaces are filled with air, as frequently happens when lungs are fixed by over-inflating them, there are only a few connective tissue fibrils. Thus, the perivascular spaces in oedema should be mostly free fluid.

Guyton: It seems as though perivascular oedema disrupts the gel matrix, if there is one around the vessels, as I presume there is.

Staub: Yes, it is pulled apart at those points.

Crosbie: Didn't Moss (1972), using an electron-opaque precipitate stain, demonstrate collections of sodium in the interstitium of primate lungs after the production of hypovolaemic shock? He showed that the precipitation matter was found close to the collagen fibres and the deposition was related to blood pH.

Staub: Yes, he did say that. But the electron micrographs in his paper show that the sodium precipitates as small clumps. Dr Robin (Robin *et al.* 1972) found the electrolyte composition of oedema fluid to be very similar to that of plasma.

Fishman: In haemodynamic oedema, which is the simplest model, one can observe that a tracer moves into the interstitium when pulmonary capillary pressures are raised. Earlier (pp. 29–38) I showed the passage of the tracer into the interstitial space and also the presence of tracer in the alveoli. Dr Pietra has provided an additional figure that pertains to the movement of tracer from the interstitial space into alveoli (Fig. 1). This figure illustrates both the tracer in the alveolus and a possible route by which it reached the alveolus.

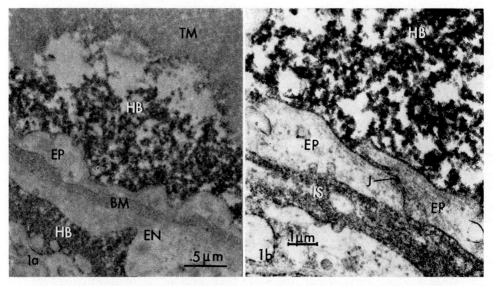

FIG. 1 (Fishman). *Left:* Accumulation of haemoglobin reaction product (HB) in the basement membrane (BM) between endothelium (EN) and squamous epithelium (EP). Reaction product is also seen in the alveolar space between the epithelium (EP) and a layer of tubular myelin (TM) of surfactant. Only those epithelial plasmalemmal vesicles that open on the basement membrane and alveolar space contain tracer. Dog perfused for 5 min with haemoglobin solution at 50 mmHg.

Right: Reaction product has escaped from the interstitial space (IS) into the alveoli, apparently through an epithelial junction (J). The dark discoloration of the epithelial cytoplasm in the vicinity of the junctional region could represent epithelial damage.

These two electron micrographs are consistent with the hypothesis that tracer has entered the alveoli via epithelial junctions, lifting the surfactant layer in the process.

There seems to be little mystery any more about how macromolecules leave the pulmonary capillaries during haemodynamic pulmonary oedema. One route is clearly via interendothelial junctions; if pinocytosis plays a role in the transendothelial transport in the lungs, its contribution seems to be small. But whether there are other undetected avenues, e.g. 'large pores', is unclear. Nor is it known whether the routes taken during resorption of oedema fluid are the same as those originally traversed by the macromolecules. It is also uncertain whether tracers of the dimensions of haemoglobin or albumin enter the interstitial space from the alveoli exclusively by pinocytosis or via interalveolar junctions. These questions are, however, quite clear and are being examined experimentally in several different laboratories.

Strang: I think the big question is whether these enormously high protein concentrations can get through any kind of physiologically adapted epithelium. In other words, can these junctions open again once they have shut or is there actual destruction? I tend to think that this could only happen when there is a tearing or destruction of some kind.

Fishman: There need not be any destruction. The bronchial venular pores are, in fact, open for only a brief while after histamine. The pulmonary capillary endothelial pores appear to remain open as long as capillary pressures are high. Less certain, as Dr Schneeberger has pointed out, is the reversibility of the opening of the alveolar junctions.

I should also point out that alveolar liquid may vary in macromolecular composition in the course of pulmonary oedema. This is well known to clinicians, who have even seen red blood cells in oedema fluid in patients with severe pulmonary oedema. Our own experience suggests that early in experimental haemodynamic pulmonary oedema the concentration of protein in alveolar fluid collected in the bronchi may be quite low but that in time the concentration of protein increases.

Staub: But in your experiments you diluted the circulating blood plasma with so much saline that the protein concentration was very low; therefore the alveolar fluid also had a very low protein concentration.

Fishman: Another type of evidence along the same line has been provided by Robin and associates (1972), using dextrans of different molecular weights. Although electrolytic composition may be the same in the plasma and oedema fluid, the pulmonary capillaries show differential permeability to macromolecules as oedema progresses.

Olver: Are the fluid cuffs the same size in the experimental and controls animals, Dr Staub?

Staub: I don't know.

Olver: If there were bigger fluid cuffs in the experimental situation it would increase the length of the diffusion pathways; one would therefore expect to get a lower apparent permeability.

Staub: At the end of our experiments the protein concentration in the cuffs was less than half that in the alveolar fluid. We calculated that all of the protein taken up into the circulating plasma could be accounted for by the volume and change of protein concentration in the cuff fluid.

References

GILLESPIE, W. J. & LEE, G. de J. (1967) Vascular and lymphatic absorption of radioactive albumen from the lungs. *Cardiovasc. Res. 1*, 42-51

MACKLIN, C. C. (1954) *Acta Anat. 23*, 1-33

MASON, J. C., MICHEL, C. C. & TOOKE, J. E. (1973) The effect of plasma proteins and capillary pressure upon filtration coefficient of frog mesenteric capillaries. *J. Physiol. (Lond.) 229*, 15-16P

MOSS, G. S. (1972) Pulmonary involvement in hypovolaemic shock. *Annu. Rev. Med. 23*, 201

NICOLAYSEN, G. & STAUB, N. C. (1975) *Microvasc. Res. 9*, 29-37

RADFORD, E. P. (1964) Static mechanical properties of mammalian lungs, in *Handb. Physiol.* Section 3: *Respiration*, American Physiological Society, Washington, D.C.

ROBIN, E. D., CAREY, L. C., GRENVIK, A., GLAUSER, F. & GAUDIO, R. (1972) Capillary leak syndrome with pulmonary edema. *Arch. Intern. Med. 13*, 66-71

STAUB, N. C., NAGANO, H. & PEARCE, M. L. (1967) Pulmonary edema in dogs, especially the sequence of fluid accumulation in lungs. *J. Appl. Physiol. 22*, 227-240

Intracellular and subcellular oedema and dehydration

EUGENE D. ROBIN and JAMES THEODORE

Stanford University School of Medicine, Stanford, California

Abstract Changes in intracellular water content appear to be common abnormalities induced by a wide variety of pathogenic mechanisms. Such changes in cell water produce changes in the water in various subcellular organelles bound by semipermeable membranes. Cell and subcell functions then alter in their turn.

In isolated alveolar macrophages (rabbit), intracellular and intramitochondrial oedema reduces mitochondrial O_2 utilization. Metabolic control is maintained because lactate production reverses (Pasteur effect). On reconstitution, O_2 utilization and lactate production return towards normal, indicating reversibility. Cellular and intramitochondrial dehydration also reduces mitochondrial O_2 utilization but metabolic control is lost because lactate production also decreases. Osmotic reconstitution does not reverse the abnormality.

Exposure to hypotonic media leads to release of lysosomal enzymes (β-glucuronidase, EC 3.2.1.31) to the extracellular phase of isolated alveolar macrophages. Some of this release is caused by exocytosis although, at low osmotic concentrations, intralysosomal oedema ultimately ruptures lysosomes, with extensive discharge of enzyme. In turn, lysosomal enzymes may injure more normal cells.

Impairment of energy metabolism caused by hypoxia leads to intracellular oedema, because Na^+ accumulates in the cells when ATP is no longer available for the sodium pump.

Continued studies of the disorders in cell physiology caused by changes in cell and subcell water should provide important new insights into a wide variety of disease states (including pulmonary oedema).

The limiting membranes of cells and subcellular organelles are generally semipermeable, with high permeability to water. In consequence, increases in cellular and subcellular water (intracellular and subcellular oedema) and decreases in cell and subcell water (cellular dehydration) are common pathophysiological disturbances.

Studies of pulmonary oedema have emphasized shifts in water that affect the interstitial and intra-alveolar spaces of the lung. In such studies, alveolar epithelial cells are regarded as more or less passive conduits for water and solute movement. Little attention has been paid to the potential abnormalities caused by cellular and subcellular oedema. In this paper, the following areas will be covered:

(1) Potential mechanisms causing lung cell and subcell oedema and dehydration
(2) Effects of cell oedema and dehydration on subcell water content
(3) Potential mechanisms of injury caused by cell oedema and dehydration
(4) Specific examples of altered cell and subcell pathophysiology related to altered water content:
   (*a*) Mitochondrial O_2 utilization and metabolic control
   (*b*) Lysosomal enzyme release
   (*c*) ATP impairment
(5) Future directions

POTENTIAL MECHANISMS CAUSING LUNG CELL AND SUBCELL OEDEMA AND DEHYDRATION

Currently available data can be used for *a priori* analyses of potential mechanisms causing lung cell and subcell oedema or dehydration. Such an analysis could generate a variety of lists. One such list indicates four major causes (Table 1). Although the precise make-up of such a list is somewhat

TABLE 1

Mechanisms of altered lung cell and subcell water content[a]

I   *Osmotic alterations*
   (1) Fresh water drowning
   (2) Sea water drowning

II *Altered cell membrane permeability*
   (1) Physical agents—ionizing radiation, temperature, ultrasonic, ultraviolet radiation
   (2) Exogenous toxins—inhaled, circulating, infections
   (3) Endogenous toxins—immunological, mediators
   (4) Osmotic alterations—hypotonic, hypertonic

III *Altered energy metabolism leading to ATP limitation*
   (1) Decreased Na^+ pump
   (2) Decreased Ca^{2+} pump

IV *Altered extracellular composition*
   (1) Water excess and dehydration
   (2) Altered plasma Na^+
   (3) Altered plasma Ca^{2+}

---

[a] Altered Starling forces not included because these involve groups of cells.

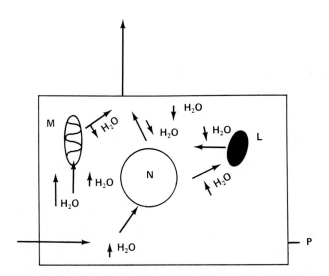

F<small>IG</small>. 1. The effect of intracellular oedema and dehydration on water content of subcellular organelles. Intracellular oedema leads to subcellular oedema. Intracellular dehydration leads to subcellular dehydration. N = nucleus. P = plasma cell membrane. L = lysosome. M = mitochondria.

arbitrary, it is clear that a wide variety of different aetiological factors can result in alterations in cell water. This undoubtedly accounts for the finding (as indicated by structural studies) that cell oedema appears to be an almost universal response to cell injury in most cell types. Obviously this is true of most pulmonary cell types as well.

EFFECTS OF CELL OEDEMA AND DEHYDRATION ON SUBCELL WATER CONTENT

Given alterations of cell water, what are the effects of these on subcellular water? To state the obvious, changes in cell water activity will lead to corresponding changes in the water activity of all subcellular components whose limiting structures possess high permeability for water (Fig. 1). With intracellular oedema, the activity of water in the cytosol will be higher than in a given organelle. Water will pass down its activity gradient until osmotic equilibrium is achieved. Cellular dehydration will lead to the opposite change. At equilibrium, subcellular osmotic pressure, cytosol osmotic pressure and extracellular osmotic pressure are presumably equal. Thus, the general rule may be stated that intracellular oedema leads to subcellular oedema and intracellular dehydration leads to subcellular dehydration. Although systematic

TABLE 2

Mechanisms of injury caused by cell oedema and dehydration

---

(1) Volume changes producing alterations of surface–volume relationships

(2) Cell or subcell rupture with extensive increases in volume

(3) Altered macromolecular physical state and properties

(4) Concentration changes

(5) Inflammatory changes

(6) Biochemical alterations

---

data are not available for all subcellular organelles, there are specific studies which show that two subcellular organelles, cell nuclei (Churney 1942) and mitochondria (Tedeschi & Harris 1955), do act as osmometers. The ultimate characterization of the consequences of changes in cell water will require evaluation of intramitochondrial oedema, intranuclear oedema, intralysosomal oedema, etc.

POTENTIAL MECHANISMS OF INJURY CAUSED BY CELL OEDEMA AND DEHYDRATION

Given an increase or a decrease in cell and subcell water content, the question arises as to the mechanisms by which secondary alterations of cell function occur. Using *a priori* analysis, it is again possible to generate a somewhat arbitrary but useful list of potential mechanisms responsible for the injury caused by alteration in cell water content (Table 2). Swelling (with ultimate lysis) and shrinkage are obvious sequelae of altered water content. The nature of the changes in volume produced by alterations in water content are quite complex in biological units. A simplifying concept that has been widely used is that of a 'perfect' osmometer, defined as a biological unit which obeys the Boyle–Van't Hoff law (osmotic pressure × cell volume = constant). This cannot be extensively discussed in this paper. However, most biological units show only small deviations from 'perfection' and linear volume–osmotic pressure curves have been described for a variety of cell types (House 1974) and for isolated mitochondria (Tedeschi & Harris 1955). Some cell types (for example, macrophages), show major deviations from the Boyle–Van't Hoff law (L. O'Brien, J. Theodore & E. D. Robin 1975, unpublished work). In cells which operate as tightly bound units, for example alveolar epithelial cells, the changes in volume are probably even more complex. Ultimate physicochemical characterization of changes in volume as a function of alterations of water

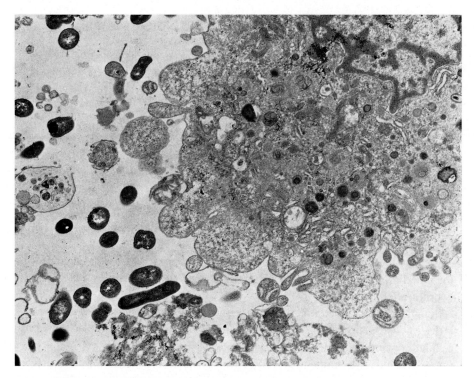

FIG. 2. Sediment from alveolar macrophages exposed to distilled water for 4.5 min and then reconstituted in isotonic medium. Note essentially intact cell. Numerous intact lysosomes are seen. Mitochondria are enlarged and distorted. No nuclei seen. ($\times$ 10 000)

content in a given biological unit (cell or subcell) would require at least knowledge of: (1) Osmotic compliance of the unit (volume–osmotic pressure curve); (2) Resistance of the limiting membrane to osmotic rupture (osmotic fragility); (3) Resistance of the limiting membrane to mechanical rupture (mechanical fragility). Various cell types and subcellular organelles show a wide variability in all three properties. For example, Fig. 2 shows an electron micrograph of macrophages studied by Professor Klaus Bensch of our Department of Pathology. Alveolar macrophages were placed in distilled water for 5 min, then reconstituted in isotonic media and studied by electron microscopy. Fig. 2 shows that under these conditions many lysosomes are still intact. Some mitochondria are still visible but abnormal. Nuclei have largely disappeared. It can be seen that an occasional intact cell may have such high resistance to osmotic rupture that even exposure to distilled water for 5 min does not rupture the cell (super cells). Clearly, then, there is wide variation in the physical behaviour of individual cells as well as a wide spectrum of differences in different subcellular organelles with increasing water content.

Osmotic lysis is itself a complex process and even simple cells like erythrocytes do not merely burst with increased volume as does a balloon overdistended with air (Seeman 1974). Alterations in macromolecular physical state and properties related to variable degrees of hydration have been suggested by several lines of work. Specific data are available concerning the relation between water content and the structure of various proteins, including collagen (Berendsen & Migchelsen 1966), silk fibroin (Berendsen & Migchelsen 1965), gramacidin S (Warner 1961), and tobacco mosaic virus protein (Warner 1964). Studies of haemoglobin have shown that proteins possess complex osmotic properties and that osmotic effects may result from changes in the osmotic coefficients of proteins (Adair 1929). It has been suggested that the cytosol may have the properties of an elastic gel (Sigler & Janacek 1971) in which variable degrees of swelling or shrinkage could involve proteins *per se*. It thus appears that the function of proteins at a molecular level is influenced by the state of hydration.

Significant increases or decreases in water content alter the concentrations of all cell constituents. This, in turn, can modify various intracellular and subcellular concentration-dependent phenomena.

Changes in water content of various intracellular organelles may cause the release of various chemical mediators which are then capable of producing various types of inflammatory changes within the cell. Biochemical alterations may occur because of alterations to some of the factors listed above, such as alterations in geometry and changes in enzyme and substrate concentrations, as well as changes in diffusion distances and other factors.

SPECIFIC EXAMPLES OF ALTERED CELL AND SUBCELL PATHOPHYSIOLOGY RELATED TO ALTERED WATER CONTENT

Having dealt with some general aspects of changes in cell water, we would now like to illustrate some of these by specific examples. During the past 10 years, a number of the alterations caused by shifts of intracellular water and electrolytes have been studied in our laboratory. One group of studies was of the changes in cellular energy metabolism caused by changes in cell water content. These studies were conducted by Dr Norman Lewiston of our Department of Pediatrics. Isolated rabbit alveolar macrophages were used as the cellular model and changes in water content were produced by modifying the osmolality of the extracellular medium with impermeant solutes and also by modifying [Na^+]. Osmolalities ranged from severely hypotonic values

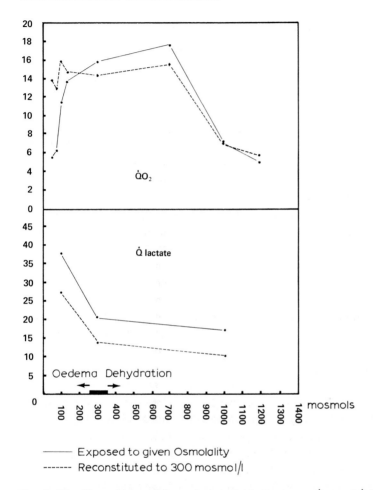

Fig. 3. The effects of intracellular oedema and dehydration on $\dot{Q}O_2$ and $\dot{Q}$ lactate in alveolar macrophages. Oedema reduces $\dot{Q}O_2$ and increase $\dot{Q}$ lactate (Pasteur effect.) These changes reverse with osmotic reconstitution. Dehydration reduces $\dot{Q}O_2$ and $\dot{Q}$ lactate. These changes are not reversible. Ordinates: $\dot{Q}O_2$ (above) measured in μl min^{-1} mg^{-1} protein, and $\dot{Q}_{lact}$ (below) measured in μmol min^{-1} mg^{-1} protein.

(50 mosM) causing intracellular oedema, to severely hypertonic values (1300 mosM) causing intracellular dehydration. Measurements of O_2 consumption ($\dot{Q}O_2$) and lactate production ($\dot{Q}_{lact}$) were made during exposure to a given osmolality and after osmotic reconstitution in an isotonic medium (Fig. 3).

Exposure of cells to hypotonic medium (mosM < 300) or to hypertonic media (mosM > 700) produced significant decreases in $\dot{Q}O_2$. Increasing degrees of cellular oedema or of cellular dehydration led to increasing reductions of cellular O_2 consumption. Moreover, this reduction must have involved primarily a reduction in mitochondrial O_2 utilization, since approximately 85% of total O_2 consumption in this cell represents mitochondrial O_2 consumption. Osmotic reconstitution of cells exposed to hypotonic media leads to a return of O_2 consumption towards normal, indicating that the mitochondrial lesion caused by intracellular oedema is reversible. In the oedematous cell, metabolic control remains intact since decreasing mitochondrial O_2 utilization is associated with a rise in lactate production (Pasteur effect). As mitochondrial O_2 utilization returns towards normal with osmotic reconstitution, the rate of glycolysis likewise changes towards normal. However, after intracellular dehydration, osmotic reconstitution does not reverse the decrease in mitochondrial O_2 utilization. In addition, normal metabolic control is lost, since the rate of anaerobic glycolysis as reflected by lactate generation decreases rather than increases (absent Pasteur effect), and remains persistently low with osmotic reconstitution. Cellular dehydration appears to produce more profound and less easily reversed alterations of cell and mitochondrial function. Although these studies involve extreme alterations of water content, it is clear that changes in cell (and mitochondrial) water content are accompanied by profound changes in energy metabolism.

It is of some interest that similar changes occur during experimental pulmonary oedema. Young has shown that in the isolated perfused rat lung, pulmonary oedema, whether produced by increased pulmonary capillary pressure or by altered capillary permeability, is accompanied by increased lactate production, whereas simple isotonic saline filling of the lung produces no significant changes in lactate production (S. L. Young et al. 1973, unpublished). A major difference between the oedematous lung and the saline-filled lung is, of course, that the former is associated with intra-alveolar epithelial oedema, whereas the latter is not. It appears that the rate of glycolysis is increased by intracellular oedema, both in the isolated cell system and in the intact organ.

We have already indicated that an important mechanism of cell injury during pulmonary oedema may be the development of inflammatory changes. Dr David Sachs in our laboratory has been studying the sequence of subcellular injury produced by osmotic alterations in isolated alveolar macrophages. The approach depends on the extracellular appearance of various macromolecular markers which are found in specific intracellular compartments. Fig. 4 shows observations made with β-glucuronidase (EC 3.2.1.31), an enzyme localized in lysosomes. These studies were done on isolated rabbit alveolar macrophages and two levels of osmotic exposure (0 mosm [distilled water] and 20 mosm) were used. Control cells were exposed to buffers containing 300 mosmol/l.

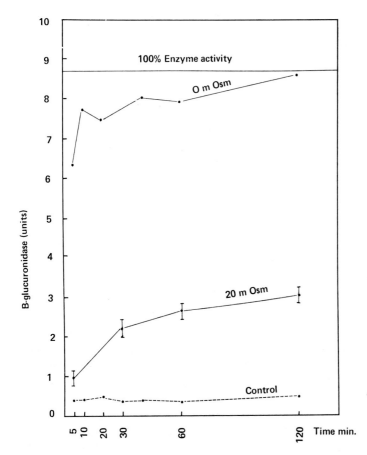

FIG. 4. The effect of hypotonic media on lysosomal enzyme (β-glucuronidase) release to the extracellular phase.

One hundred per cent of enzyme activity represents the total activity found in cell ultrasonicates. Both in distilled water and in 20 mosм, β-glucuronidase activity increases progressively with time in the extracellular phase. There is substantial extracellular leak of the lysosomal enzymes in the 20 mosм study, even at a time when the plasma membranes of most cells are still intact. This suggests that lysosomal enzymes may enter the extracellular phase without total cell disruption (presumably entering by exocytosis). In distilled water, lysosomal leak continues to increase long after most cells are completely ruptured (4–5 min). This suggests that osmotic resistance of the lysosome is high, so that complete rupture of lysosomes takes several hours even in distilled water. This suggestion is consistent with the observations made by electron

TABLE 3

Energetics of active Na$^+$ transport in rabbit alveolar macrophages (AM) versus human erythrocytes

	AM	Erythrocytes
'Active' Na$^+$ efflux (mequiv. kg^{-1} h^{-1})^a	200	1
Calories kg^{-1} h^{-1}	56	6

^{a} kg = kg cell water

microscopy indicating high osmotic resistance by lysosomes. Intracellular oedema then leads to lysosomal oedema, triggering a release of lysosomal enzymes. These, in turn, may leak extracellularly, either by exocytosis or because of ultimate rupture of the membrane of the cell with rupture of the lysosomal membrane. Lysosomal enzymes, in turn, may produce injury to more normal cells as well as producing an inflammatory response.

The final example illustrates the concept that impairment of energy metabolism may lead to intracellular oedema by impairing the active transport of Na$^+$. Dr Jan Smith in our laboratory has shown (Table 3) that alveolar macrophages have a high rate of active Na$^+$ transport and thereby need large amounts of ATP to maintain intracellular Na$^+$ concentration and intracellular H$_2$O at normal values. As compared to human erythrocytes, the rate of ouabain-sensitive active transport is 200 times greater in the alveolar macrophages than the erythrocyte and the energy requirement is almost 10 times higher (Robin et al. 1971). Given a high energy requirement, it would be predicted that ATP depletion should lead to intracellular Na$^+$ accumulation and oedema. This turns out to be the case. Dr Anthony Tanser, working in our laboratory, has studied the effect of limiting ATP supply to alveolar macrophages by impairment of oxidative phosphorylation. The impairment of ATP supply was accomplished by exposure of the cells either to approximately 100% N$_2$ or to high concentrations of NaCN, thereby blocking the mitochondrial electron transport chain at the cytochrome c oxidase (EC 1.9.3.1) step (Table 4).

Impairment of ATP supply leads to substantial increases in intracellular Na$^+$ accompanied by substantial increases in intracellular water content. Although admittedly the cells under these conditions are exposed to profound alterations of energy supply, it is reasonable to extrapolate that less severe degrees of ATP depletion would result in less dramatic but still significant intracellular and subcellular oedema.

TABLE 4

The effect of inhibition of ATP generation from oxidative phosphorylation on intracellular (Na^+) and water content of alveolar macrophages

	Control	$100\% \ N_2$	NaCN
(Na^+)mequiv./kg cell H_2O	83	120	135
H_2O (%)	80	85	88
'P'		<0.01	<0.001

FUTURE DIRECTIONS

A number of mechanisms have evolved which closely regulate cell and subcell water content. Alterations of these lead to changes in cellular and subcellular water content and produce important abnormalities of cellular and subcellular function and structure in most cell types. This is true not only of cells generally but also of alveolar epithelial cells and other lung cells. An important segment of the pathophysiological alterations which accompany pulmonary oedema must depend on the alterations in alveolar epithelial water which frequently accompany clinical pulmonary oedema. Future studies which spell out the osmotic compliance characteristics of various cells and subcellular organelles, which describe and correlate physical changes with metabolic and structural changes, and which define the details of the sequence of subcellular injury associated with alterations of lung cell water should provide important new insights into pulmonary oedema and into cellular pathophysiology.

ACKNOWLEDGEMENT

This work was supported by a grant from the National Institute for Occupational Safety and Health (2 RO1 OH00352).

References

ADAIR, G. S. (1929) *Proc. R. Soc. (Lond.) 126*, 16
BERENDSEN, H. J. C. & MIGCHELSEN, C. (1965) *Ann. N. Y. Acad. Sci. 125*, 365
BERENDSEN, H. J. C. & MIGCHELSEN, C. (1966) *Fed. Proc. 25*, 998
CHURNEY, L. (1942) *Biol. Bull. (Woods Hole) 82*, 52
HOUSE, C. R. (1974) *Water Transport in Cells and Tissues*, Edward Arnold, London
ROBIN, E. D., SMITH, J. D., TANSER, A. R., ADAMSON, J. S., MILLEN, J. E. & PACKER, B. (1971) *Biochim. Biophys. Acta, 241*, 117
SEEMAN, P. (1974) *Fed. Proc. 33*, 2116
SIGLER, K. & JANACEK, K. (1971) *Biochim. Biophys. Acta, 241*, 528

Tedeschi, H. & Harris, D. L. (1955) *Arch. Biochem. Biophys. 58*, 52
Warner, D. T. (1961) *Nature (Lond.) 190*, 120
Warner, D. T. (1964) *J. Theor. Biol. 6*, 118

Discussion

Fishman: In watching pulmonary oedema forming it is impressive to see how nicely the endothelial cells are preserved. Apparently there need not be any swelling. How do you relate these observations to the dramatic cell swelling that you showed?

Robin: These changes in the isolated cell system would be similar to those found with fresh water drowning (an important but relatively uncommon form of pulmonary oedema). The degree of swelling of the alveolar epithelial cells must also be limited by the elastic framework in which they are enmeshed. I would guess that alveolar epithelial cells have a low osmotic compliance and that a large osmotic pressure change would be needed to produce a large change in the cell volume. Moreover, there is now evidence suggesting that there is an important metabolic component in pulmonary oedema. The studies by Young *et al.* (1973) to which I referred (p. 280) seem to demonstrate in the whole organ the kind of changes that we have shown in isolated cells. Extensive changes in alveolar epithelial cell volume may not happen often in clinical pulmonary oedema. On the other hand, if the permeability of alveolar epithelial cells is altered, there may be profound metabolic changes. The altered permeability which then activates lysosomes may explain why pulmonary oedema can be associated with extensive tissue injury. Our observations indicate that alterations to cell water are an important aspect of general cell injury and that oedema of intra-alveolar epithelial cells is one of the critical components of clinical pulmonary oedema.

Strang: How do you obtain these cells and how do you know what they are? I have always been uncertain about alveolar macrophages.

Robin: They can be obtained in one of two ways. One is by pulmonary lavage. If you pick your species carefully—for example, the rabbit—over 90% of the cells obtained by lavage are alveolar macrophages. Purity is 'ensured' by the fact that they have a more or less specific appearance in the electron microscope, and that the cells are phagocytic and are recognized by the company they keep. No one can guarantee that they are 100% pure but by good histological and functional criteria they are reasonably pure. Another property which permits purification is that macrophages (unlike other cells) stick to glass. Thus isolation methods based on this property have been developed. And it is now possible to maintain them in tissue culture.

Strang: Are they specifically lung cells or are they the same as macrophages from anywhere else?

Robin: In the lung they have highly specialized characteristics which include the following: they have a high oxygen consumption as compared, for example, with peritoneal macrophages; their mitochondria are much more numerous than macrophages from elsewhere; their concentration of glycolytic enzymes is much lower than that of other macrophages; and they have a high concentration of superoxide dismutase, which we think is an important marker enzyme. These biochemical differences are dramatic. What is not clear is whether the differences are due to alveolar macrophages that develop *in situ* in the lung or to alveolar macrophages which arise by adaptation, from precursor macrophages from, say, bone marrow, which 'decide' to make a new home in the lung and then undergo striking biochemical and morphological changes.

Strang: Has all room for confusion between these macrophages and type II pneumocytes now been removed, in your view?

Robin: I think so. I would like Dr Schneeberger to comment on that histologically.

Schneeberger: On purely morphological grounds, I would say there is still confusion. Some alveolar macrophages appear to have ingested lamellar bodies, so it is difficult to distinguish these cells from sloughed type II pneumocytes. There are cytochemical differences. It appears that type II pneumocytes have peroxisomes whereas alveolar macrophages do not (Schneeberger 1972).

In those species which have the enzyme, the intracellular distribution of endogenous peroxidase (EC 1.11.1.7) differs in type II pneumocytes as compared to alveolar macrophages. Endogenous enzyme markers can be used to distinguish the two types of cells. I think cytochemistry is important in the determination of what pulmonary cells one is dealing with in pulmonary lavage.

Robin: The biochemical evidence which permits characterization of type II cells goes approximately like this. Dr William Lynn at Duke University (Bhattacharyya *et al.* 1975) and Dr Richard King (King 1974) have found proteins which appear to be unique to lamellar bodies. These proteins seem to be closely associated with type II alveolar epithelial cells and not with macrophages.

Olver: Presumably one can't be sure that alveolar macrophages aren't old type II cells which have dropped off at some stage, maybe having discharged their lamellar bodies?

Robin: Then they would not only have to be drop-outs, but would also really have to acquire new functions. The alveolar macrophage is intensely phagocytic. It has a characteristic oxygen burst during phagocytosis. I can't say that anybody has looked into this with respect to type II alveolar epithelial cells. More recently, it has also been shown that type II cells, when stained by the Papanicolaou method, can easily be identified since the inclusion bodies stain deep blue (Kikkawa & Yoneda 1973).

Olver: What is the turnover of type II cells in the lung?

Fishman: That is not a simple question to answer. Dr John Aronson, working at the University of Pennsylvania, has been examining the response of these cells to injury (unpublished observations, 1975). Apparently, they have long life spans with little inclination to divide until provoked by noxious stimuli that come into contact with them. Also, type II cells are activated by injuries to the alveolar lining that destroy type I cells. Accordingly, they may remain quiet for months, performing their ordinary biological functions as generators of surfactant and as lining cells, unless stimulated to divide by local events.

However, I harbour the notion that they are entirely different in their origins from alveolar macrophages which settle in the lungs after release from the bone marrow.

Robin: A disease which provides a nice model for distinguishing between type II cells and macrophages is alveolar proteinosis, in which there is either increased breakdown or decreased removal of type II alveolar epithelial cells. Accumulations of macrophages do not give rise to either the clinical or the pathological picture of alveolar proteinosis. In fact, areas in which the material in alveolar proteinosis is richly deposited are histologically characterized by a near-absence of macrophages. They appear to shun such areas.

Maetz: Work by Ripoche *et al.* (1973) and Ripoche (1973) on the effect of cell shrinkage or swelling in membranes such as frog bladder might be relevant here. If the frog bladder is suddenly shrunk from the inside by an increase in the osmotic concentration of the internal medium by some impermeant solute, a feedback response then increases the water permeability of the cells. The reverse happens when the cells are made to swell: the permeability to water decreases. There is a kind of feedback mechanism which changes the water permeability of the apical membrane. This mechanism includes adenylate cyclase (EC 4.6.1.1) which implements feedback in the cell and regulates its permeability.

Robin: The activity of water—its increase or decrease in the cell—is undoubtedly a critical variable in cell function generally, and a wide series of regulatory mechanisms must maintain water activity at a fairly stable value. Distortions of these mechanisms are responsible for the development of intracellular oedema or dehydration.

Lee: Can one kind of oedema be distinguished from another in the cell? For instance, if fluid moved from the capillary into the interstitium but the cell membrane was not affected, one could envisage a situation in which the extracellular fluid volume increases and the cell fluid volume remains constant. But where permeability is altered by viruses, toxins and so forth, the whole system would be involved. So by looking at the different modalities of water distribution, one could get at something to do with pathogenesis.

Robin: That is possible. One may ultimately be able to say that if there is a given sequence of subcellular injury, the pathogenic mechanism must have been this or that. For example, if there is pure osmotic injury without solute movement, clearly there will be corresponding changes in the water activity of subcellular particles. If there is a permeability injury, then what happens to subcellular water activity depends on how much water has entered, as compared to how much solute. I think your analysis is quite right, but approaches to how to document and quantitate the various alterations of intracellular water and solute distribution are in their infancy.

Dickinson: Major crystalloid osmotic changes in lung liquids are uncommon clinically except after someone has drowned. What happens to permeability in the lungs after someone has drowned in salt water or fresh water?

Robin: It is not unreasonable to conclude that in addition to the primary osmotic alteration, there are secondary permeability injuries to the membranes. There is a well recognized phenomenon called late drowning or near-drowning which happens in either fresh water or salt water. The affected people or animals absorb the water to which they were initially exposed and some hours later they develop generalized pulmonary oedema. In one patient whom we studied, the pulmonary oedema fluid was of the high protein variety. If you are willing to accept this nebulous and largely clinically based evidence, then severe osmotic alterations can produce secondary alterations in the structure and function of lung cell membranes, leading to altered permeability.

Staub: Electron micrographs of the alveolar lining cells in both fresh and sea water drowning show intracellular disruption of mitochondria and other organelles (Reidbord 1967).

Dickinson: How long does the lung take to recover totally?

Donald: In many reported cases of near-drowning where some water has been aspirated, clinical recovery, checked radiologically, has taken two to seven days.

Strang: It has been claimed that even isotonic saline, never mind anything else, caused changes in air-breathing lungs which could be identified in electron micrographs.

Adamson: That is correct. Alexander's pictures show that isotonic saline destroys the lung epithelial layer (Alexander 1968).

Staub: The alveolar epithelial damage with isotonic saline was minimal compared to that of hypertonic and hypotonic fluids. I don't believe there was any actual disruption of the alveolar epithelial cell membrane.

Gatzy: What kind of release of lysosomal enzymes were you postulating, Dr Robin?

Robin: The specific enzyme we examined was β-glucuronidase. Macrophages were placed in buffered solution, 20 mosm. In that solution, more lysosomes were released than could be accounted for by the number of cells which disappeared and whose membranes had been disrupted. The argument there would be, as has been shown by Weissman *et al.* (1971), that exocytosis of lysosomal enzymes can happen without total disruption of the cell. On the other hand, if the cells were placed in distilled water, release of lysosomal enzyme continued long after almost all the cells had disappeared. We think this indicates that lysis of lysosomes is now occurring because of lysosomal oedema. That explains the fact that although 90% of the cells had disappeared within 10 min, it was 120 min before all the enzyme activity present in the lysosomes appeared in the extracellular phase.

Hugh-Jones: Are these events hormone-dependent? Is there a difference between male and female cells in their tendency to oedema or dehydration? I ask because in patients with α_1-antitrypsin deficiency, for example, one would expect an equal frequency of lung damage in males and females, yet males predominate until after the menopause, when the expected equal frequency is found. It has been postulated that this lack of female cases is because of the effect of female hormones on maintaining the stability of the lysosome membrane.

Robin: I am not certain that it would be easy to tell a male macrophage from a female macrophage. My guess would be that if there are perturbations they are relatively small. I think we are really looking at the operation of physicochemical forces that override even sexual differences.

References

ALEXANDER, I. G. S. (1968) Ultrastructure of the pulmonary alveolar vessels in Mendelson's (massive pulmonary aspiration) syndrome. *Br. J. Anaesth. 40*, 408-414

BHATTACHARYYA, M. A., PASSERO, M. A., DiAUGUSTINE, R. P. & LYNN, W. S. (1975) Isolation and characterization of two hydroxyproline-containing glycoproteins from normal animal lung lavage and lamellar bodies. *J. Clin. Invest. 55*, 914-920

KIKKAWA, Y. & YONEDA, K. (1973) Isolation of Type II epithelial cells from rat lung. *Am. Rev. Respir. Dis. 107*, 1115

KING, J. R. (1974) The surfactant system of the lung. *Fed. Proc. 33*, 2238-2247

RIPOCHE, P. (1973) Réajustements osmotiques et régulation cellulaire de la permeabilité à l'eau de la vessie de grenouille. Doctorat d'Etat Sci. Nat., Université de Paris

RIPOCHE, P., BOURGUET, J. & PARISI, M. (1973) The effect of hypertonic media on water permeability of the frog urinary bladder. *J. Gen. Physiol. 61*, 110-124

SCHNEEBERGER, E. E. (1972) A comparative cytochemical study of microbodies (peroxisomes) in great alveolar cells of rodents, rabbit and monkey. *J. Histochem. Cytochem. 20*, 180

WEISSMAN, G., BZURIER, R., SPIELER, P. J. & GOLDSTEIN, I. M. (1971) Mechanisms of lysosomal enzyme release from leukocytes exposed to immune complexes and other particles. *J. Exp. Med. 134*, 149S-165S

General discussion III

Crosbie: There are many pulmonary problems in uraemia and it may be that the lungs reflect changes in other organs in the body. The sodium pump mechanisms in red blood cells and leucocytes become abnormal in uraemia and the cells swell (Welt 1969; Patrick & Jones 1974). We have been trying to investigate whether lung cells behave in a similar manner. We looked at lung capillary function in shocked patients who become anuric and develop the advanced respiratory distress syndrome. I have been using multiple indicator dilution techniques to study the behaviour of labelled albumin, sodium, urea, adenosine triphosphate and water as they flow through the lung capillary bed in hepato-renal failure. The principle is that if an indicator is lost from the perfused system during the time of transit through the capillary bed then the amount of that indicator which is recovered will be less than the amount of labelled albumin which is recovered. I can best demonstrate our findings by showing typical curves we have obtained.

Fig. 1 shows indicator curves from a 56-year-old male with severe hepato-renal failure. The cardiac output is normal (5.5 l/min) but there is excess water in the lungs (pulmonary extravascular water [PEVW$_v$] 840 ml). But the curves for labelled sodium and urea are smaller than the labelled albumin curve, showing that these ions have been lost from the vascular compartment in this state.

The second example is a 32-year-old male who had to have 40 units of blood after severe trauma (crushed pelvis). He also had a good cardiac output (7.7 l/min) with increased lung water (PEVW$_v$ 510 ml) but he lost a lot of labelled ATP from the lung capillary bed, perhaps due to excessive uptake by the lung tissue (Fig. 2).

With these techniques it may be possible to detect metabolic changes in the lungs in these seriously ill patients; more definitive treatment could then be developed.

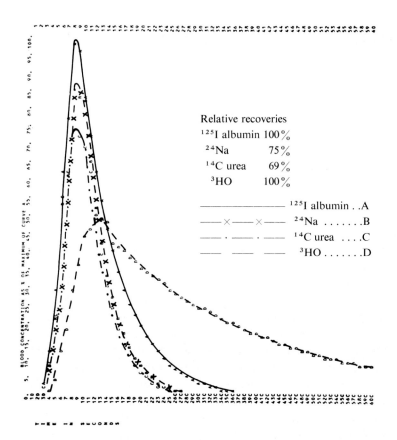

Relative recoveries
^{125}I albumin 100%
^{24}Na 75%
^{14}C urea   69%
^{3}HO 100%

——————————— ^{125}I albumin . .A
——×——×—— ^{24}Na . . . . . . .B
——.——.—— ^{14}C urea C
—— —— —— ^{3}HO . . . . . . .D

Fig. 1 (Crosbie). Multiple indicator dilution curves obtained from an anuric patient (56-year-old male) with hepato-renal failure and acute respiratory distress syndrome after gall bladder surgery. Cardiac output: 5.5 l/min. There is an increased amount of water (840 ml) in the lung capillary bed ($PEVW_V$ normal 200 ml) and chest X-ray shows bilateral parenchymal infiltration. Note the loss of labelled sodium and urea compared with the labelled albumin, indicating abnormal lung capillary permeability.

Strang: Where did the ATP come from?

Crosbie: The four indicators including the ATP were injected together into the central veins.

Staub: Is the normal recovery 100%?

Crosbie: Yes.

Hughes: The difficulties of measuring lung water have held up our understanding of the clinical situation. We haven't really got good simple methods of measuring oedema and following it as patients are treated and get better or worse. The technique Dr Crosbie has just told us about uses arterial sampling.

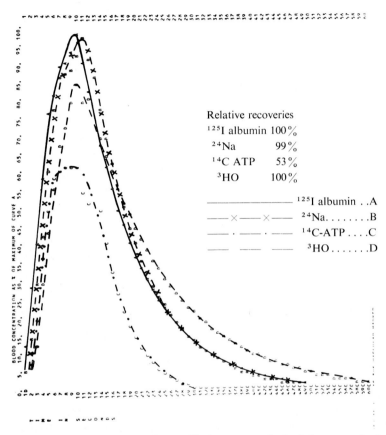

Relative recoveries
^{125}I albumin 100%
^{24}Na   99%
^{14}C ATP   53%
^{3}HO   100%

——————————— ^{125}I albumin . .A
——×——×—— ^{24}Na. . . . . . .B
——.——.—— ^{14}C-ATP C
—— —— —— ^{3}HO. . . . . . .D

Fig. 2. (Crosbie) Multiple indicator dilution curves obtained from a patient (32-year-old male, given 40 units of blood) with acute respiratory distress syndrome after severe abdomino-pelvic injury. Cardiac output: 7.7 l/min. The chest X-ray shows bilateral parenchymal infiltration. There is an increased amount of water (510 ml) in the lungs (PEVW$_V$ normal 200 ml). Note the displacement of the labelled sodium relative to the albumin and the reduced recovery of labelled ATP, indicating abnormal capillary function in the lungs.

With the abundance of isotopes from our cyclotron at Hammersmith we looked at the possibility of using some non-invasive external counting methods for quantitating oedema. We considered three possibilities. The first was the double indicator dye-dilution technique which Dr Crosbie used and which was introduced by Chinard many years ago. One indicator should be freely diffusible. We used H$_2$^{15}O, which equilibrates with the total water pool when it is injected. The other indicator was 113m-indium, which binds to transferrin and is confined to the vascular pool. Subtraction of the vascular from the total water pool gives the extravascular water pool. There are many problems with dye-dilution methods. Not all the water may be accessible to indicators which have to be put into the blood stream, and after a single passage through the lung there are various problems in analysis of the curves.

The second technique we tried was inhalation of a tracer, $C^{15}O_2$. Under-perfused areas, relatively inaccessible to an intravenous tracer, are accessible to an inhaled tracer, and there is evidence from dog lungs that that is probably true. Inhalation of CO_2 was originally used to measure regional blood flow because, as bicarbonate, it equilibrates with the total water pool of the lung. Ideally a tracer which binds avidly to haemoglobin should also be inhaled, so that an estimate of the vascular pool can be obtained and some estimate of the extravascular water made by subtraction. Carbon monoxide as ^{11}CO or $C^{11}O$ would be very suitable but its diffusion rate across the alveolar mem-brane is much slower than that of CO_2 so we can't use it as a vascular reference.

The third method is to use a steady-state infusion of diffusible and non-diffusible isotopes instead of a single injection, and count over the lung 4–6 min later as equilibrium is approached. This overcomes some of the analytical problems of single pass. Also more time is available for equilibration with vascular and extravascular water pools. The problem here of course is the chest wall. At the moment we have only tried this in isolated dog lungs, where there is no chest wall. One attractive technique would be to find isotopes with a sufficiently short half-life so that they decay before they ever reach the chest wall. For instance, ^{19}O with a half-life of 30 s could be used. It would be difficult to find a blood label with a similarly short half-life.

We are currently measuring extravascular water and its distribution in a normal man by the first technique. In Fig. 3 (F. Fazio, T. Jones, C. G. Rhodes and J. M. B. Hughes, unpublished) lung radioactivity has been recorded by external counting after intravenous injections of diffusible ($H_2^{15}O$) and non-diffusible (113m-Ind) indicators. The definition of the curves is good, the amount of extravascular water in the lung being proportional to the differences between the mean transit time for both curves. From a previous injection of indium with a counter over the heart, the Hamilton dye-dilution technique was used to estimate cardiac output. Extravascular water volume is obtained by multiplying the mean transit time difference over the lung by the pulmonary blood flow. Whether this method is going to be sufficiently sensitive to dis-tinguish early oedema, we don't yet know. In dogs there is a good relationship between the extravascular lung water, measured by external counting over the lung with these two isotopes, and the water measured from simultaneous arterial curves. There are still many problems but with very short-lived isotopes it should be possible to make sequential measurements and gain valuable information.

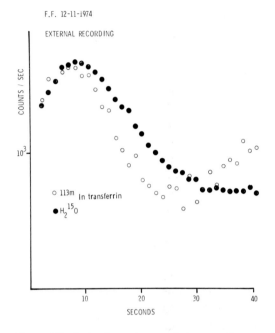

F.F. 12-11-1974

EXTERNAL RECORDING

○ 113m In transferrin

● H$_2$^{15}O

FIG. 3 (Hughes). Counts/s recorded externally over lower lobe of right lung in normal subject plotted against time after intravenous injection of indium-113m transferrin (vascular pool marker) and ^{15}O-labelled water (total water pool marker). Extravascular water volume is proportional to the mean transit time difference between H$_2$^{15}O and 113m-indium.

Dickinson: Has this been done in fetal lungs?

Strang: No.

Lee: What is the gamma energy of the inulin and its isotopic half-life?

Hughes: The half-life is about 100 min and its gamma emission energy is 390 keV. The energy of the oxygen-15 is 511 keV.

Maetz: How is the ^{15}O made?

Hughes: By deuteron bombardment of nitrogen with a 7 MeV beam (Clark & Buckingham 1975). ^{15}O has a half-life of 2.1 min.

Maetz: What about using ^{18}O at the same time? Then one would need just a mass spectrometer costing about £10 000 instead of a cyclotron at £400 000.

Hughes: Unfortunately non-radioactive isotopes would require arterial sampling unless analyses could be made in expired air.

Maetz: Is ^{11}C one of the possibilties?

Hughes: We have used ^{11}CO for labelling red cells and for measuring regional diffusion capacities. ^{11}C has a half-life of 20 min, and is a good vascular tracer, but indium is more convenient for human studies.

Strang: Does this labelled oxygen molecule exchange with oxygen in the air and in the haemoglobin? Why should it stay stuck to the water? There is a lot of oxygen in the air.

Staub: There should be no significant change within 20 s.

Dickinson: In the fetus the slow bulk flow of water out of the lung might still allow a fast water flux across the alveolar epithelium.

Strang: We have measured isotopic water flux across the pulmonary epithelium and obtained a permeability value of 3.3×10^{-6} cm/s. It is difficult to get accurate measurements because of the problem of flow limitation but in the lamb fetus we were able to make valid measurements when pulmonary blood flow was high (Normand *et al.* 1971).

Staub: Because of the large right-to-left shunt you probably couldn't measure that flux by indicator dilution curves. Most of the tracer would go through the foramen ovale or the ductus arteriosus.

Lee: May I try out an idea which Dr John Prichard and I are working on in Oxford? It is about how to estimate regional water distribution volumes, as well as changes in regional capillary permeability in the lung, using external scintillation counting methods, which we hope might ultimately be applied to man. As I see it, one big problem in the damaged whole organ is to separate oedema caused by changes in hydrostatic pressure from oedema caused by changes in capillary permeability. If we first measure the distribution volumes of the organ's tissue water (in blood, interstitium and cells: using the appropriate markers labelled with a gamma emitter), we can then follow the redistribution of a solute within these compartments over a period of time, and estimate the flux constant of that solute across the membranes separating the compartments from one another. Albumin, for example, will initially be confined for all practical purposes to the blood compartment within the distribution volume defined by the geometry of our external scintillation counting system. We can get the concentration of albumin related to count rate by assuming that the regional blood has the same concentration of albumin as the blood in a mixed venous sample taken during the count period. Next, by following the change in albumin concentration in the region under observation over two known periods of time consecutively, we are able to solve two simultaneous equations which allow us to calculate the flux rate of albumin from capillary to interstitium; and assuming that capillary permeability for back diffusion of the albumin from interstitium to capillary is the same, we can calculate this flux too. Lastly we are at liberty to estimate the rate of removal of the protein via the lymph. Fig. 4 and equations (1) to (5) indicate the principles of the method and give an example of the kind of result we obtain in the normal open-chested dog; for obviously at this stage we have to eliminate chest wall contribution to counts detected by our external scintillation detector.

Clearly there are numerous assumptions implicit in the method we are developing; moreover the work is at an early stage of its development. Hence my keenness to try it out on you before we go too far down what could well be a false trail.

Equation (1) describes the relationships when a γ-emitting isotope, labelling a solute, is injected intravenously. Its concentration in plasma (C_p) falls progressively with time, as it moves across the capillary membrane into the interstitial spaces of the body. Conversely, the interstitial concentration of the solute in the tissue being studied will rise (C_i). At any time 't' after the injection the count rate external to the tissue will be:

$$R(t) = K \cdot V_v \cdot C_p(t) + K \cdot V_i \cdot C_i(t) \tag{1}$$

where R is external count rate detected by the scintillation counter,
    K is the geometric calibration of the detector system,
    V_v is the vascular volume being studied,
    V_i is the interstitial volume of the tissue being studied,
    C_p is the plasma concentration of the solute, and
    C_i is the interstitial fluid concentration of the solute

and
$$V_e = V_i + V_v \tag{2}$$

where V_e is the extracellular space.

We have assumed as a first approximation that the transcapillary fluxes of solute obey Fick's law and that the solute concentrations of interstitial fluid and lymph are the same. The rate at which solute accumulates within the interstitial space will be the sum of the fluxes forth and back across the capillary membrane between plasma and interstitial fluid, as well as that removed via the lymphatics. Thus:

$$\frac{d}{dt}(C_i \cdot V_i) = f_c \cdot A_c \cdot C_p(t) - f_c \cdot A_c \cdot C_i(t) - f_L C_i(t) \tag{3}$$

Where A_c is the area of capillary wall through which solute movement takes place,

    f_c is the capillary constant relating solute flux to solute concentration,
    f_L is the lymphatic flux of solute, and
    C_p, C_i and V_i are as already stated for equation (1)

Next, integrating over a period of time, t_o–t_1:

$$C_i(t_1) = \frac{f_c \cdot A_c}{V_i} \int_0^{t_1} C_p(t)dt - \frac{f_c \cdot A_c}{V_i} \int_0^{t_1} C_i(t)dt - \frac{f_L}{V_i} \int_0^{t_1} C_i(t)dt \qquad (4)$$

and again, integrating over a longer period of time, t_o–t_2:

$$C_i(t_2) = \frac{fc \cdot A_c}{V_i} \int_0^{t_2} C_p(t)dt - \frac{fc \cdot A_c}{V_i} \int_0^{t_2} C_i(t)dt - \frac{f_L}{V_i} \int_0^{t_2} C_i(t)dt \qquad (5)$$

allows one to solve for both $(f_c \cdot A_c)$ and (f_L).

Fig. 4 shows the dynamics of ^{125}I-labelled albumin obtained from the interstitium of the lung of an anaesthetized ventilated dog whose chest wall had been removed.

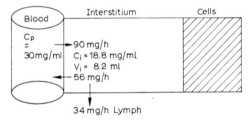

FIG. 4 (Lee). ^{125}I-labelled albumin dynamics: dog lung interstitial space per 100 ml inflated lung.

Staub: We are using a similar approach. Instead of iodinated albumin, we use red cells labelled with technetium-99 and transferrin labelled with indium-113 to measure the relative blood volume and the rate of protein transfer from plasma to lung interstitium, respectively. Our results are quite similar to yours, Dr Lee, except that we can use the intact chest wall. We have compared the interstitial accumulation of transferrin by our external counting procedure with the simultaneous direct sampling of lung lymph in sheep. The time courses are identical. The half-time of transferrin accumulation in normal sheep is about $2\frac{1}{2}$ hours (almost the same as for albumin). After we had infused *Pseudomonas* bacteria into the sheep to increase pulmonary vascular permeability, the half-time of the tracer protein turnover was reduced to about 1 h for both the external counting and lung lymph comparison. These new non-invasive methods offer considerable promise for a sensitive clinical approach to measuring changes in lung vascular permeability (Gorin *et al.* 1976).

Lee: The chest wall contributes about 30% of the counts detected externally. There may be tricks we can play in the future that will allow us to subtract the contribution of gamma emission coming from solute marker in chest wall from that in the lung. This involves using a radioactive isotope to label our solute marker, which has two energy peaks widely different from one another. In particular, one peak must lack sufficient energy to penetrate externally from the deep tissue under study. This may allow us to use subtraction techniques to estimate the distribution of the marker in the organ under study independently of its distribution in superficial tissues, such as the chest wall.

Strang: If you can use two or more different molecules at the same time, the amount of information obtained begins to rise a lot.

Lee: That will obviously come, but it is no good doing this sort of study unless the concepts are right.

Strang: The problems are mainly technical, aren't they?

Crosbie: The problem of arterial sampling isn't quite so acute in intensive care units, especially with patients on dialysis who already have shunts in place. The measurements can be done in 5 min.

Staub: Permeability cannot be measured in that time. You measure sodium loss and urea loss, which may well have something to do with permeability.

Crosbie: With computerized techniques an hour is enough.

Staub: You can get the initial up-slope of the permeability curves, but the longer you continue the better the results will be.

Michel: Dr Lee, you are making one big assumption, that is that there is uniformity of concentration in the three compartments. This may be an unreasonable assumption when you are dealing with the interstitial space, for the pericapillary space might have a different concentration of protein from other parts. There are also relatively long diffusion distances between the pericapillary space and the lymphatics.

Lee: If an isotope with a sufficiently long half-life is used in a quasi-steady-state condition, namely a resting animal that is healthy, won't there be uniform distribution with time, if the time is long enough?

Michel: You could have gradients running across the interstitial space in the steady state.

References

CLARK, J. C. & BUCKINGHAM, P. D. (1975) *Short-Lived Radioactive Gas for Clinical Use,* ch. 5, Butterworth, London

GORIN, A. B., WEIDNER, J. & STAUB, N. C. (1976) *Am. Rev. Respir. Dis.* in press

NORMAND, I. C. S., OLVER, R. E., REYNOLDS, E. O. R. & STRANG, L. B. (1971) Permeability of lung capillaries and alveoli to non-electrolytes in the foetal lamb. *J. Physiol. (Lond.)* *219*, 303-330

PATRICK, J. & JONES, M. F. (1974) Cell sodium potassium and water in uraemia and the effects of regular dialysis as studied in the leucocyte. *Clin. Sci. Mol. Med. 46*, 583

WELT, L. G. (1969) A further evaluation of erythrocyte sodium transport in control subjects and uraemia. *Nephron 6*, 406

Clinical disorders of lung liquid

C. J. DICKINSON

Medical Unit, University College Hospital Medical School, London

Abstract Clinical pulmonary oedema is often persistent and of sudden onset, suggesting a vicious circle, i.e. positive feedback. It is difficult to produce in animals by any haemodynamic manoeuvres, but the important neurogenic component can be illustrated by acutely increasing cerebrospinal fluid pressure of rabbits to 300 mmHg (40 kPa). Breathing stops virtually at once, and restarts when cerebrospinal fluid pressure is again reduced. With cerebral ischaemia lasting for up to 2 min, all is well; with longer times pulmonary oedema is almost invariable and often eventually fatal, although the animals may otherwise apparently recover. Comparable events sometimes follow subarachnoid haemorrhage in man. A few hypotheses on the pathogenesis of pulmonary oedema in man are offered.

A clinician discussing pulmonary oedema at the end of a symposium devoted to the fundamental aspects of physiology of lung liquids is like a man who has listened to a technical discussion about the fine points of the design of motor car engines and then tries to switch the discussion so that he can offer hypotheses that explain bad driving. I am afraid the physiologists at this meeting will find my naive clinical remarks almost equally incongruous. My excuse for talking about pulmonary oedema is that it remains one of the great unsolved problems of clinical medicine, and one which those present may be uniquely qualified to solve.

It is not possible to produce pulmonary oedema in the rabbit, or in any other mammal as far as I know, by any obstruction to the left side of the heart, even with a ligature tied round the proximal aorta. All that happens is that the animal dies of acute circulatory failure—what used to be described as 'forward failure' of the heart. The lungs are not pathologically engorged with blood at necropsy. Partial degrees of left ventricular or aortic obstruction are

* *Present address:* Department of Medicine, St Bartholomew's Hospital Medical College, London no more successful. Pulmonary oedema can nonetheless easily be produced in the rabbit, as in other mammals, by sufficiently large and rapid infusions of blood, plasma or saline—most easily with saline. It is remarkably difficult to induce pulmonary oedema by the infusion of noradrenaline or adrenaline, probably because of reflex adjustments of circulatory capacitance by the autonomic nervous system.

During an investigation in which W. P. Cockshott and I were trying to produce a critical degree of ischaemic cerebral damage, we subjected a number of rabbits to sudden and complete stoppage of the cerebral circulation for periods between a few seconds and $3\frac{1}{4}$ minutes. The animals were anaesthetized with pentobarbitone, the larynx was intubated and a fine needle was inserted into the cisterna magna. The cerebrospinal fluid pressure was acutely elevated by the rapid infusion of sterile isotonic saline into the cisterna magna at a pressure of 300 mmHg (40 kPa). Breathing stopped within a few seconds, but respiratory excursions which were approximately normal were maintained by artificial ventilation. At the end of a timed period of complete ischaemia, the pressure bottle was disconnected and pressure was acutely reduced to atmospheric. Providing the ischaemia time had not been prolonged much beyond 3 min, the animals almost at once started to breathe again spontaneously. However, as Fig. 1 indicates, there was a sharp distinction between those animals with cerebral ischaemia lasting less than 2 min and those whose ischaemia time was greater than this. Virtually every animal in the latter group showed signs of respiratory distress, i.e. tachypnoea and wheezing, and was cyanosed. In some cases the dyspnoea only lasted a few minutes, but in others it lasted several hours, even though the animals had recovered consciousness by this time and were walking about, eating and drinking. The figure demonstrates that a number of animals subjected to prolonged cerebral ischaemia eventually died despite having apparently fully recovered from the anaesthetic. At necropsy every one of these animals showed the most florid pulmonary oedema with intra-alveolar flooding.

Though this method of producing acute pulmonary oedema is in some ways novel, 'neurogenic' pulmonary oedema has been recognized for a very long time. Its closest clinical counterpart is the sometimes fatal oedema which may follow a sudden large subarachnoid haemorrhage in man. This can cause death from pulmonary oedema in a previously fit young person despite the lack of prior expansion of the blood volume and despite the lack of any clinical or pathological evidence of heart disease. Presumably in such cases the immediate cause of the pulmonary oedema is a massive constriction of capacitance reservoirs of the circulation, leading to a rise in mean systemic pressure and to a comparable rise in pulmonary capillary pressure large enough to stretch endothelial and

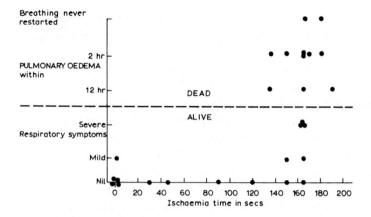

FIG. 1. Respiratory effects in rabbits subjected to complete cerebral ischaemia for the time indicated on the abscissa (see text).

eventually epithelial pores, and large enough eventually to overcome the natural defence mechanisms which we heard about earlier in this symposium.

I have used this simple example to introduce the topic of pulmonary oedema. There is something of a mystery about the breakdown of total integrated circulatory and respiratory control systems during an attack of pulmonary oedema. Most typically a sufferer may be woken from sleep in the early hours of the morning, finding himself unable to breathe freely and having to sit up or even stand with rapidly increasing dyspnoea. This may be accompanied by a falling arterial Po_2.

Standing up normally translocates some 800 ml of blood into the legs and lower abdomen and might be expected to produce instant relief of pulmonary oedema, but the relief is usually not all that dramatic. This suggests that some vicious circle has been initiated and in some way perpetuates the condition.

There are various possible explanations and I will simply mention a few of these as talking points for further discussion. For example, the occurrence of pulmonary oedema interferes with the matching of ventilation to perfusion. The resulting hypoxaemia dilates much of the vascular bed and may also strongly activate the sympathetic nervous efferent system, constricting the circulatory reservoirs and increasing venous return. This may then shift more blood into the lungs and aggravate the oedema. The strong sympathetic reflex component of pulmonary oedema can easily be demonstrated by its frequently dramatic relief by the use of a small dose of a ganglion-blocking agent, such as 5 mg intravenous hexamethonium. Morphine and its derivatives are almost specific remedies for pulmonary oedema, though they are not much used nowadays. This is also surprising since, as a respiratory depressant, morphine might appear liable to reduce alveolar ventilation and hence intensify hypoxaemia.

Another aetiological factor that we might consider is the stimulation of some intrapulmonary neural receptor mechanism by the accumulation of interstitial oedema. Churchill & Cope (1929) first observed that the tachypnoea induced by pulmonary oedema was a reflex phenomenon stimulated by intra-pulmonary receptors. These receptors were subsequently identified by Paintal (1969) as juxta-pulmonary capillary ('type J') receptors. They can be stimulated by CO_2 and various drugs but can also be stimulated by pulmonary oedema. The reflex effects include tachypnoea, inhibition of spinal stretch reflexes, and, when intense, bradycardia. Possibly the tachypnoea so characteristic of pulmonary oedema worsens the inevitable hypoxaemia by reducing the effective alveolar ventilation, thus again perpetuating a vicious circle.

There are other possibilities, at present theoretical, such as constriction of pulmonary veins. Such a mechanism might seem physiologically inappropriate, but it is possible to envisage a physiologically plausible mechanism adapted to preventing overdistension of the left ventricle by restricting its filling.

Amongst other contributors to the vicious circle, the reflex rise in systemic arterial pressure, which is often seen clinically, presumably may reduce the output of the left heart and lead to a further damaging rise in left ventricular end-diastolic pressure, and hence in pulmonary capillary pressure.

It would be easy to multiply hypotheses of the total physiological derangement in pulmonary oedema. Indeed, there may be many ingredients of the total vicious circle.

Pulmonary oedema gives us a very nice lead-in to the subject of the regulation of the volume of each compartment of lung liquid. We have spent some time here discussing the balance of forces between the blood stream and the inter-stitial space across a semi-permeable membrane. The lymphatic system draining the interstitial space provides a buffer against unduly excessive accumulation of liquids. Perhaps we now understand the regulation of interstitial fluid volume. However, I might draw attention to the clinical fact that, in my experience at least, clinical pulmonary oedema is extremely rare in conditions of gross hypoalbuminaemia such as are found in the nephrotic syndrome and in cirrhosis of the liver. These conditions would be interesting to study from the point of view of pulmonary interstitial volume and pressure, and of pulmonary lymph flow.

Patients who suffer from pulmonary oedema, especially over long periods of time, tend to develop pleural effusions though they may have no signs of systemic circulatory failure such as engorged neck veins or liver. This suggests that some component of the raised pulmonary capillary pressure which is normally present in clinical pulmonary oedema plays a part in the dynamic balance of forces across the parietal pleura. If time permits, we might profitably also discuss the formation of pleural fluid.

References

CHURCHILL, E. D. & COPE, O. (1929) The rapid shallow breathing resulting from pulmonary congestion and edema. *J. Exp. Med. 49*, 531-537
PAINTAL, A. S. (1969) Mechanism of stimulation of type J pulmonary receptors. *J. Physiol. (Lond.) 203*, 511-532

Discussion

PULMONARY OEDEMA

Michel: You referred to pulmonary oedema as an all-or-nothing phenomenon, whereas for much of the time we have been thinking in terms of gradual processes, the interstitium filling with fluid, followed by alveolar flooding. What were you referring to when you talked about pulmonary oedema?

Dickinson: In the rabbit experiments I was referring to intra-alveolar flooding. The lungs were solid and pink froth was pouring out of them at the time of death. I see this occasionally in patients. Most patients with these symptoms die but a few recover. I was really referring to a combination of clinical symptoms and signs, X-ray signs and other evidence suggesting that there is too much liquid in the lungs.

Michel: So you were including both interstitial and alveolar oedema?

Dickinson: I don't know what causes the sensation of breathlessness. It seems to be a graded process. My guess now is that the perivascular cuffing that Dr Staub described may happen very early indeed. As far as I know, no nervous receptors can be assigned yet to the pulmonary vasculature itself. On the other hand, there are receptors in the pulmonary interstitium ('type J' receptors) which are stimulated by increased interstitial fluid volume. The symptom of breathlessness on exertion and the more severe dyspnoeic symptoms in disease may arise from stimulation of these receptors in the first instance. Then there are later signs associated with changing gas tensions.

Olver: Were you suggesting that neurogenic pulmonary oedema is mediated by a mechanism other than a raised left atrial pressure and increased pulmonary capillary pressure?

Dickinson: No. I presume it results from very severe translocation of blood into the lungs.

Strang: The existence of 'neurological' lung oedema has been disputed. Perhaps Dr Staub could give us the latest opinions about this.

Staub: I have not studied neurogenic pulmonary oedema. Many investigators can produce it by raising cerebrospinal fluid pressure or by injecting irritating substances into the fourth ventricle. It is a distinct entity.

However, I do take issue with the claims that the oedema accumulates very rapidly. This would be against it being a simple form of hydrostatic oedema (Staub 1974). The measured elevations of left atrial pressure are not high enough to produce such rapid oedema. There must be additional factors.

Donald: Is there a rise in blood pressure in these cases?

Dickinson: Yes. I have often observed blood pressure much above normal levels in patients admitted in acute pulmonary oedema.

Staub: But it is not sufficient to cause the rapid oedema that has been reported.

Olver: When you say you haven't produced pulmonary oedema yourself, Dr Staub, do you mean that you haven't tried to produce it?

Staub: That is correct.

Fishman: About 30 years ago, circulatory physiologists were deeply involved with the question of neurogenic pulmonary hypertension. The centre of attention was the mysterious increase in pulmonary capillary permeability which was presumed to occur as intracranial pressure was raised to inordinate levels. Over the years, using systemic vasodilators to prevent the rise in arterial blood pressure that accompanies raised intracranial pressure, it was shown that 'neurogenic' pulmonary oedema was a misnomer. Indeed, it proved to be secondary to severe and sudden haemodynamic overload on the left ventricle. In essence, the so-called 'permeability' pulmonary oedema was really a form of haemodynamic pulmonary oedema.

This is not to discount completely the idea of neurogenic or reflex pulmonary oedema. How else can one explain the generalized pulmonary oedema that may occur after discrete pulmonary emboli?

Dickinson: Is there any evidence of an acute effect of the nervous system on the permeability of the alveolar epithelium?

Robin: There is evidence of an indirect effect on permeability. Dr James Theodore and I have written a paper (Theodore & Robin 1975) which puts the facts about neurogenic pulmonary oedema in a reasonable framework. One clear-cut fact is that in experimental animals, overwhelming pulmonary oedema can be induced in an incredibly short time, even shorter than the period you report, Dr Dickinson. For example, if mice or rats are hit on the head with a measured force, then even if the blow is instantaneously fatal, the lungs are found to be filled with pulmonary oedema fluid and blood (MacKay 1950; Bean & Beckman 1969). The same thing is reported in humans. Overwhelming pulmonary oedema may be found after instantaneously fatal gunshot wounds of the brain (Weissman 1939).

Another experimental technique associated with pulmonary oedema is the production of electrolytic lesions in the hypothalamus. Lesions in the basal portion of the preoptic nucleus or midline destruction involving the periventricular system caudal to the preoptic region were associated with 100% development of pulmonary oedema in rats (Reynolds 1963). Interestingly enough, in these forms of experimental pulmonary oedema, if the animal has been pretreated with either alpha-blocking agents or high doses of central nervous system depressants, pulmonary oedema does not develop (MacKay 1950).

A third line of evidence, which is less documented but seems nevertheless to be certain, is that once the pulmonary oedema has evolved, systemic and pulmonary haemodynamics are normal. There is no increase in left atrial or pulmonary wedge pressure, cardiac output is normal, and so on. On the other hand, when pulmonary oedema first forms, haemodynamics are transiently but profoundly altered. For example, Sarnoff & Sarnoff (1952) placed thrombin and fibrinogen on the floor of the fourth ventricle. This caused an extraordinarily sharp rise in pressures of both segments of the circulation—the systemic circulation, aortic pressure, arterial pressure, venous pressure, and in the pulmonary circulation as well as on the left side of the circulation. These rises in pressures were transient and subsided within minutes. It looks as if the oedema persists after the initial haemodynamic insult. Finally, a few measurements on the fluid of neurogenic pulmonary oedema suggest that it has a high protein content from the beginning and that it has many of the characteristics of pulmonary oedema fluid caused by alterations of pulmonary capillary permeability (Cameron & De 1949).

These facts suggest that neurogenic pulmonary oedema is a two-phase lesion; the initial phase is a massive sympathetic discharge from the central nervous system, hypothalamically mediated, which then produces a striking shift of blood from the systemic to the pulmonary circulation, and increased pressures. The interstitial space and intra-alveolar space, and often the bronchial tree, are flooded with liquid. The increases in pressure and fluid redistribution are so extensive that pulmonary vessels (capillaries) are injured and capillary permeability is altered, leading to pulmonary oedema fluid with a high protein content. This alteration of capillary permeability results in persistent pulmonary oedema, even though haemodynamics have become normal (phase two).

Olver: Is it so surprising, after this catalogue of catastrophes, that the liquid is not absorbed rapidly? If large gaps are formed in the alveolar epithelium the osmotic reflection coefficient for albumin is going to be zero, and anyway the liquid on both sides of the epithelium will contain large amounts of protein. The other point which Dr Dickinson touched on is that perfusion is going to be markedly reduced in those areas that are fluid-filled and absorption would be slow for that reason too.

Dickinson: We probably have a consensus that there isn't anything magical about neurogenic pulmonary oedema, and like other types of clinical pulmonary oedema it appears to be due to a rise in pulmonary capillary pressure. It would be straying too far from our brief to discuss high altitude pulmonary oedema, which is still an unsolved problem.

Guyton: Dr Dickinson has asked that, in this final discussion, I should present a few additional thoughts on pulmonary oedema in the light of the papers and discussions of the past few days. I would like to begin by expanding some of the thoughts that Dr Dickinson has expressed in his talk.

Like Dr Dickinson, we too have developed a large total circulatory model that we run on a computer. Several years ago, while the model was running, the simulated 'patient' went into pulmonary oedema. This 'patient' had already had a weak left ventricle for weeks or years, but had not previously had pulmonary oedema. Then an extra work load was placed on the heart for about one hour, after which a typical episode of developing pulmonary oedema ensued, leading to death. It was very easy to trace in the model the cause of the initiation of the pulmonary oedema and also the cause of its progression to death. The sequence of events was the following: during the period of extra work load on the heart, a small amount of extra fluid filtered into the lungs. Next, the arterial oxygen saturation began to fall. Then the decreased oxygen delivery to the peripheral tissues caused peripheral vascular dilatation. This in turn increased the venous return to the heart. Also, a slight tendency for the arterial pressure to fall elicited sympathetic stimulation, which contracted the veins and further exacerbated venous return. The right heart pumped this extra venous return into the lungs but, unfortunately, the failing left heart could not pump the increased quantities of blood. Therefore, the left atrial pressure rose slightly more, and still more fluid filtered into the lungs, leading to a second cycle of decreasing arterial oxygen saturation, further increase in peripheral vasodilatation, additional venous return, and further rise in left atrial pressure. Thus, the computer 'patient' went into a vicious cycle from which he could not recover without drastic 'therapy'. Since these events are so reminiscent of acute pulmonary oedema in the human patient, there is much reason to believe that a similar vicious cycle occurs in many if not most instances of acute pulmonary oedema. A better understanding of all these sequential events would perhaps be valuable in increasing the effectiveness of therapy.

Now I would like to change the subject entirely and raise a thought that has occurred to me more and more often during the meeting. This is the possibility that the epithelial lining of the alveoli is not important, except for the surfactant that it secretes, in determining whether the alveoli will be filled with fluid or will be dry. If we simply assume that the interstitial spaces of the lungs operate at a subatmospheric pressure low enough to overcome the surface tension effect in the airways, any abnormal fluid that should appear in the alveoli would immediately be absorbed into the interstitial spaces. From here the fluid would either enter the lymphatics or be absorbed through the capillary walls into the blood capillaries.

One might suspect that lack of an epithelial lining would also allow air to enter the interstices of the pulmonary tissues. However, the surface tension of tissue fluid at its interface with alveolar air is so great that air would fail to be pulled by the negative interstitial fluid pressure into the minute tissue interstices. Indeed, calculations show that a negative pressure of several thousand millimetres of mercury would be needed in the interstitial spaces to cause air to be sucked into the tissues.

On the other hand, denuded tissues are highly susceptible to infection, for which reason it would be preferable to have the surfaces of the alveoli covered with a cell barrier, the alveolar epithelial cells. Furthermore, special cells are needed to secrete surfactant so that the surface tension of the alveolar fluid will be low. And other cells are needed to provide detoxifying functions, bactericidal functions, and so forth. Thus, the purpose of the epithelial barrier may have nothing whatsoever to do with providing a barrier between the fluid of the interstitial spaces and the air of the alveoli, but, instead, entirely different functions.

We have heard in several of the papers, particularly in the studies of Dr Egan, that simple mechanical forces can increase the permeability of the alveolar epithelial membrane. This suggests that some of the junctions between epithelial cells can be ruptured by mechanical stretching. For instance, over-expansion of the lungs could perhaps open the seams between at least some of the epithelial cells. Likewise, appearance of a positive fluid pressure in the interstitial fluid spaces could swell these spaces and push rifts between the epithelial cells.

Therefore, I would like us to consider the following idea: so long as the interstitial fluid pressure is far enough below atmospheric pressure to keep the alveoli dry, and so long as the lungs are not unduly overstretched, a normal epithelial lining can presumably be maintained in the alveoli. However, there is reason to believe that even a very minute increase in the interstitial fluid pressure, to a value slightly greater than the surface tension pressure of the alveolar fluid (about -2 to -4 mmHg [-0.27 to -0.53 kPa]), can open the seams between the epithelial cells and allow fluid to pour from the interstitial spaces into the alveoli. This would give a very simple view of pulmonary oedema: so long as the interstitial fluid pressure is sufficiently subatmospheric, pulmonary oedema will not occur. On the other hand, whenever the interstitial fluid pressure rises to a value that is slightly positive to the pressure of the fluid in the alveoli (as determined by the surface tension of the fluid and by the radii of the alveoli), then fluid will collect in the alveoli and cause pulmonary oedema. In this mechanism the alveolar epithelial cells play only a passive role.

Strang: I can see that these systems work so long as there is indeed a subatmospheric pressure in the interstitial area. Of course, if fluid is flowing through the interstitial space there must be another part of the system with an even lower pressure. There must be a still lower pressure in that part of the lymphatic channel which lies distal to the first valve. The pressure must get lower and lower until a lymphatic valve is reached. I suppose there is no reason why that shouldn't be so. There are circumstances in which these spaces change in shape and become distended with fluid, as shown histologically. Physiologically, for example, as opposed to pathologically, this takes place a few hours after birth. These spaces become larger at that time and develop convexities. It is a little difficult to believe that at that time the pressure doesn't rise above the usual pressure. This makes me feel that a system like this wouldn't provide sufficient protection against fluid accumulation unless there was something to back it up in the shape of the epithelium.

Donald: Don't some neonates develop a very strong negative pressure at this stage, a few hours after birth?

Strang: They take breaths and they get low pleural pressures, certainly. Nevertheless these spaces become distended so that the negative pressure, the driving force, creates a situation where the volume is actually taken up with a space filler which must then diminish the initial driving pressure again.

Guyton: If we assume that tensile forces in the alveolar walls, such as forces caused by surface tension of the alveolar fluid, cause the alveolar epithelium to pull away from the perivascular spaces, these spaces could then collect large amounts of fluid without completely losing their negative pressure.

Staub: Why do you think that alveolar fluid clears so slowly when interstitial fluid clears so rapidly in the lung? Obviously the alveolar membrane is there in life and it would be difficult to do an experiment to strip it off without damaging the underlying tissue.

Guyton: The alveolar membrane would certainly make a difference to the rapidity of fluid absorption from the alveoli, but I am talking about the equilibrium state. If a gel that has been dehydrated down to a negative pressure of -7 mmHg $(-0.93$ kPa) (which is what we think is the case in most peripheral tissues) is then expanded by 30–50%, all of the negative pressure, or 'imbibition pressure', of the gel will be lost. If one then expands it beyond that volume, the gel breaks up. If tensile forces occur in the alveolar walls to pull them away from the perivascular spaces, after a critical degree of swelling one would then expect pockets of free fluid (free of gel) to appear in the perivascular spaces.

Egan: There are pathological conditions in which the epithelium seems to be broken but without the production of what we would clinically call pulmonary oedema. In paediatrics we see it in hyaline membrane disease, where histologically the epithelium is not intact. Indeed plasma proteins are seen in the alveolar space though no massive amounts of liquid were there. I think the same thing is seen in what they call the adult respiratory distress syndrome. So I guess it is conceivable that a negative pressure in the interstitial space, as described by Dr Guyton, could keep water out of the alveolar space even if the alveolar epithelium is disrupted. We might see something like that in some clinical conditions.

Fishman: I too am only prepared to offer a personal view. In contrast to the circumspect biophysical analysis that has just been provided by Dr Guyton, my concern will be with the relationships between some of the physiological observations that we have heard and clinical pulmonary oedema.

At the outset, I should like to be sure that we agree that pulmonary oedema simply signifies an excess of water in the lungs, the hallmark of a disproportion between outflow and inflow. It is generally agreed that this water contains crystalloids and other water-soluble ingredients of plasma in about the same concentrations as in plasma. Much less consensus exists concerning the concentration of proteins in this oedema fluid; it may vary not only with the type and duration of the pulmonary oedema but also from locus to locus within the lung. Finally, the water content of the lung must fluctuate during the day even in normal subjects. But, rarely in the normal subject does an expanded water volume reach the level of clinical awareness.

How does one recognize clinically that the lungs contain too much water? This is not easy unless considerable flooding has occurred. Methods for early detection of excess water have not been easy to apply and modest increments in lung water have proved difficult to detect in man. How much water is 'excess'? Ordinarily the quantity of interstitial water in adult man is estimated to be of

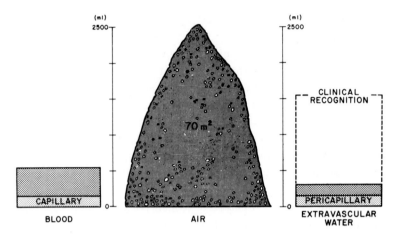

FIG. 1 (Fishman). Schematic representation of the compartments of the lung in a young adult with a normal functional residual capacity (2500 ml). The gas-exchanging surface area is depicted as approximately 70 m². The corresponding blood volume is about 600 ml, of which some 100 ml is in the capillaries. The extravascular water space is small, about 300 ml. The pericapillary water space is about the same size as the capillary blood volume.

Extravascular water volume may increase sixfold before the stage of clinical signs and symptoms is reached.

the order of 100 ml, i.e. of the same magnitude as the capillary blood volume (Fig. 1). This small volume is spread over the enormous expanse of interstitial space, forming an infinitesimally thin film. Clearly, unless puddling were to occur, considerable interstitial oedema would be required to thicken this film appreciably.

There is some opportunity for puddling since the distribution of the interstitial volume is exceedingly non-uniform. This inhomogeneity begins with the eccentric disposition of the interstitial space at the level of the alveolar capillaries: a distinct space is confined to one side of the capillary whereas the opposite side is exceedingly thin. This arrangement protects the gas-exchanging portions of the capillaries by directing excess water to the thick side and, from there, to pulmonary lymphatics.

When the water space of the lungs is greatly enlarged, interstitial oedema becomes apparent clinically. It is generally held that excess water in the interstitial space is clinically *inapparent* until the total interstitial water volume has increased five- to sixfold (Fig. 1). The respiratory rate increases and X-ray evidence of interstitial pulmonary oedema begins to appear: the lungs look cloudy; vascular shadows lose their sharp boundaries; Kerley 'septal' lines, reflecting collections of water in interlobular septa, become discernible. Sensitive pulmonary function tests, such as closing volumes, may provide supportive evidence that interstitial oedema surrounds terminal bronchioles. In states of chronic pulmonary congestion, as in left ventricular failure, the water content of the lungs may be chronically increased. Despite this reset, the lungs may continue to do well in gas exchange. Unless the excess water manages to overflow alveolar boundaries and reach the terminal bronchioles, râles are absent. Only the sustained increase in respiratory frequency—a sign to which little heed is paid in clinical medicine—may signal to the physician that the patient has come closer to the verge of clinical pulmonary oedema. Dr Waaler (pp. 65–71) pointed out that as pulmonary capillary pressures increase interstitial and capillary pressures may automatically achieve a new relationship, thereby re-establishing a new balance of transvascular hydrostatic and osmotic forces which prevents inordinate increments in the water input into the interstitial space. Clinical pulmonary oedema may represent a failure of this automatic control mechanism. And, once this mechanism becomes ineffective, the stage appears to be set for positive feedback that will perpetuate the pulmonary oedema.

Clearly my thinking so far has been along the lines of Starling's law of transcapillary exchange. But not all transcapillary exchange obeys this law. For example, in the elasmobranch (J. A. Fishman & Pietra 1973) gill capillaries appear to be freely permeable to plasma proteins, so Starling's law cannot work. In this species, the important barrier to exchange between the ambient environment and plasma is the epithelium that separates the interstitial fluid from the outside world. A homologous situation appears to obtain in the lung where the tight alveolar junctions allow considerable interstitial oedema to occur before there is any overflow into the alveoli.

It would be misleading to consider pulmonary oedema solely in terms of the *input* of water, solutes and proteins into the interstitial spaces of the lungs. Clearly there must be an adequate drainage system. As far as we now know, drainage is the responsibility of the pulmonary lymphatics: an ingenious architectural arrangement at the level of the capillaries directs the interstitial fluid to lymphatic capillaries in the vicinity of the terminal bronchioles; once in the lymphatics, the liquid is on its way out of the lungs. But there is no assurance that the protein content of the lymph remains unchanged as it moves towards the exits from the thorax. Indeed, how the protein concentration of the lymph relates to interstitial protein concentration in the vicinity of the pulmonary capillaries is still unsettled.

Bronchial venules and lymphatic vessels lie side by side on the walls of the airways; conceivably, a change in the permeability of one could affect the operation of the other. The administration of histamine and bradykinin causes interstitial pulmonary oedema by causing the bronchial venules to leak.

Whether this increase in bronchial venular permeability is of clinical importance is unknown. However, endotoxinaemia also causes bronchial venules to leak (Pietra *et al*. 1974), suggesting that noxious agents in the circulation may promote water accumulation in the lungs in a variety of different ways.

How clear are clinical distinctions between *haemodynamic* and *permeability* oedema? In terms of simple models, the distinction is quite straightforward: *haemodynamic* oedema is a consequence of high hydrostatic pressures in the pulmonary capillaries; *permeability* oedema is the result of injury to the capillary barrier which allows inordinate quantities of protein to enter the interstitial space. Unfortunately, if we accept these rigid definitions, it proves difficult to explain unusual forms of clinical oedema, such as the oedema of high altitude, shock lung and narcotic overdosage (Fishman 1972).

Explanations become a bit less contrived once it is recognized that 'stretched pores' have blurred this distinction. Thus, high capillary pressures in the lungs (haemodynamic mechanism) not only increase the rate of bulk flow into the interstitial spaces, but also widen interendothelial junctions so that molecules of the size of albumin also gain ready access to the interstitial space (permeability mechanism). Thus, in common clinical disorders involving volume overload of the circulation, increased 'permeability' of the pulmonary capillaries to blood proteins may be a consequence of haemodynamic upset rather than of primary damage to capillary walls. This awareness has important practical implications for disorders such as 'the adult respiratory distress syndrome' ('shock lung'): anyone who gives hyperoncotic solutions to such patients, who may have 'stretched pores' in the lungs as well as damaged capillary endothelium, runs the risk of aggravating pulmonary oedema by promoting the entry of plasma proteins into the interstitial space.

Experimental models of 'permeability' pulmonary oedema are often too extreme to relate meaningfully to clinical disorders. One such fearful model is that produced by alloxan which denudes alveolar-capillary walls, leaving only the basement membrane as a skeleton (Cottrell *et al*. 1967). Recovery from this disastrous form of injury is unlikely. In contrast, clinical forms of injury, such as oxygen toxicity, are generally much more modest and full recovery is often achievable. Between these two extremes is a form of severe pulmonary capillary damage which allows large proteins to accumulate in the interstitial spaces. Recovery from oedema may then be followed by respiratory insufficiency due to organization of the interstitial exudate. A common example of this untoward consequence is the interstitial fibrosis of the lung bases in patients with chronic left ventricular failure.

Once it is appreciated that enhanced permeability need not be only a consequence of capillary injury, other traditional concepts also become suspect.

How conclusive is the evidence that histamine causes pulmonary capillaries to leak? There is little convincing evidence to support this popular notion. Indeed, as yet only the *bronchial venules* have shown increased permeability to macro-molecular tracers after histamine. The same is true for bradykinin and endo-toxin. Nor does hypoxia increase pulmonary capillary permeability. How important is the fact that many of these substances are extensively inactivated by pulmonary capillary endothelium as they traverse the lungs (Fishman & Pietra 1974)?

Important beginnings have been made in clarifying the topics mentioned above. But new insights are still needed. What accounts for the familiar 'butterfly oedema' in which the distribution of pulmonary oedema appears to defy gravity, as though excess fluid were accumulating in the 'medulla' of the lung while the 'cortex' is spared? Is uraemic pulmonary oedema primarily haemodynamic in origin or does it depend on permeability? Is it true that a tiny pulmonary infarct may elicit *bilateral* pulmonary oedema? This list of enigmas in clinical pulmonary oedema could certainly be continued. But perhaps those that have been mentioned will serve to illustrate not only the complexity of the clinical disorders in pulmonary water balance but also the fresh insights into pathogenesis that physiology is being called upon to supply.

Lee: How fast does water move across the capillary membrane? One thing that has not been considered much in this symposium is that the lung preserves, under virtually all circumstances, its pulsatile capillary blood flow. In systole, the capillary pressure rises and there will be a flux of water out into the inter-stitial space. During diastole, the intracapillary pressure will fall below the osmotic pressure and there will be a considerable period of time for water to get back into the capillary again. Next, if heart rate is increased, say by exercise, the local net flux in parts of the lung will tend to be outwards, the compliance of the tissue would fall, fouling up the J receptors, and the person would become breathless and stop exercising. The heart rate would then come down again and there could thus be a beautiful mechanism for keeping the lungs dry, just because of this pulse through the capillaries. However, if water moves slower than the time constant set by the heart rate, then this hypothesis is obviously wrong.

Widdicombe: If the J receptors are monitoring interstitial fluid volume they should respond fast enough to have a pulsatile rhythm, but none of them do (Paintal 1973).

* * *

Strang: I will restrain myself from trying to say a last word about so many topics and just confine myself to a few prejudices. I sometimes wonder what the physiology of the lung would have looked like if it had been known to the early investigators that the whole respiratory surface was covered by an epithelium. Most of the classical work in lung physiology was done before this structure was definitely known to exist. It was not finally demonstrated until Low & Daniels (1952) applied the electron microscope to studying the lung.

Lung physiologists have been mainly concerned with the transfer of respiratory gases and inert gases across the epithelium, but they have given little thought to how the gas molecules actually get through the epithelial structures. I suppose the truth is that they have never had to bother much about this question, because the permeability of the pulmonary epithelium to respiratory gases is so high that these transfers are ordinarily flow-limited. But flow-limited transfer is only one kind of transfer across this epithelium and when studying the transfer of water and polar solutes the physiologist becomes much more involved in how the individual substances get through the barrier.

I suppose I look on the lung primarily as a very large area of epithelium—it is about 10^6 cm^2 in adult man. Perhaps this epithelium matters most to a fetal physiologist who is interested in the movement of liquid and solutes, but it has some general importance for the whole subject of lung physiology. Lung epithelium, to my way of looking at things, has two functions. One is to let the respiratory gases through and the other is to stop solutes from the blood from getting through. Respiratory gases have oil/water partition coefficients greater than unity (Lawrence et al. 1946) and the lung epithelium has been shown to be very permeable to lipid-soluble substances such as thiourea and ethylthiourea (Normand et al. 1971).

For the lung to work as it does, a vast flow of blood has to go through it, and the capacity to sustain gas exchange is always threatened by the possible escape of solutes from the circulation into the air spaces. As we know, that happens from time to time. But the lung can't really work as a primary gas exchanger unless these movements of liquid are strictly controlled. It seems to me very likely, and I think we have heard evidence here to suggest it is so, that the most important function of the pulmonary epithelium is to protect the small air spaces from penetration by water and solutes.

In conclusion, I would remind you that the lung begins in embryonic life as an out-pouching of the foregut epithelium. About 28 days after ovulation, in the human, the first rudiment is recognizable as an outgrowth of epithelium into the mesoderm on either side of the heart; and later development in both fetal and postnatal life consists mainly of its growth by branching and differentiation.

References

BEAN, J. W. & BECKMAN, D. L. (1969) Centrogenic pulmonary pathology in mechanical head injury. *J. Appl. Physiol. 27*, 807-812

CAMERON, G. R. & DE, S. N. (1949) Experimental pulmonary edema of nervous origin. *J. Path. Bact. 61*, 375-387

COTTRELL, T. S., LEVINE, O. R., SENIOR, R. M., WIENER, J., SPIRO, D. & FISHMAN, A. P. (1967) *Circ. Res. 21*, 783-797

FISHMAN, A. P. (1972) Pulmonary edema. The water exchanging function of the lung. *Circulation 46*, 390-408

FISHMAN, A. P. & PIETRA, G. G. (1974) The handling of bioactive substances by the lung. *N. Engl. J. Med. 291*, 884-890, 953-959

FISHMAN, J. A. & PIETRA, G. G. (1973) *Bull. Mt. Desert Isl. Biol. Lab. 13*, 36-38

LAWRENCE, J. H., LOOMIS, W. F., TOBIAS, C. A. & TURPIN, F. H. (1946) Preliminary observations on the narcotic effect of xenon with a review of values for solubilities of gases in water and oils. *J. Physiol. (Lond.) 105*, 197-204

LOW, F. N. & DANIELS, C. W. (1952) Electron microscopy of rat lung. *Anat. Rec. 113*, 437

MACKAY, E. M. (1950) Experimental pulmonary edema. IV. Pulmonary edema accompanying trauma to the brain. *Proc. Soc. Exp. Biol. Med. 74*, 695-697

PAINTAL, A. S. (1973) Vagal sensory receptors and their reflex effects. *Physiol. Rev. 53*, 159-227

PIETRA, G. G., SZIDON, J. P., CARPENTER, H. A. & FISHMAN, A. P. (1974) Bronchial venular leakage during endotoxin shock. *Am. J. Pathol. 77*, 387-402

NORMAND, I. C. S., OLVER, R. E., REYNOLDS, E. O. R. & STRANG, L. B. (1971) Permeability of lung capillaries and alveoli to non-electrolytes in the foetal lamb. *J. Physiol. (Lond.) 219*, 303-330

REYNOLDS, R. W. (1963) Pulmonary edema as a consequence of hypothalamic lesions in rats. *Science (Wash. D.C.) 141*, 930-932

SARNOFF, S. J. & SARNOFF, L. C. (1952) Neurohemodynamics of pulmonary edema. I. Autonomic influence on pulmonary vascular pressures and the acute pulmonary edema state. *Circulation 6*, 51-62

STAUB, N. C. (1974) Pulmonary edema. *Physiol. Rev. 54*, 678-811

THEODORE, J. & ROBIN, E. D. (1975) Pathogenesis of neurogenic pulmonary edema. *Lancet 2*, 938-939

WEISSMAN, S. J. (1939) Edema and congestion of the lungs resulting from intracranial hemorrhage. *Surgery (St Louis) 6*, 722-729

Closing remarks

C. J. DICKINSON

As a non-specialist in this field I have enjoyed this meeting and have learnt a lot. I hope that the others present, despite being specialists themselves, have also found the meeting interesting.

During our first day's discussions I was struck by the general agreement between ultrastructure and ultrafunction. Anatomically and physiologically the capillary endothelium is a reasonably permeable membrane. By contrast the alveolar epithelium, at least in its unstretched state, is not. We were not entirely agreed whether alveolar epithelium could become more permeable under special conditions, apart from extreme conditions such as shock lung. Clearly it is tightly sealed during fetal life. This allows alveolar liquid to maintain a pH quite strongly acid relative to plasma. The unusual composition of the liquid is also maintained by a remarkably high active secretion rate and it seems that alveolar liquid may have a pressure slightly positive to that in the fetal pleural space. The larynx evidently provides some degree of sealing, and fluid is normally expelled intermittently. We speculated briefly that a hollow organ might need to secrete fluid to develop normally.

What happens to the lungs at birth is still not entirely clear to me. Strenuous inspiratory movements of diaphragm and chest wall will suck air quite rapidly to the level of alveolar ostia. As Dr Guyton clearly pointed out, even with high surfactant concentration some appreciable negative pressure is needed to maintain air in the alveoli, and this pressure needs to be most negative in the corners of the alveoli. Probably a negative pressure between -5 and -15 mmHg (-0.67 to -2 kPa) is required. Since most fetal alveolar liquid is reabsorbed into the blood after birth it must be sucked into the interstitial spaces. This might be due in part to hydraulic forces aided by the lymphatic pump. My guess, however, if I may be allowed one as a Chairman's privilege, is that at birth the stretching of alveolar epithelium might open up pores through which alveolar fluid passes in across a gradient established by the difference in colloid osmotic pressure between interstitial fluid and lung liquid. The process can continue because lymph flow rapidly, though temporarily, increases. This cannot of course explain the complete clearing of alveolar spaces, because protein concentration would increase. There must be some active transport mechanism as well.

I do not think we were able to agree whether the apparently sudden switch from alveolar fluid production to rapid absorption might be mediated by some hormonal means rather than by an effect of mechanical stretch—though the striking ability of the teleostean gill to switch its active transport systems from absorption to excretion of electrolytes and water allows us to hypothesize that the mammalian lung lining might retain some vestiges of teleostean transport-reversing function.

In the adult lung we are hampered by the difficulty of studying the composition of alveolar lining fluid and measuring the dynamics of its exchange. We do not know whether adult alveolar fluid is secreted slowly, or secreted rapidly and leaked back almost as rapidly. Fluids introduced into the adult lung pass rapidly into the circulation. Whether actual structural change needs to take place to allow this is not certain, but it seems certain that any leaks in alveolar epithelium can be repaired very rapidly. Dr Staub argued persuasively in favour of leaks upstream in the airways. Increased endothelial permeability also probably occurs when intravascular pressure is increased, and in pulmonary oedema large free interstitial fluid cuffs develop. If intravascular pressure is high enough, protein-rich fluid fills the alveolar spaces. Whether this high permeability to protein is a normal property of the adult alveolar epithelium seems doubtful.

Since fetal alveolar liquid has some resemblance to gastric juice, we have considered the coupled movement of water and electrolytes in gastric mucosa, which brought up interesting questions about the maintenance of an endogenous osmotic gradient within a membrane, and about the function and distribution of carbonate dehydratase (carbonic anhydrase). Dr Farhi showed us that storage of carbon dioxide by the lung made some measurements by respiratory physiologists difficult to interpret. But he also showed that carbonate dehydratase was not needed for adequate gas exchange. Comparative studies, about which Dr Maetz reminded us frequently and helpfully, suggest that acetazolamide has actions apart from inhibition of carbonate dehydratase. However, despite much interesting discussion I remain as uncertain as I was about the function of carbonate dehydratase in the lung, either in fetal or adult life.

Although we have not devoted much time to discussing pleural liquid it has gradually dawned on me that the pleural liquid can be regarded as a natural

Guyton capsule, in which pressure and liquid composition seem to be closely similar to those of the interstitial fluid of the lung. The protein content is low. We have been reminded of the potential protein-concentrating ability of lymphatic pumps—which means that the high protein content of lung lymph does not necessarily reflect a similarly high interstitial fluid content. The pleural pressure is negative (though to different degrees in different regions) to about the same degree as measurements and theoretical calculations suggest that interstitial fluid pressure has to be negative to atmospheric pressure. It appears that fluid can move very freely between lung interstitium and pleural space.

I hope this naive analogy will not provoke too much disagreement, especially as there is no time left for others to protest! I believe we have now a much clearer understanding of the events in the lung which underlie clinical pulmonary oedema. We still do not understand all the ingredients of what appears to be a vicious circle by which pulmonary oedema is more easily maintained than spontaneously resolved. We probably need more cooperative studies of haemodynamics and lung function to get all the answers.

Index of contributors

*Entries in **bold** type indicate papers; other entries refer to discussion contributions*

Indexes compiled by William Hill

Subject index